Pediatric and Adolescent Plastic Surgery for the Clinician

Aleksandar M. Vlahovic • Emir Q. Haxhija

Pediatric and Adolescent Plastic Surgery for the Clinician

Springer

Aleksandar M. Vlahovic
Department of Plastic Surgery and Burns
Institute for Mother and Child Health Care
of Republic Serbia
University of Belgrade
New Belgrade
Serbia

Emir Q. Haxhija
Department of Pediatric and
Adolescent Surgery
Medical University Graz
Graz
Austria

ISBN 978-3-319-56003-8 ISBN 978-3-319-56004-5 (eBook)
DOI 10.1007/978-3-319-56004-5

Library of Congress Control Number: 2017941188

Printed on acid-free paper

This Springer imprint is published by Springer Nature
The registered company is Springer International Publishing AG
The registered company address is: Gewerbestrasse 11, 6330 Cham, Switzerland

I dedicate this book to my sons Maksim and Vuk and to my wife Natasa.

Aleksandar M. Vlahovic

Preface

Pediatric plastic surgery is a specific field of surgery which includes reconstructive and aesthetic procedures in children.

The majority of procedures in pediatric plastic surgery are reconstructive in nature. Purely aesthetic procedures in children are rare.

Pediatric plastic surgeons are involved in the treatment of a wide spectrum of congenital lesions.

The treatment of patients in pediatric plastic surgery often requires a multidisciplinary approach including different specialties (pediatricians, dermatologist, vascular surgeons, orthopedic surgeons, maxillofacial surgeons, otorhinolaryngologist, anesthesiologist, etc.) and other medical caregivers.

For most of the patients with clefts, malignant tumors, complicated hand anomalies, and breast anomalies, long-term evaluation is required, very often in adulthood.

Health practitioners in their clinical practice are often dealing with these patients, and this book should serve as a guide in their everyday practice.

This book includes 16 years of my personal experience in this field.

Belgrade, Serbia — Aleksandar M. Vlahovic
Graz, Austria — Emir Q. Haxhija

Contents

Abbreviations

AD	Autosomal dominant
AER	Apical ectodermal ridge
AM	Arterial malformation
AMN	Acquired melanocytic nevi
ASN	Atypical spitzoid neoplasm
ASZ	Alcoholic solution of zein
BA	Branchial anomaly
BAA	Branchial arch anomaly
BH	Breast height
BRBN	Blue rubber bleb nevus
BW	Breast width
CCBR	Cervical chondrocutaneous branchial remnant
CCBS	Congenital constriction band syndrome
CL	Cleft lip
CLOVES	Congenital lipomatous overgrowth, vascular malformations, epidermal nevi and scoliosis, skeletal or spinal anomalies
CLP	Cleft lip and palate
CLVM	Capillary-lymphatic-venous malformation
CM	Capillary malformation
CMCJ	Carpometacarpal joint
CMN	Congenital melanocytic nevi
CNLN	Congenital nevus-like nevus
CNs	Cranial nerves
CNS	Central nervous system
CO_2	Carbon dioxide
CP	Cleft palate
CSS	Cultured skin substitutes
CT	Computerized tomography
DFSP	Dermatofibrosarcoma protuberans
DHEA	Dehydroepiandrosterone
DIC	Disseminated intravascular coagulation
EPC	Endothelial progenitor cell
EVLT	Endovenous laser treatment
EXIT	Ex utero intrapartum treatment

FGFR	Fibroblast growth factor receptor
FGFs	Fibroblast growth factors
FNAB	Fine needle aspiration biopsy
FS	Fibrosarcoma
FTSG	Full-thickness skin graft
GLUT1	Glucose transporter protein
GPP	Gingivoperiosteoplasty
GVM	Glomuvenous malformation
GW	Gestational week
HemEPCs	Hemangioma-derived endothelial progenitor cells
HL	Hodgkin lymphoma
IF	Infantile fibrosarcoma
IHs	Infantile hemangiomas
IMD	Inframammary distance
IMF	Inframammary fold
IPJ	Interphalangeal joint
KHE	Kaposiform hemangioendothelioma
KMP	Kasabach-Merritt phenomenon
KTP	Potassium titanyl phosphate
LAHSHAL	Lip, alveolus, hard and soft palates
LCH	Langerhans cell histiocytosis
LDH	Lactate dehydrogenase
LIC	Localized intravascular coagulopathy
LM	Lymphatic malformation
LMWH	Low molecular weight heparin
LUMBAR	Lower body infantile hemangioma, urogenital anomalies and ulceration, myelopathy, bony deformities, anorectal malformations and arterial anomalies, renal anomalies
LVM	Lymphaticovenous malformation
MC	Metacarpal
MCPJ	Metacarpophalangeal joint
MIBG	Metaiodobenzylguanidine
MMPs	Matrix metalloproteinases
MRI	Magnetic resonance imaging
NAC	Nipple-areola complex
NB	Neuroblastoma
NCM	Neurocutaneous melanosis
Nd:YAG	Neodymium-doped yttrium aluminum garnet
NDCS	Nasal dermoid cyst and sinus
NF	Neurofibroma
NHL	Non-Hodgkin lymphoma
NICH	Noninvoluting congenital hemangioma
OMENS	Orbital asymmetry, mandibular hypoplasia, ear deformity, nerve involvement, soft tissue deficiency
OOM	Orbicularis oris muscle

OOPS	Operation on placental support
PAL	Power-assisted liposuction
PDL	Pulsed-dye laser
PG	Pyogenic granuloma
PHACES	Posterior fossa malformations, hemangioma, arterial anomalies, cardiovascular anomalies, eye abnormalities, sternal clefting
PMM	Pectoralis major muscle
PNAM	Presurgical nasal and alveolar molding
pPNET	Peripheral primitive neuroectodermal tumor
PSIO	Presurgical infant orthopedics
PT	Prothrombin time
PTT	Partial thromboplastin time
RICH	Rapidly involuting congenital hemangioma
RMS	Rhabdomyosarcoma
SHBG	Sex hormone-binding globulin
Shh	Sonic hedgehog protein
SLN	Sentinel lymph node
SpLN	Speckled lentiginous nevus
SS	Synovial sarcoma
SSN	Suprasternal notch
STS	Sodium tetradecyl sulfate
STSG	Split-thickness skin graft
TA	Tufted angioma
TGDC	Thyroglossal duct cyst
TSH	Thyroid-stimulated hormone
TTM	Topical timolol maleate
UAL	Ultrasound-assisted liposuction
US	Ultrasound
UV	Ultraviolet
VASER	Vibration amplification of sound energy at resonance
VEGF	Vascular endothelial growth factor
VH	Verrucous hemangioma
VM	Venous malformation
VPI	Velopharyngeal insufficiency
WHO	World Health Organization
Wnt	Wingless type
ZPA	Zone of polarizing activity

1 Introduction

The primary goal of this book is to share our experience in field of pediatric plastic surgery with health practitioners who are involved in primary practice and for all others who are involved in treatment of these patients.

Some fields of pediatric plastic surgery such as clefs, benign and malignant tumors, and vascular anomalies are difficult to present in short chapter, or even in one a book, because of their complexity, especially that they are already described by many other authors. Our idea was to present most important topics in pediatric plastic surgery through 14 chapters with general information about the clinical presentation, diagnostic procedures, treatment options, and complications.

Correction of prominent ears is presented because it is the most commonly performed aesthetic procedure in pediatric population, performed by different specialists. Microtia is in opposite extremely difficult to correct, and it is usually performed in specialized centers by highly experienced surgeons. Treatment of these patients by inexperienced surgeons can lead to devastating consequences.

Breast anomalies are common in pediatric population, with aesthetic and reconstructive goals tightly connected. Breast augmentation in pediatric population has to be performed with high precautions, and these patients are best to treat at the end of adolescence. There is high variety of breast anomalies and there is no adequate classification yet. Fortunately breast tumors in pediatric population are mostly benign. Gynecomastia is the most commonly treated breast anomaly in male pediatric population and in most cases with minimally invasive procedures.

Cleft patients are probably the most complicated group of patients in pediatric plastic surgery, and in this field multidisciplinary approach is extremely important, as well as the long-term follow-up. Hand surgeons are mainly dealing with hand problems (congenital or acquired), but often pediatric plastic surgeons have to perform surgery, especially for congenital hand anomalies.

Benign and malignant skin and soft tissue tumors belong to an extremely wide field, and it is almost impossible to classify them. We point out to the most important and most common benign and malignant skin and soft tissue tumors in pediatric

A.M. Vlahovic, E.Q. Haxhija, *Pediatric and Adolescent Plastic Surgery for the Clinician*, DOI 10.1007/978-3-319-56004-5_1

population. Pigmented lesions are often seen in pediatric population; fortunately they are in vast majority benign. Congenital melanocytic nevi are specific for pediatric population, and along with melanoma they have most attention in our book. Vascular anomalies are not in general part of aesthetic surgery; however, they are described in this book because of their high incidence and they often present indication for reconstructive surgery.

Our intention with this book is to bring basic information and to help the medical caregivers who are dealing with these patients in their everyday practice. We included figures of author's patients for almost all entities that are mentioned in the book. We hope that this book will be of great help to our colleagues and other health practitioners.

Otoplasty 2

2.1 Introduction

Surgical correction of prominent ears (otoplasty) is a cosmetic procedure commonly performed in the pediatric population, mostly by plastic and pediatric surgeons, and otorhinolaryngologists [1–13]. Children with prominent ears older than 5 or 6 years are generally complaining of being teased about their ears and usually style their hair to camouflage their deformity [3, 4, 10].

There is almost unlimited number of procedures for correction of the prominent ear [1, 5–14]. Parents are often the initiators of the idea for ear correction, and in most cases they have to bring a decision about the surgical treatment for their children [2]. The understanding between the surgeon, child, and parents has to be well established, and it is very important that the child cooperates with the surgeon (most surgeons wait until awareness of the deformity arises) [3, 10, 13]. Psychological aspect of this procedure and its impact on the child are also extremely important [2–4, 13].

Different terminologies have been used for this deformity: prominent ears, "bat" ears, apostasis otis, prominauris, etc. [4, 6, 8–13].

2.1.1 Epidemiology

The incidence of prominent ears is different among different population (5% among the Caucasian population) [11, 13, 14]. Familial history is noted in 8% of those patients, with males and females equally affected [13, 14].

2.1.2 Embryology

At about 40 days of gestation, the auricle is derived from the mesoderm of the first two branchial arches (six hillocks of His) [4, 10–12, 15–17]. During the third month of gestation, the auricle's protrusion increases, and by the end of the

A.M. Vlahovic, E.Q. Haxhija, *Pediatric and Adolescent Plastic Surgery for the Clinician*, DOI 10.1007/978-3-319-56004-5_2

sixth month, helix and antihelix are nearly completely formed [15]. The auricle is fully shaped at birth, approximately 85% of auricular growth is finished at 3 years of life and nearly adult size is achieved by age 5 or 6 years [4, 6, 11, 12, 15]. At 6 years, the ear size values are nearly the same for both sexes: 34 mm width in boys and girls, 55 mm length in boys and 54 mm in girls, and 22 mm protrusion in boys and 20 mm in girls [10, 12, 13]. Ear length is definitive by age of 15 years in boys and by age of 13 years in girls (60–65 mm), and ear width is complete by age 10 in girls and age 13 in boys (35 mm) [10–12]. Otoplasty in children aged 5–8 years has no significant influence on later auricular growth [4, 12].

2.1.3 Anatomy

The structures that formed the auricle are the helix, the antihelix, the antihelical scapha, the antihelical crura, the tragus, the antitragus, the cavum conchae, the cymba conchae, and the lobule (Fig. 2.1) [4, 9–11]. Fibroelastic auricular cartilage is medially covered by connective tissue and skin and laterally by skin only [4, 12]. The lobule is mainly composed of adipose and connective tissue [4, 16]. Several intrinsic and extrinsic muscles and ligaments influence the auricular shape [12]. The arterial supply to the auricle is derived from the posterior auricular, superficial temporal, and occipital arteries, and sensory innervation is provided by the auriculotemporal and great auricular nerve and branches of cranial nerves (CN) VII, IX, and X [11, 12, 15].

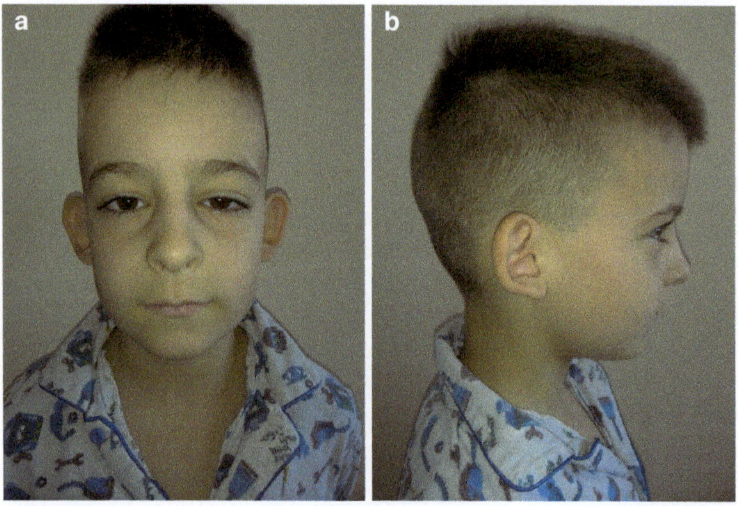

Fig. 2.1 Reconstruction of bilateral prominent auricle with suture technique: (**a**–**d**) preoperative view; (**e**–**h**) postoperative view

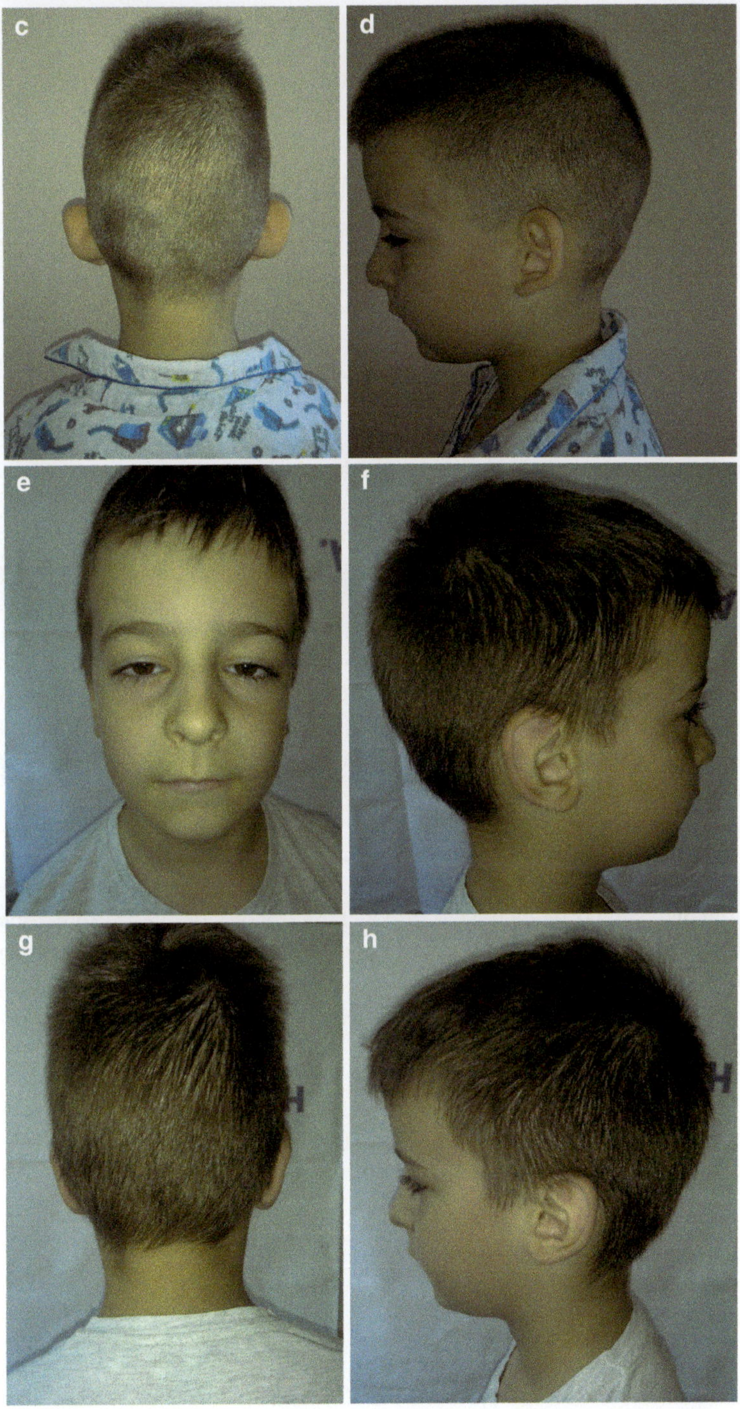

Fig. 2.1 (continued)

2.2 Psychosocial Aspects

Children have to be well motivated for correction of protruding ears because it can provoke long-term emotional consequences, and there is also parental responsibility since they give the consent for their children (if they are in preschool or in early school age) [2, 3]. The decision about surgery should be based on the needs of the child, not on pressure from the parents [2–4]. Children usually have better quality of life after correction of prominent ears, but an operation cannot guarantee that the child will be happier afterwards, even if the quality of surgical correction is good [1–4, 18].

2.3 Preoperative Evaluation

The precise anamnestic data should be taken (especially about excessive bleeding and poor wound healing) [1, 4, 12]. If there is a history of previous surgery and hypertrophic scarring or keloids, surgery has to be performed with maximum precautions [4, 14]. Both the patient and parents have to be well informed about every detail of the surgical procedure along with potential risk and complications [4, 6, 19]. The patient has to be intellectually and emotionally mature enough to cooperate [4, 12]. Otoplasty is contraindicated if patient has unrealistic expectations or if the patient is judged to be noncooperative postoperatively [3, 4, 13]. General anesthesia is recommended for children under 14 years of age (risks should be explained), and for teenagers local anesthesia with sedation can also be an option [4, 6, 11].

A careful preoperative examination of the auricles by thirds has to be performed, and any pre-existing asymmetry should be presented to patients [1, 4, 6, 8, 10, 13].

Cartilage consistency and thickness with the other ear abnormalities and associated anomalies should be evaluated; preoperative photography has to be obtained (for evaluation of the ear from the lateral direction, the patient should be in Frankfort horizontal plane) [4, 6, 8]. Distance between the lateral helical rim and the mastoid region is usually 17–21 mm, and the angle between mastoid and the auricle is approximately 30° [4, 6, 11–13, 18, 20].

The most common deformity seen in prominent ears is an underdeveloped (unfurled) antihelical fold, increased angle between the mastoid and concha (prominent concha), and protruding earlobe presenting as a single deformity or as a combination [4, 8, 9, 14, 18, 19, 21, 22].

2.4 Treatment Options

The goal of otoplasty is to restore normal anatomic features: however, perfection is hard to achieve [7, 8, 12, 13]. The decision about the technique that will be used depends of the deformity of the ears, patient demands, technical equipment, and surgeon's experience [2–4, 6, 7, 9–13, 19–21, 23–27].

2.5 Time of Otoplasty

Surgery can be performed as early as 3–6 years (before school age) since 85% of growth is finished at that time [9, 12, 13, 22]. Mostly, surgery is performed after 5 years of age [4, 12, 13, 24].

2.6 Techniques of Otoplasty

The basic goals of otoplasty according to Mc Dowell are as follows: all trace of protrusion of the upper one third of the ear must be corrected; from the front view, the helix of both ears should be seen beyond the antihelix; the helix should have a smooth and regular line through; the postauricular sulcus should not be markedly decreased or distorted; the ear should not be placed too close to the head; and the position of two ears should match fairly closely—to within 3 mm at any given point [6, 8, 12].

There are between 100 and 200 procedures that have been published for correction of prominent ears [4–12, 14, 16, 20, 22–27]. Surgical methods can be essentially divided into pure stitching techniques, pure incision techniques, and combined stitching-incision techniques (also are divided in cartilage-breaking and cartilage-spearing techniques) [1, 6, 12, 14, 27]. There has been increasing criticism of cartilage-cutting techniques [7, 19, 20, 27].

2.6.1 Pure Stitching Techniques

2.6.1.1 Mustardé Technique

This is one of the most widely used techniques to correct the prominent ear [4–6, 8, 11, 12]. Mustardé described an otoplastic technique which is suitable for folding an antihelical fold [4, 6, 22, 25]. The mattress sutures (nonabsorbable, transparent or white) are placed using a retroauricular access through the auricular cartilage and the perichondrium, without penetrating the ventral skin [22, 25]. This technique mainly addresses the superior third of the ear, it is suitable for soft or thin cartilage, and it can be combined with a lobulopexy and/or cavum rotation [4, 6, 12, 13, 25].

2.6.1.2 Furnas Technique

Furnas described a technique for overdeveloped conchal bowl and well-formed antihelical fold [4–6, 10, 12, 27]. Nonabsorbable sutures which penetrate entirely through both the auricular cartilage and the mastoid periosteum create a lasting correction of the conchal prominence [5, 6, 10]. It can be also used in conjunction with Mustardé mattress sutures for correction of antihelical fold underdevelopment [5, 6, 12]. Narrowing of external auditory canal is a complication of this technique described in literature if the mastoid sutures are placed too anteriorly [6, 12].

2.6.1.3 Horlock, Misra, and Gault Technique

In this technique, the concept of posterior concho-scaphoid and concho-mastoid suturing is used, with a posterior subcutaneous tissue elevated as a fascial flap in order to prevent complications of the sutures (Fig. 2.1) [7, 19, 20, 27].

2.6.2 Pure Incision Techniques

2.6.2.1 Chongchet Technique

Chongchet technique is based on Gibson and Davis work (cartilage incision on one side has the ability to warp to the opposite side) [4, 7, 11, 16]. Weakening of the anterior auricular cartilage is performed by multiple partial-thickness incisions in order to restore normal curvature of antihelical fold and soften the external contour of the corrected prominent ear [4, 7, 16, 18, 20].

2.6.2.2 Stenstrom Technique

The Stenstrom technique is also based on Gibson-Davis principles; the excision of the skin is performed on the posterior side of the ear, and superficial cartilage scoring is made by a special instrument on the lateral side of the ear [4, 10, 11, 26]. The author stated that the technique is adequate for insufficient folding of the antihelix and excessive cupping of concha [26].

2.6.2.3 Nordzell Technique

This technique is based on the skin incision on the medial side of the ear, entering to the anterior surface of the cartilage with abrasion of the antihelix and superior crus [11].

2.6.3 Combined Incision-Suture Techniques

Combination of techniques is often performed by surgeons, yet these techniques are complex to perform [4, 10–12]. There are several combination techniques described in the literature [4, 6, 10, 12, 13].

2.6.3.1 Converse Technique

This technique is suitable for patients with stiff cartilage [4, 6]. The cartilage incisions are placed parallel to the helical rim and the base of the antihelix, including a superior crus, using a retroauricular approach, followed by tubing of the cartilage with placement of sutures to secure the position [4, 10–12]. This technique is complicated, and sharp and undesirable edges in antihelical area frequently occur [4].

2.6.3.2 Farrior Technique

This technique may include cartilage scoring for the creation of antihelical fold (multiple incisions perpendicular to the direction of antihelical fold), suturing, and conchal setback techniques [6, 12]. Several other procedures may be included according to local anatomical findings such as longitudinal, partial-thickness wedge excisions of cartilage, horizontal mattress sutures, trimming of the cauda helicis, and excision of postauricular elliptical dumbbell skin segment [12].

2.6.3.3 Weerda Technique

By this technique, the auricular cartilage is weakened by diamond drill immediately above and below the intended new antihelical fold and the antihelical crus, using a retroauricular access with additional, full-thickness mattress sutures used to fix the antihelix in the intended position [4].

2.6.4 Lobuloplasty

There are several techniques for correction of protruding lobule, including in most cases skin excision on medial part of lobule and suture to a posterior part of concha [4, 9–11, 21–23].

2.6.5 Nonsurgical Correction of Protruding Ears

Auricular molding has been reported to be a simple, effective, and inexpensive treatment for correction of all kinds of congenital auricular deformities [4–8, 11, 12, 28–30]. There are various ear splinting materials and methods [11, 28–30]. Splints can be easily placed by plastic (pediatric) surgeons, nurses, and parents [24]. Correction is most effective within first 96 h (cartilage is soft since maternal estrogens are highest in the first 3 days of birth), and maximum age that splinting should be applied until 3 or 6 months of age [6, 12, 15, 28, 29]. If there is no result after 4 weeks, it should be stopped [29]. Minimal invasive otoplasty recently has become popular, but long-term data are not yet available [4].

2.6.6 Complications of Otoplasty

Up to 10% of each of the three categories of otoplasty techniques can result in complications, and they are well described in the literature [1, 4, 6, 12, 13, 21]. Ear deformation after primary otoplasty such as overcorrection, undercorrection, visible cartilage irregularities or unnatural contours, and unpleasing shape of the ear requires revision surgery [9, 13, 19]. Severe complication requires ear reconstruction with autologous costal cartilage [1, 14, 18, 19]. Complications can be divided into two categories: early (within first 14 postoperative days) and late (14 days after surgery) [1, 4, 6, 8, 9, 12–14, 18].

2.6.6.1 Early Complications

Hematoma can occur because of inadequate hemostasis and coagulation disorders (that were not recognized preoperatively) or if local anesthetic with vasoconstrictor is used, and it requires prompt reaction (Fig. 2.2a, b) [1, 6, 13, 21]. *Infection* is rare in pediatric population, it can be provoked by placing the fingers in the auricle area because of pruritus, and it usually requires antibiotics with local treatment (Fig. 2.3a–c) [1, 4, 6]. *Pressure ulcers* can occur on the skin of the auricle and on

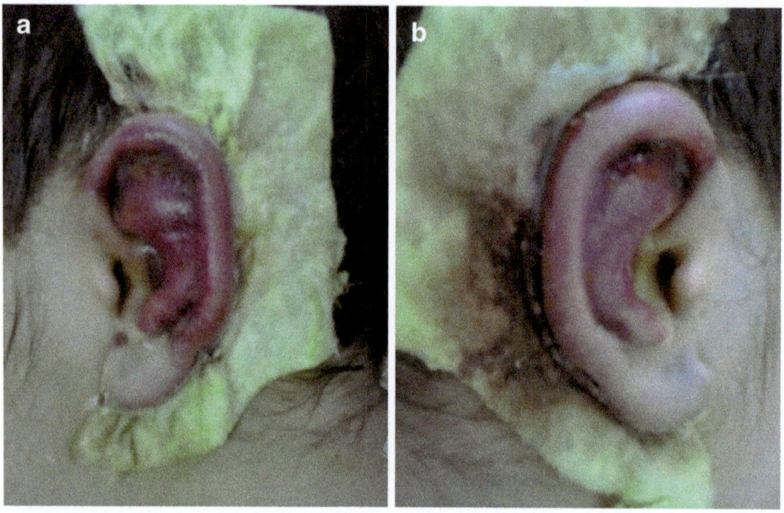

Fig. 2.2 Hematoma on both ears after otoplasty as the result of coagulation disorder revealed after the surgery: (**a**) left ear; (**b**) right ear

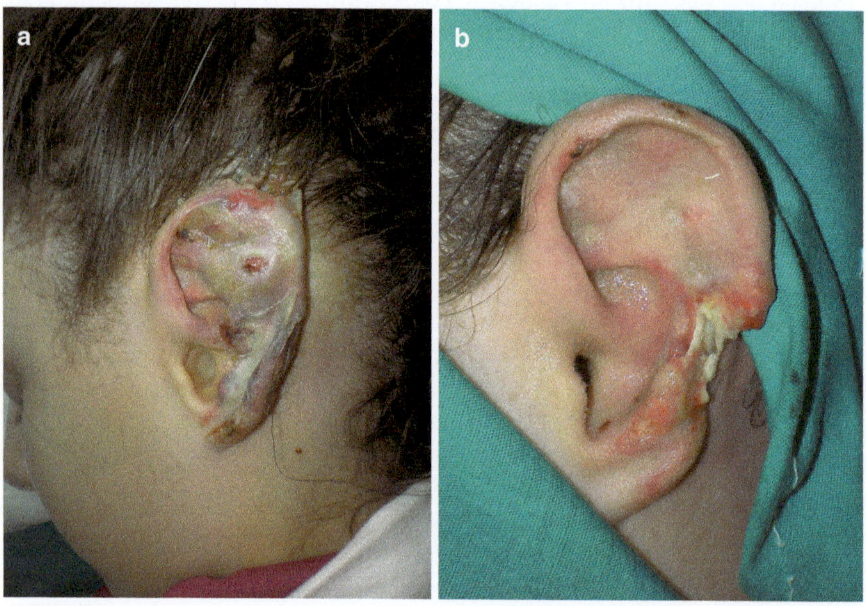

Fig. 2.3 Ear necrosis (child scratches the ear): (**a**) preoperative view; (**b**) necrectomy performed; (**c**) postoperative view

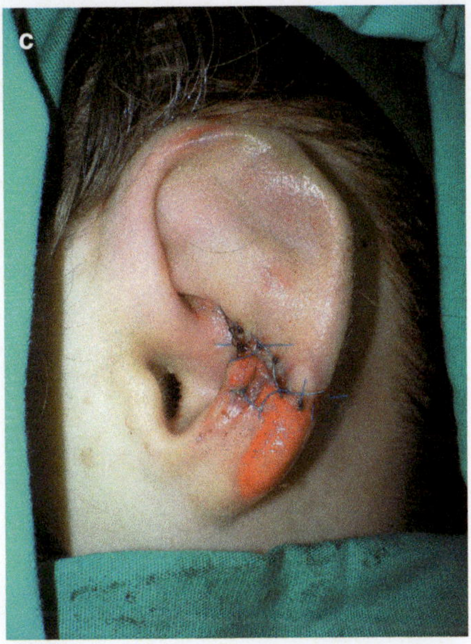

Fig. 2.3 (continued)

the ear cartilage as a result of pressure necrosis if the head bandages are too closely fitting [1, 13, 21]. *Asymmetry of auricles* in comparison with the sides in early postoperative period is usually iatrogenic [1, 13].

2.6.6.2 Late Complications

Recurrence is the most common complication observed following otoplasty, and it occurs frequently with incision techniques [1, 4, 6, 12–14]. *Suture complications*, such as protrusion through the posterior skin (fistulae), are quite common, and the stitching material should be completely removed [1, 4, 6, 8, 9, 13]. *Telephone ear* occurs if overcorrection of the middle part of the ear is performed with the protrusion of the upper part of the helix and of the earlobe (Fig. 2.4) [1, 8, 9, 13]. *Excessive edge formations* usually occur with pure cutting techniques, and it can be corrected by careful abrasion of the cartilage (Fig. 2.5) [1, 10, 14]. *Overcorrection* (mostly occurs because of excessive excision of retroauricular skin) can be corrected by using free full-thickness skin graft or conchal cartilage grafting, and *undercorrection* is usually corrected by suture revision and conchal reduction (Fig. 2.6a–f) [1, 9, 12, 14, 19, 21]. A *hypertrophic scar* and *keloid* formation are late complication of otoplasty, and there are several treatment options, including local injection of triamcinolon and excision (Fig. 2.7a, b) [1, 2, 12–14, 21].

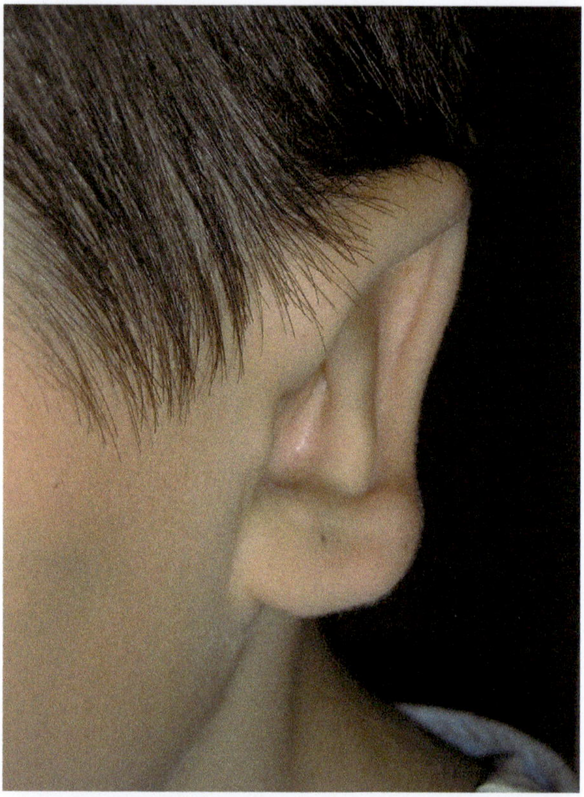

Fig. 2.4 Overcorrection of the middle third of the ear: "telephone ear" deformity as a complication of the otoplasty

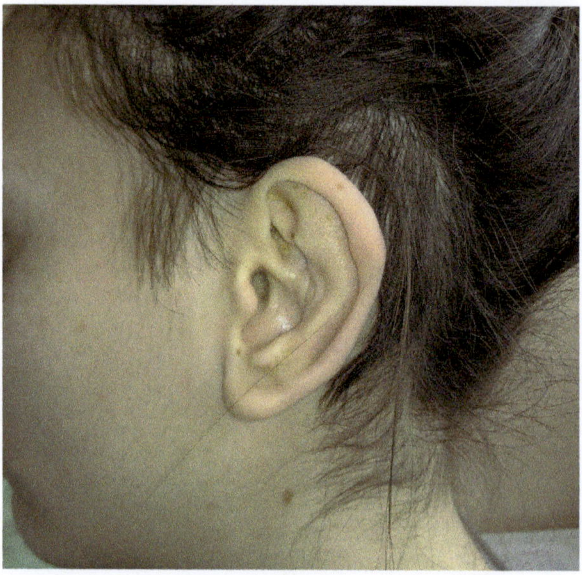

Fig. 2.5 Excessive ear edges as a complication after otoplasty

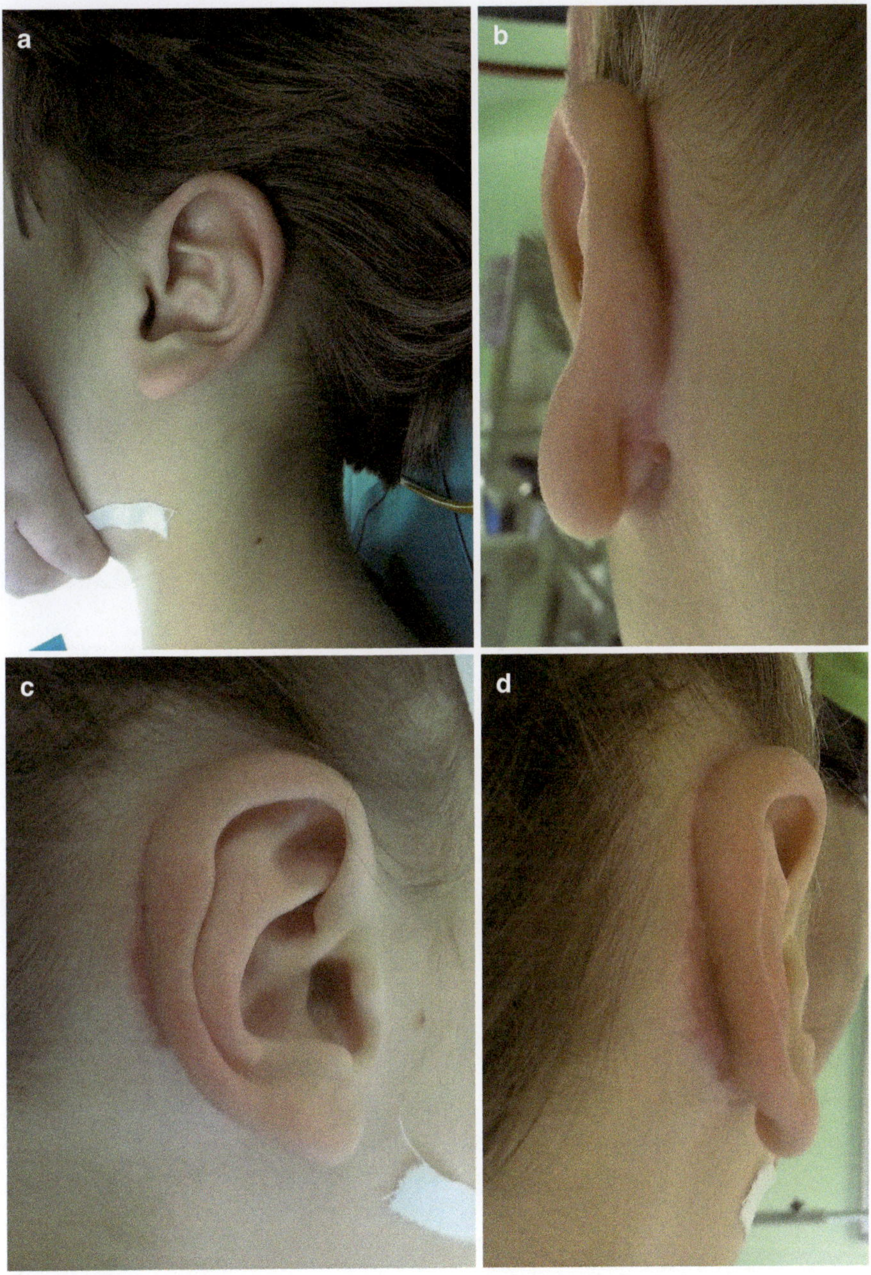

Fig. 2.6 Overcorrection of both ears caused by excessive skin excision: (**a**–**d**) preoperative view; (**e**, **f**) postoperative result after reconstruction with skin grafts

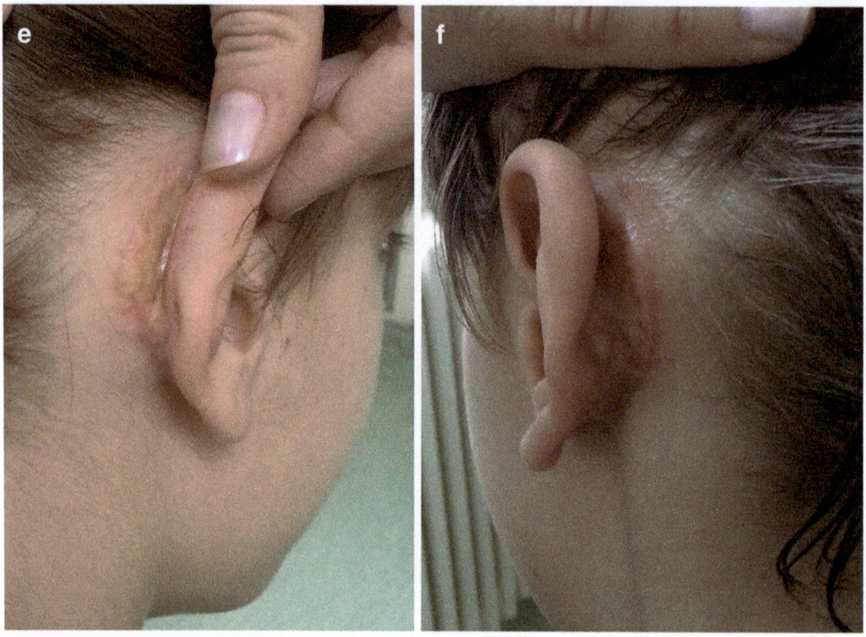

Fig. 2.6 (continued)

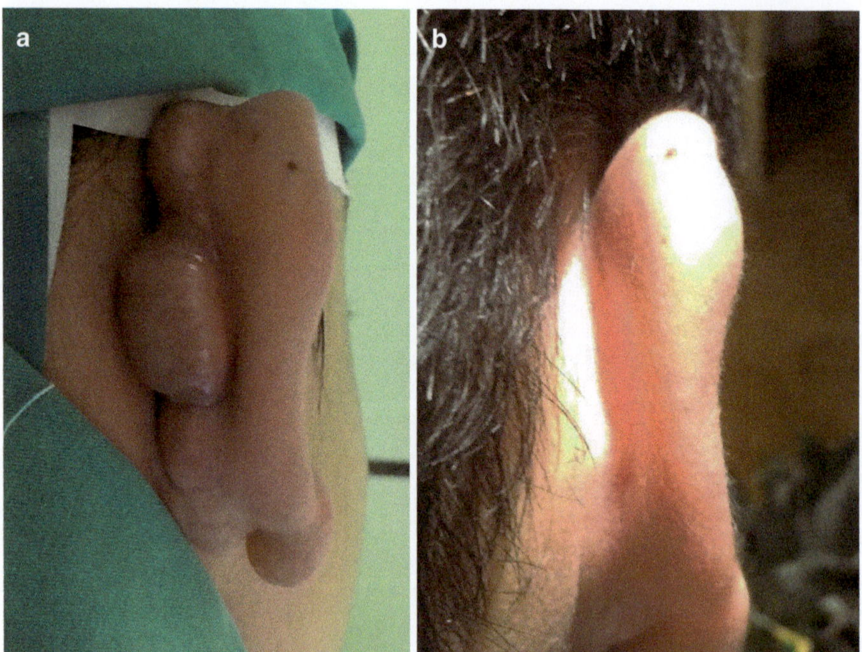

Fig. 2.7 Ear keloid: (**a**) appearance after previous otoplasty and three excisions of hypertrophic scars in other institutions; (**b**) 4 years after our reconstruction

2.7 Postoperative Care

The concavities of the ear are packed with cotton to maintain positioning and correct healing [4, 6]. The purpose of the dressing is to protect the repair and it should be retaining bandage [1, 9]. For pediatric patients the first dressing is performed on the first or second postoperative day to evaluate any early complication [1, 4].

Standard head bandage is usually recommended for 4–5 or 7–8 days after the procedure [1, 8, 18, 20]. If nonabsorbable sutures are used, they are removed after the seventh postoperative day, and a forehead bandage worn at night for 6 weeks is recommended [4, 9, 20]. Sustaining of physical activities is also recommended.

References

1. Staindl O, Siedek V. Complications of auricular correction. Curr Top Otorhinolaryngol Head Neck Surg. 2007;6:Doc 3.1–13.
2. Hong P, Gorodzinsky AY, Taylor BA, Chorney JM. Parental decision making in pediatric otoplasty: the role of shared decision making in parental decisional conflict and decisional regret. Laryngoscope. 2016;126(Suppl 5):S5–S13.
3. Bradbury ET, Hewison J, Timmons MJ. Psychological and social outcome of prominent ear correction in children. Br J Plast Surg. 1992;45:97–100.
4. Naumann A. Otoplasty-techniques, characteristics and risks. Curr Top Otorhinolaryngol Head Neck Surg. 2007;6:Doc 04.1–14.
5. Furnas DW. Correction of prominent ears by conchamastoid sutures. Plast Reconstr Surg. 1968;42(3):189–93.
6. Nazarian R, Eshraghi AA. Otoplasty for the protruding ear. Sem Plast Surg. 2011;25(4):288–93.
7. Mandal A, Bahia H, Ahmad T, Stewart KJ. Comparison of cartilage scoring and cartilage sparing otoplasty—a study of 203 cases. J Plast Reconstr Aesthet Surg. 2006;59(11):1170–6.
8. Thorne CH, Wilkes G. Ear deformities, otoplasty and ear reconstruction. Plast Reconstr Surg. 2012;129:701e–16e.
9. Thorne CH. Otoplasty. In: Neligen PC, Grotting JC, editors. Plastic surgery. 3rd ed. St Louis: Elsevier/Saunders; 2013. p. 485–93.
10. Furnas DW. External ear. In: Jurkiewitz MJ, Krizek TJ, Mathes SJ, Ariyan S, editors. Plastic surgery. Principles and practice. St Louis: Mosby; 1990. p. 171–206.
11. Preuss S, Eriksson E. Prominent ears. In: Achauer BM, Eriksson E, Guyuron B, Coleman III JJ, Russell RC, Craig A, Kolk V, editors. Plastic surgery, indications, operations, and outcomes. St Louis: Mosby; 2000. p. 1057–64.
12. Petersson RS, Friedman O. Current trends in otoplasty. Curr Opin Otolaryng Head Neck Surg. 2008;16:352–8.
13. Limandjaja GC, Breugem CC, Mink van der Molen AB, Kon M. Complications of otoplasty: a literature review. J Plast Reconstr Aesthet Surg. 2009;62(1):19–27.
14. Firmin F, Sanger C, O'Toole G. Ear reconstruction following severe complications of otoplasty. J Plast Reconstr Aesthet Surg. 2008;61:S13–20.
15. Tan ST, Gault DT. When do ears become prominent? Br J Plast Surg. 1994;47(8):573–4.
16. Chongchet V. A method of antihelix reconstruction. J Plast Surg. 1963;16:268–72.
17. Bartel-Friedrich S, Wulke C. Classification and diagnosis of ear malformations. GMS Curr Top Otorhinolaryngol Head Neck Surg. 2007;6:Doc05.
18. Jeffery SLA. Complications following correction of prominent ears: an audit review of 122 cases. Br J Plast Surg. 1999;52(7):588–90.
19. Szychta P, Orfaniotis G, Stewart KJ. Revision otoplasty: an algorithm. Plast Reconstr Surg. 2012;130(4):907–16.

20. Schaverien MV, Al-Busaidi S, Stewart KJ. Long-term results of posterior suturing with post-auricular fascial flap otoplasty. J Plast Reconstr Aesthet Surg. 2010;63(9):1447–51.
21. Calder JC, Naasan A. Morbidity of otoplasty: a review of 562 consecutive cases. Br J Plast Surg. 1994;47(3):170–4.
22. Mustardé JC. Protruding or lop ear deformity. In: Mustardé JC, editor. Plastic surgery in infancy and childhood. Edinburgh: E. & S. Livingstone; 1971. p. 292–313.
23. Spira M, McCrea R, Gerow FJ, Hardy SB. Correction of the principal deformities causing protruding ears. Plast Reconstr Surg. 1969;44(2):150–4.
24. Webster GV. The tail of helix as a key to otoplasty. Plast Reconstr Surg. 1969;44(5):455–61.
25. Mustardé JC. The correction of prominent ears using simple mattress sutures. Br J Plast Surg. 1963;16:170–8.
26. Stenstrom SJ. A "natural" technique for correction of congenitaly prominent ears. Plast Reconstr Surg. 1963;32(5):509–18.
27. Horlock N, Misra A, Gault DT. The postauricular fascial flap as an adjunct to Mustardé and Furnas type otoplasty. Plast Reconstr Surg. 2001;108(6):1487–90. Discussion 1491.
28. Brown FE, Colen LB, Addante RR, Graham Jr JM. Correction of congenital auricular deformities by splinting in the neonatal period. Pediatrics. 1986;78(3):406–11.
29. Van Wijk MP, Breugem CC, Kon M. Non-surgical correction of congenital deformities of the auricule: a systematic review of the literature. J Plast Reconstr Aesthet Surg. 2009;62:727–36.
30. Anstadt EE, Johns DN, Kwok AC, Siddiqi F, Gociman B. Neonatal ear molding: timing and technique. Pediatrics. 2016;137(3):1–4.

3 Microtia and Other Congenital Auricular Deformities

3.1 Introduction

A child with malformed ear often attracts attention from curious playmates (usually at 4 or 5 years of age when body image relating to face develops), and very often the child faces rejection, teasing, and name-calling [1, 2]. Early surgery for the deformity is desirable for the child psyche, but it is in vast majority of cases technically impractical [1].

Ear deformities can be classified into *anotia*, complete hypoplasia or *microtia* (with or without atresia of external auditory canal), *hypoplasia of middle third* of the auricle, *hypoplasia of superior third* of the auricle (constricted ear, cryptotia, hypoplasia of entire superior third), and *prominent ear* [1, 3]. Other ear anomalies also occur with variable incidence and different treatment options [1, 3–9].

3.2 Embryology

The auricle, the auditory canal, and the middle ear originate from the first and second branchial arches [1]. At the end of the fifth and the beginning of the sixth embryonic week, mesenchymal proliferation of the first and second branchial arches develops six surface irregularities (hillocks) which fuse into the definitive ear [1, 4]. In case of incomplete fusion, malformation of the external and/or middle ear can occur [1, 3, 4]. External and middle ear has same embryonic origin (microtia is accompanying with anomalies of middle ear), and the inner ear is almost always normal in patients with microtia since it has different embryonic development [3]. The hearing loss in microtia/atresia is conductive in nature [1, 3, 6].

A.M. Vlahovic, E.Q. Haxhija, *Pediatric and Adolescent Plastic Surgery for the Clinician*, DOI 10.1007/978-3-319-56004-5_3

3.3 Anatomy

The structures that formed the auricle are helix, the antihelix, the antihelical scapha, the antihelial crura, the tragus, the antitragus, the cavum conchae, the cymba conchae, and the lobule [3, 7–9]. Fibroelastic auricular cartilage is medially covered by the connective tissue and skin and laterally covered by skin only, and the lobule itself is mainly composed of adipose and connective tissue [3].

3.4 Microtia

Microtia is severe hypoplasia of external ear with variable deformation of auditory canal [1–4, 7, 8, 10–18].

The incidence of microtia is between 1 in 6000 and 8000 live births [2, 8, 12]. The incidence is low among Caucasians and it's high in Japanese and among American Indians [1, 8, 15]. Microtia is unilateral in vast majority of cases (80–90%); the right side is involved more often than the left, and boys are affected more often than girls [1, 2, 7, 8].

Microtia is probably multifactorial in etiology with environmental and genetic factors involved, and it counts as a part of the spectrum of hemifacial microsomia deformities (maldevelopment in the first and second branchial arches) [1, 7, 12]. Microtia can be associated with other deformities such as facial skeletal asymmetries, facial nerve paralysis, cleft lip and palate, cardiac anomalies, and urinary tract anomalies [1, 3, 7, 8, 15].

Gilles is credited with the first use of rib cartilage for construction of an auricular framework in 1920, and Tanzer reintroduced the technique of autogenous costal cartilage grafts as a method of auricular reconstruction in 1959 [2, 11, 12]. Brent and Nagata techniques are most widely used for auricular reconstruction, followed by Firmin, Park, and Siegert modifications of these techniques [1, 3, 7, 8, 12, 13, 15–17].

Patients with unilateral microtia/atresia usually have normal hearing on the contralateral ear, and hearing rehabilitation in these patients can include observation, band-retained bone conduction sound processor, osseointegrated implant-retained bone conduction sound processor (after 5 years of age), and atresiaplasty [1, 3, 6–8, 15]. Patients with bilateral microtia/atresia usually have serviceable hearing, and these patients should be fitted with a bone-conduction hearing aid as early as possible in life [1, 3, 6–8, 15]. Computerized tomography (CT) of temporal bone has to be performed at about 4 years of age prior to surgical treatment [15].

Canal construction (atresiaplasty) and tympanoplasty in children with microtia should be performed only in cases with hearing loss in the contralateral ear or in cases of bilateral microtia, and it is performed in most cases after the microtia reconstruction [1, 7, 15]. Recently some authors proposed that atresiaplasty can be performed before or simultaneously with the microtia reconstruction [15].

3.4.1 Classification

The microtia deformity itself is enormously variable [3]. The most common variety of microtia involves an irregular cartilage remnant with an associated small vertical earlobe with absent auditory canal [1, 3, 4, 8]. There are several classification of microtia derived from any authors: Nagata, Brent, Fukuda, Muerman-Marks, Asse, Firmin, and Marx (Rogers modification) [1, 3, 8, 12, 15].

According to Nagata classification, there are five types of microtia: *lobule type* (the patient has an ear remnant and malpositioned lobule but has no concha, acoustic meatus, or tragus), *concha type* (the patient presents with ear remnant, malpositioned earlobe, concha, tragus, and antitragus with an incisura antitragica), *small concha type* (the patient presents with an ear remnant, malpositioned earlobe, and a small indentation instead of concha), *anotia* (the patient is present with no, or only a minute, ear remnant), and *atypical microtia* (the patient presents with deformities that do not fit into any of the above categories) (Fig. 3.1a–d) [1, 7, 8, 12, 15]. There is a four-grade classification proposed by Marx (modified by Rogers), detailed classification of microtia proposed by

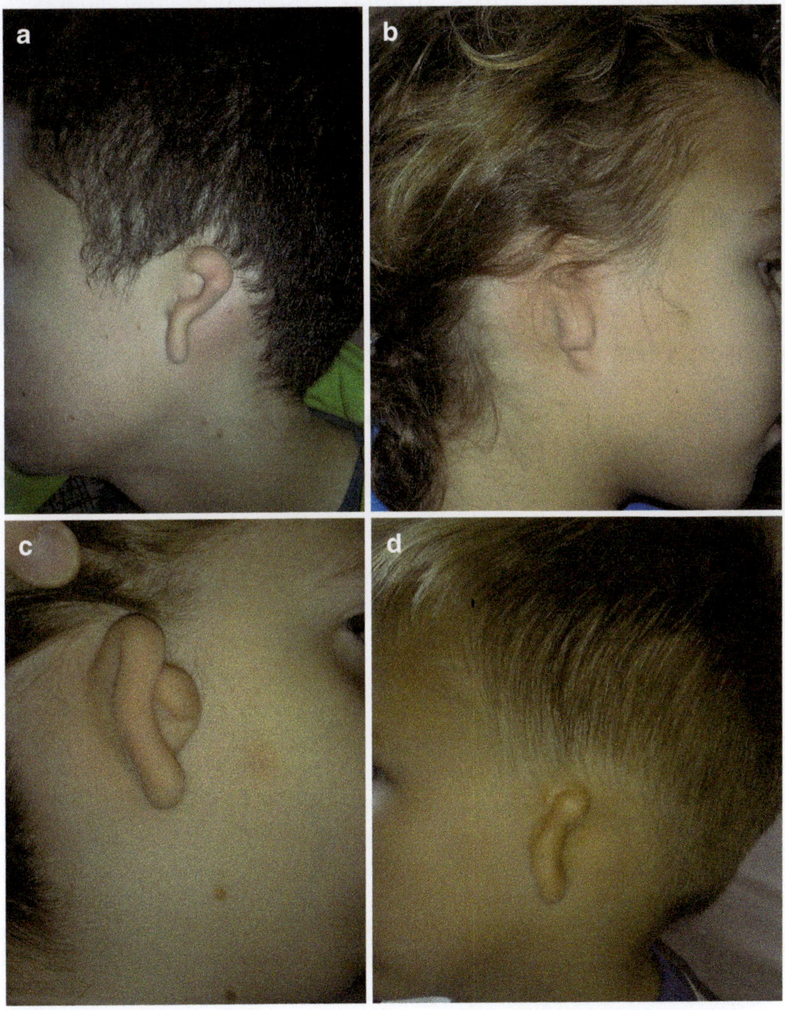

Fig. 3.1 Different types of microtia: (**a**) lobule type; (**b**) anotia; (**c**, **d**) atypical microtia

Firmin, and also a classification of hemifacial microsomia associated with microtia proposed by Mulliken et al., named OMENS (Orbital asymmetry, Mandibular hypoplasia, Ear deformity, Nerve involvement, Soft tissue deficiency) [7, 11, 15].

3.4.2 Patient Evaluation

These patients are usually seen within the first 12 months of age, and parents are instructed to return annually until the age for surgery [8]. The recommended age for surgery is at least 6 years, and in most cases, it is around 10 years of age [6, 8, 15]. Alloplastic reconstruction is possible from 3 years of age [15]. Preoperative photographs are obtained, and normal ear side is evaluated (position and anatomy of normal ear), since it is the model for opposite side [1, 3, 7, 8, 14, 15]. At opposite side with microtia, we examine the skin quality, presence of external auditory canal, hair line position, and scar presence [7, 8, 14]. During the exam, the chest wall has to be checked in every detail, and we need to establish any deformity that may complicate chondral graft taking [1, 3, 7, 11, 15]. Treatment options should be discussed with the patient and parents [3, 8, 15].

3.4.3 Surgical Reconstruction

Indications for surgical treatment are aesthetic, functional, and psychosocial [15]. Reconstruction of the architectural structure of the auricle and the projection of auricle are two important topics in this surgery [1–3, 6–8, 10–15]. There are three options for auricular reconstruction of microtia: autogenous reconstruction, composite autogenous/alloplastic reconstruction (using an alloplastic ear framework), and prosthetic reconstruction [1–4, 6–8, 10–18]. Reconstructed ear in the long term is usually more bulky with lack of the flexibility of the normal ear [7].

3.4.3.1 Autogenous Reconstruction

This is the most widely used approach [1–3, 7, 8, 11, 13, 15, 17]. Two techniques for autogenous reconstruction of the auricle, using a rib cartilage framework, described by Brent and Nagata were dominant for a long period of time [1, 3, 7, 8, 12]. Firmin adopted Nagata's two-stage approach and modified it, and Park used a three-stage procedure for patients with microtia, with tissue expansion during the first stage [7, 11–13, 18]. Siegert and colleagues also described a technique for microtia reconstruction [15]. The Brent technique involves four stages: creation and placement of a rib cartilage auricular framework, rotation of malpositioned ear lobule into the correct position, elevation of the reconstructed auricle, and deepening of the concha with creation of the tragus [3, 7]. The Nagata technique encompasses two stages [3, 8, 15]. The first stage is performed not earlier than 10 years of age (chest circumference at the level of the xiphoid has to be at least 60 cm) [8, 12]. In the first stage, creation of costal cartilage framework is performed, including the rotation of the lobule into the correct position [7, 8, 12, 15]. The second stage involves elevation of the reconstructed ear and creation of retroauricular sulcus [7, 8, 12, 15, 18].

3.4.3.2 Preoperative Marking

The location of the earlobe on the normal side is transferred to the affected side (reconstructed ear has to be in symmetrical position with unaffected ear) [7, 8, 14]. The normal ear is traced on the x-ray film, thin plastic film, or paper pattern and sterilized, and by using these tracing, a template of the desired framework is fashioned, it's reversed, and framework pattern is designed for the new ear [3, 7, 8, 14, 15]. An acrylic or plaster replica of normal ear can also be used (Fig. 3.2a–c) [3]. The exact location and orientation of the desired auricle are drawn on the patient

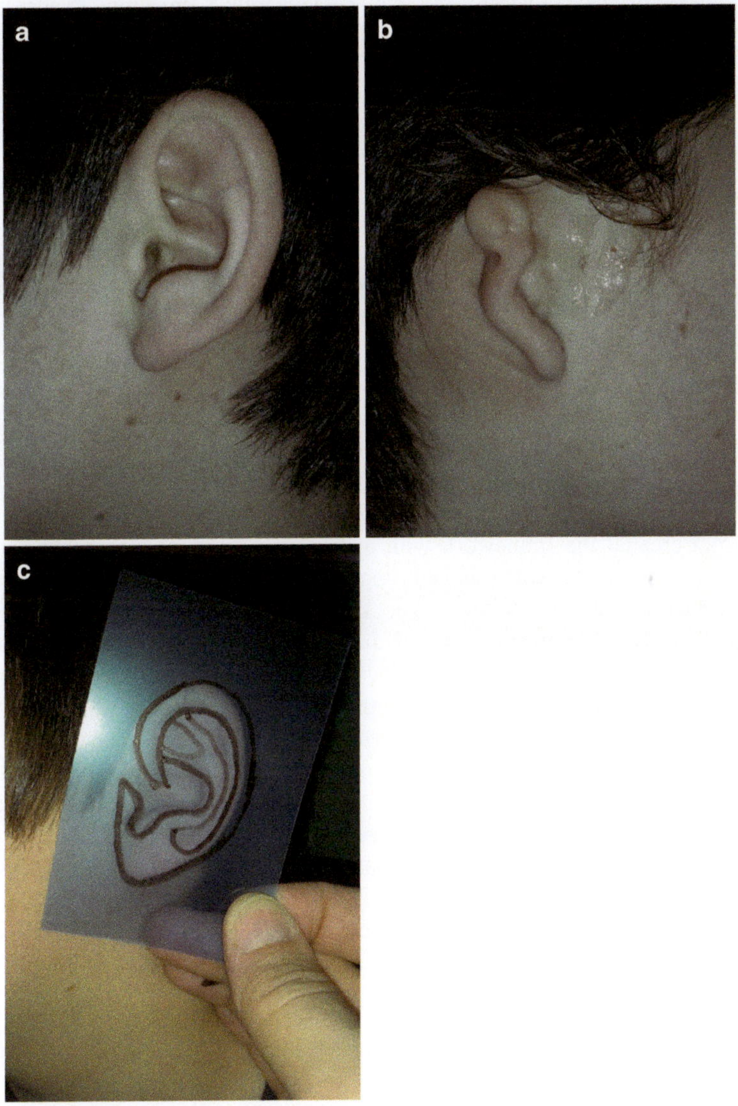

Fig. 3.2 Preoperative marking: (**a**) normal ear; (**b**) contralateral ear deformity; (**c**) normal ear traced on a plastic film

[3, 7, 8, 11]. Different incisions on the skin are made depending on the technique that is used; cartilage remnant is removed preserving the skin, and the pocket is dissected beyond the outline of the eventual auricle [3, 7, 8, 11, 13, 15–18].

3.4.3.3 Chest

Incision on the chest can be transverse or oblique, allowing access to the fifth to ninth ribs [1–3, 7, 8, 12–18]. The cartilage can be harvested in subperichondrial plane or with perichondrium, leaving the posterior perichondrium intact [7, 10, 12]. For Brent technique, synchondrosis of the sixth to seventh rib is taken as well as a free part of the eighth rib for the helical rim, and in Nagata technique, three more pieces of cartilage have to be taken: for antihelix/triangular fossa, a piece for tragus/antitragus and a piece to be banked for the second stage [3, 7, 10]. The donor area is closed by primary suture with excess cartilage placed superficially to rectus muscle [7, 13, 15].

3.4.3.4 3D Graft Fabrication

Different numbers of pieces are needed, and that depends on the technique that is used, and details are spliced together by using nylon or wire sutures [1–3, 7, 8, 11, 15–18]. The antihelix/triangular fossa piece is attached, followed by the helical rim in a similar way in both techniques and finally the tragus/antitragus piece in Nagata technique [3, 7, 8, 15]. The framework is inserted into the pocket [1–3, 7, 8, 10–18]. Once the closure has been accomplished, the auricular convolutes are packed with Xeroform bolster or with Vaseline gauze over the skin and into cavities, bulky non-compressive dressing is applied, and closed suction drains are used [1–3, 7, 8, 12, 15, 16]. Tubes are frequently changed (to provide skin coaptation and hemostasis) and removed after there is no drainage (usually after 5 days) [3, 7, 10, 15]. A piece of cartilage is banked in the chest or in the scalp region [3, 7, 15].

Firmin created the framework with at least six different pieces: the base, the antihelix, the helix, the tragus and antitragus, the projection piece, and a spare piece stored under thoracic skin to reconstruct the posterior wall of the concha during the second stage [11, 13]. Firmin et al. distinguish three types of microtia concerning carving of the framework: (1) microtia without tragus; (2) microtia with tragus, but without antitragus; and (3) microtia with a good tragus-antitragus complex [11]. Authors have been adding a piece of cartilage deep to the root of the helix and the tragus, bridging the two improving 3D contour, and they also devised an algorithm to manage the skin remnants depending on skin potential [11, 13, 18]. Park technique is consisted of two or three stages [12, 16–18]. In the first stage, tissue expander is inserted in the mastoid region, and after the expansion is completed, the second stage is performed with cartilage frame harvesting from the contralateral rib followed by placement of framework into position [12, 16, 18]. In some cases, the third stage is performed for additional shaping of framework [12, 16].

3.4.3.5 Elevation of Framework

The elevation of framework is performed at least 6 months after grafting [10, 11]. This is the second stage in Nagata technique and the third stage in Brent technique [3, 7, 8, 12, 15, 18]. The framework is elevated, and the retroauricular sulcus is resurfaced with retroauricular scalp and full-thickness graft [1–3, 7, 8, 11, 15, 16, 18]. Nagata adds a piece of rib cartilage covered with the temporoparietal flap, while Brent and Firmin use turnover "book flap" of occipitalis fascia to cover this wedge of rib cartilage [3, 7, 8, 11, 13, 15, 17, 18]. Hydroxyapatite can be used as an alternative to cartilage to sustain the angle of elevated concha [10]. For the second stage, when small amount of projection is needed, Firmin used advancement of retroauricular skin with split thickness skin graft (STSG) from the scalp, for moderate projection piece of cartilage into tunnel behind the framework, and for reconstruction of entire posterior wall, modified Nagata technique is used [11]. After elevation of the framework and placing skin graft, sutures are tied over a bolster for a tamponade [1, 3, 7, 8, 15].

3.4.3.6 Rotation of Lobule

The rotation of lobule has to be done from vertical to horizontal position, and in Nagata and Firmin techniques, it is performed at the first stage and in Brent technique during the second stage [3, 7, 8, 11, 12, 15, 18].

3.4.3.7 Brent Technique 4 Stadium: Creation of Tragus

Conchal composite graft is taken from the posterior conchal wall of the contralateral ear, and through L incision, insertion of graft is performed [3, 7]. Conchal excavation and contralateral otoplasty can be performed during this stage [3].

3.4.4 Complications

Cartilage exposure, infection, and skin necrosis are the most often complications [2, 3, 7, 15]. Antibiotic is applied locally along with systemic therapy [3, 12, 15]. In case of exposition of the cartilage framework, an exposed area is more than 1 cm, and urgent covering with temporoparietal flap and skin graft is required [3, 7]. Nylon and wire sutures may become visible [3, 7]. Distortions due to the frame, contracture of conchal cavity, and displacement of helical cartilage are complications described in the literature [2, 15]. The most common acute complications related to obtaining a cartilage graft are pneumothorax and atelectasis, and late complications include unsatisfactory scars and chest contour deformities [3, 19].

3.4.5 Composite Autogenous/Alloplastic Reconstruction

An auricular framework composed of high-density porous polyethylene is used as an alternative option to costal cartilage [7, 12, 15, 17, 20, 21]. Ear reconstruction can be completed in one stage, and it can be done before the school age [12, 15]. There is a high rate of frame exposition, but if temporoparietal flap for covering the framework is used, complications are less common [7, 12, 15, 17].

3.4.6 Prosthetic Reconstruction

The ear prosthesis (epithesis) is an alternative to plastic surgery [7, 12, 15, 17]. The retention of prosthesis is achieved by osseointegration using titanium implants to integrate prosthesis into living bone [7, 12]. Children are poor candidates for prostheses (they need to maintain adequate hygiene, and the daily removal and the replacement of the prosthesis serve as a constant remainder of the deformity) [7, 12, 15]. Prostheses have to be changed in approximately every 5 years which is more expensive in the long term than autogenous reconstruction [12, 15]. Tissue engineering is the future option for construction of precisely shaped cartilage implant without donor site morbidity [17].

3.5 Constricted Ear

The constricted ear (known as cup or lop ear canoe ear, cockle shell ear) is a congenital ear deformity of variable severity characterized in all types by lidding of the helix and compression of narrowing of the scapha and fossa triangularis and with protrusion of the ear and low ear position in moderate and severe cases (Fig. 3.3a–c)

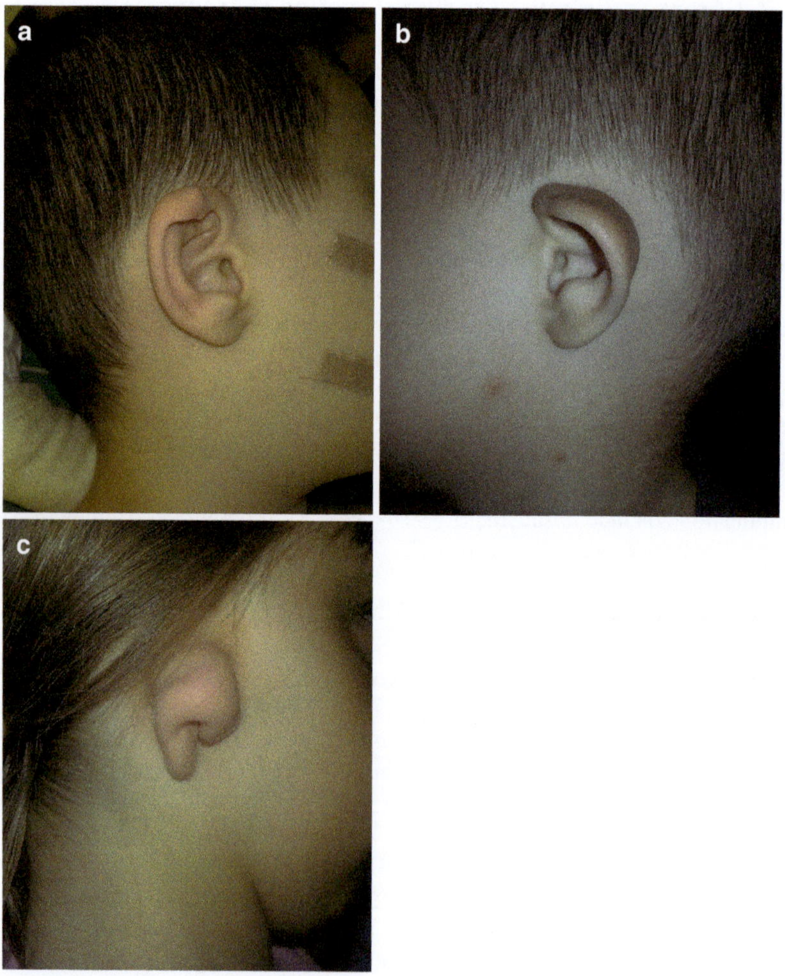

Fig. 3.3 Constricted ear: (**a**) minor case; (**b**) moderate case; (**c**) severe case

[1, 3, 5, 7, 22–24]. Most cases occur sporadically [22]. Tanzer coined the term "constricted ear" to minimize the confusion of a multitude of descriptive terms and categorized the constricted ear into three groups [1, 3, 22, 23]. Park divided the constricted ear into four graded types with different surgical approaches depending on the constricted ear type [21]. There are several surgical procedures described for the correction of this abnormality [1, 3, 5, 7, 22–24]. The repair must be individualized for each patient; however, they all have to include the lengthening of the helix [3–5, 7]. In group I (minimal height discrepancy), there is involvement of helix and scapha, and they are amenable to refashioning of cartilage lidding and placement of modified Mustardé sutures [1, 22]. In group II, there is involvement of helix and scapha [1, 23]. For IIa deformity shaping of cartilage is required without skin supplement, and IIb deformity has to be corrected by cartilage maneuvers (banner flap) and in most cases with importation of skin [1, 3, 22, 23]. Extreme cupping deformity (type III) with height deficiency of 1.5 cm requires a major auricular reconstruction using a costal cartilage framework (similar to microtia) [1, 3, 5, 21, 22]. A major problem of surgical correction of moderately severe constricted ears is recurrence of cupping of the upper ear [5, 21, 22].

3.6 Cryptotia

In cryptotia, the cephaloauricular sulcus is obliterated, and the superior pole of ear is hidden beneath the temporal scalp [1, 3, 7, 25]. Cryptotia is uncommon in Western countries, and the incidence is high in Orientals (in Japan 1:400 births) [1, 25]. Hirose stated that contraction of intrinsic auricular muscles in the neonatal period is responsible for cryptotia [1]. Nonsurgical treatment methods include splinting of the ear in children younger than 6 months [3]. There are several surgical techniques for correction of cryptotia including skin grafts and different flaps (Z plasties, V-Y advancement flaps, rotation flaps, and when there is lack of cartilage, additional techniques are used) [1, 3, 7, 25].

3.7 Stahl's Ear

Stahl's ear is characterized by abnormal bar of cartilage (third crus), running from the inferior crus (antihelix) to the upper pole of helical rim (Fig. 3.4a, b) [1, 7, 26, 27]. There is a high incidence among Asian people, near 20% is bilateral, and the male-female ratio is equal, as the left-right ratio [1]. There are a large number of techniques proposed for surgical correction of this deformity, but in general, treatment is very difficult [26, 27]. A "Z" plasty of the third crus alone may be effective for mild cases [1]. For more severe cases, there are several options such as excision of the third crus with mattress sutures in the antihelix, augmentation of the deficient superior crus with excised piece of cartilage, and technique with periosteal sling, and there is a technique with remodulation of auricular cartilage which is previously returned to amorphous state [7, 26, 27].

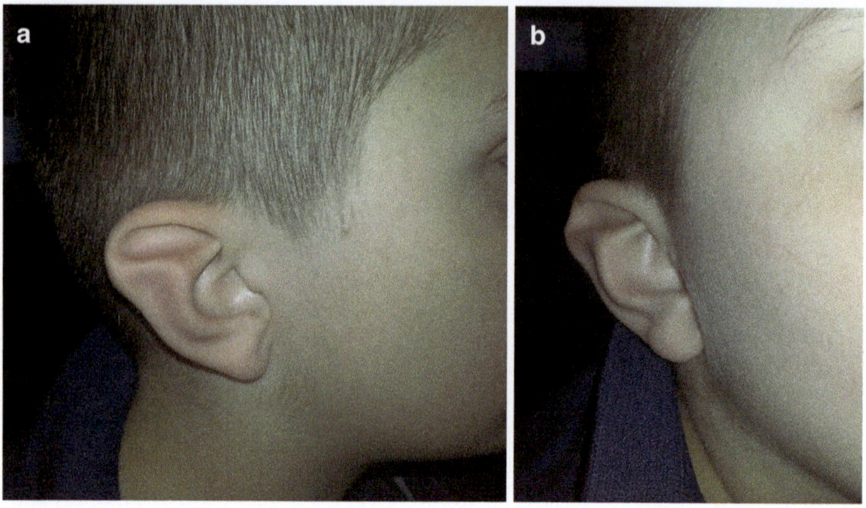

Fig. 3.4 Stahl ear: (**a**) lateral view; (**b**) oblique view

References

1. Furnas DW. External ear. In: Jurkiewitz MJ, Krizek TJ, Mathes SJ, Ariyan S, editors. Plastic surgery. Principles and practice. St Louis: Mosby; 1990. p. 171–206.
2. Tanzer RC. Microtia. Clin Plast Surg. 1978;5(3):317–36.
3. Brent B. Reconstruction of the ear. In: Neligen PC, Grotting JC, editors. Plastic surgery. St Louis: Elsevier/Saunders; 2013. p. 186–225e5.
4. Rogers BO. Microtic, lop, cup and protruding ears: four directly inheritable deformities? Plast Reconstr Surg. 1968;41(3):208–31.
5. Al-Qattan MM. An alternative approach for correction of constricted ears of moderate severity. Br J Plast Surg. 2005;58(3):389–93.
6. Fukuda O. The microtic ear: survey of 180 cases in 10 years. Plast Reconstr Surg. 1974;53(4):458–63.
7. Thorne CH, Wilkes G. Ear deformities, otoplasty, and ear reconstruction. Plast Reconstr Surg. 2012;129(4):701e–16e.
8. Nagata S. Microtia: auricular reconstruction. In: Achauer BM, Eriksson E, Guyuron B, Coleman III JJ, Russell RC, Craig A, Kolk V, editors. Plastic surgery, indications, operations, and outcomes. St Louis: Mosby; 2000. p. 1023–54.
9. Matsuo K, Hirose T, Tomono T, Iwasawa M, Katohda S, Takahashi N, Koh B. Nonsurgical correction of congenital auricular deformities in the early neonate: a preliminary report. Plast Reconstr Surg. 1984;73(1):38–51.
10. Tai Y, Tanaka S, Fukushima J, Kizuka Y, Kiyokawa K. Refinements in the elevation of reconstructed auricles in microtia. Plast Reconstr Surg. 2006;117(7):2414–23.
11. Firmin F, Marchac A. A novel algorithm for autologous ear reconstruction. Semin Plast Surg. 2011;25(4):257–64.
12. Baluch N, Nagata S, Park C, Wilkes GH, Reinisch J, et al. Auricular reconstruction for microtia: a review of available methods. Plast Surg (Oakv). 2014;22(1):39–43.
13. Siegert R, Weerda H, Magritz R. Basic techniques in autogenous microtia repair. Facial Plast Surg. 2009;25(3):149–57.
14. Converse JM. Construction of the auricle in congenital microtia. Plast Reconstr Surg. 1963;32:425–38.

15. Bly RA, Bhrany AD, Murakami CS, Sie KC. Microtia reconstruction. Facial Plast Surg Clin North Am. 2016;24(4):577–91.
16. Park C. Subfascial expansion and expanded two-flap method for microtia reconstruction. Plast Reconstr Surg. 2000;106(7):1473–87.
17. Park C, Yoo YS, Hong ST. An update on auricular reconstruction: three major auricular malformations of microtia, prominent ear and cryptotia. Curr Opin Otolaryngol Head Neck Surg. 2010;18(6):544–9.
18. Bauer BS. Reconstruction of microtia. Plast Reconstr Surg. 2009;124(1 Suppl):14e–26e.
19. Thomson HG, Kim TY, Ein SH. Residual problems in chest donor sites after microtia reconstruction: a long-term study. Plast Reconstr Surg. 1995;95(6):961–8.
20. Cronin TD. Use of a silastic frame for total and subtotal reconstruction of the external ear: preliminary report. Plast Reconstr Surg. 1966;37(5):399–405.
21. Ohmori S, Sekiguchi H. Follow-up study of the reconstruction of microtia using Silastic frame. Aesthet Plast Surg. 1984;8(1):1–6.
22. Horlock N, Grobbelaar AO, Gault DT. 5-year series of constricted (lop and cup) ear corrections: development of the mastoid hitch as an adjunctive technique. Plast Reconstr Surg. 1998;102(7):2325–32.
23. Kim YS, Chung S. A simplified method for correcting Tanzer's group II constricted ears: construction of the superior crus as a strut with cartilage expansion grafting. J Plast Reconstr Aesthet Surg. 2016;69:e71–6.
24. Park C, Park JY. Classification and algorithmic management of constricted ears: a 22-year experience. Plast Reconstr Surg. 2016;137(5):1523–38.
25. Ono I, Gunji H, Suda K, Tateshita T, Kaneko F. A new operative method for treating severe cryptotia. Plast Reconstr Surg. 1995;96(2):461–8.
26. Nakayama Y, Soeda S. Surgical treatment of Stahl's ear using the periosteal sling. Plast Reconstr Surg. 1986;77:222–6.
27. Noguchi M, Matsuo K, Imai Y, Furuta S. Simple surgical correction of Stahl's ear. Br J Plast Surg. 1994;47(8):570–2.

Breast Augmentation in Children

4

4.1 Introduction

Breast augmentation is the most popular cosmetic surgery procedure performed worldwide [1–5]. Teenage patients may account for up to 4% of breast augmentation [6, 7]. Breast surgery for cosmetic reasons is not commonly performed on patients under 18 years of age, and it should be performed only after careful discussion with the patient and family [6].

4.2 Embryology

Breast begins to form at 5–7 weeks of fetal development as a bilateral thickening of the ectoderm (mamillary line) which extends from the axilla to the groin and involutes shortly after forming [8–10]. The limited portion in the thoracic region of the embryo remains (at the level of the fourth intercostal space) and forms the basis for development of the neonatal breast [8–11]. The connective tissue of breast is derived from the mesoderm [10]. During normal development, the breasts remain quiescent until puberty (grows at the same rate as the body), and the growth begins usually at an average age of 11 years (8–13 years) [6, 8, 9]. Breast development (five stages by Tanner) is generally completed by 16 to 18 years of age [3, 6, 8, 11].

4.3 Breast Anatomy

In adults, breasts are in position between the second and third and seventh and eighth rib; medially there is sternal edge and laterally midaxillary line [9, 10]. The portion of breast that projects into the axilla is termed the tail of Spence [9]. The nipple is normally located over IV intercostal space, laterally from the midclavicular line [1–3, 9, 10]. Beside the skin and subcutaneous tissue, the breast is made up of parenchymatous and stromal tissue [3, 9, 10].

A.M. Vlahovic, E.Q. Haxhija, *Pediatric and Adolescent Plastic Surgery for the Clinician*, DOI 10.1007/978-3-319-56004-5_4

The breast is supplied by a vascular network consisting of the internal mammary, lateral thoracic, intercostals arteries, subscapular, and thoracodorsal arteries [1, 3, 9, 10]. Sensory innervation has three major nerve distributions (anterolateral intercostals, medial intercostals, and the cervical plexus) [1, 3, 9, 10]. Multiple groups of lymphatics drain the breast, and it is parallel with venous drainage [9, 10].

4.4 Patient Evaluation

Psychological and developmental characteristics of each patient have to be evaluated [3, 5, 6]. A careful medical history (earlier breast problems, breast Ca, allergic reactions) and physical examination (chest wall deformity, spinal curvature, asymmetry of breast size, nipple and inframammary fold (IMF) position) has to be performed for each patient [1–5]. Indications for augmentation mammaplasty in pediatric population are breast hypoplasia (unilateral and bilateral), breast deformity as a part of Poland's syndrome, tuberous breasts, and failure of breast development due to a trauma [8, 11, 12]. Cosmetic indications are extremely rare [6].

Preoperative markings are made with the patient in the upright position, using the IMF, the nipple areola complex (NAC), and the suprasternal notch as key landmarks [2, 4]. The breast width (BW), the breast height (BH), the distance from the NAC to the inframammary fold, the distance from the suprasternal notch (SSN) to the NAC, and the intermammary distance (IMD) have to be measured [2].

Both the patient and the parents have to be informed about the risks, benefits, and treatment alternatives [1–3]. Pediatric patients in most cases want to have natural appearance of the breasts [6–8, 12].

4.5 Implant Selection

There are two implant materials: saline- and silicone-filled implants [1, 2, 4, 5, 13]. Implants are round and anatomical, with wide variety in width, height, and projection [2, 4, 5, 13]. Essentially there are two types of round implant shell: smooth and textured [2, 4, 5]. Anatomic implants are all textured by design (to minimize malrotation) [2, 5].

4.6 Treatment Option

Breast augmentation in pediatric population can be performed for either unilateral or bilateral deformity, and basic approach is similar to adults [1–6, 8, 12]. There are four distinct variables requiring decision in the preoperative process: implant type, implant size, incision location, and pocket plane [1–5, 14]. Three types of incision are commonly employed in breast augmentation, transaxillary, inframammary, and periareolar, and each approach has its own advantages and disadvantages [1–5, 14]. Transumbilical approach is only possible with empty implants that are inflated [2, 4, 5, 14].

The inframammary approach is most popular since it permits complete visualization of the implant pocket (for both subglandular and subpectoral plane), and it allows any type of secondary surgery (Fig. 4.1a–e) [1–5, 14]. The incision should be placed in the predicted location of the new inframammary fold, mostly lateral to

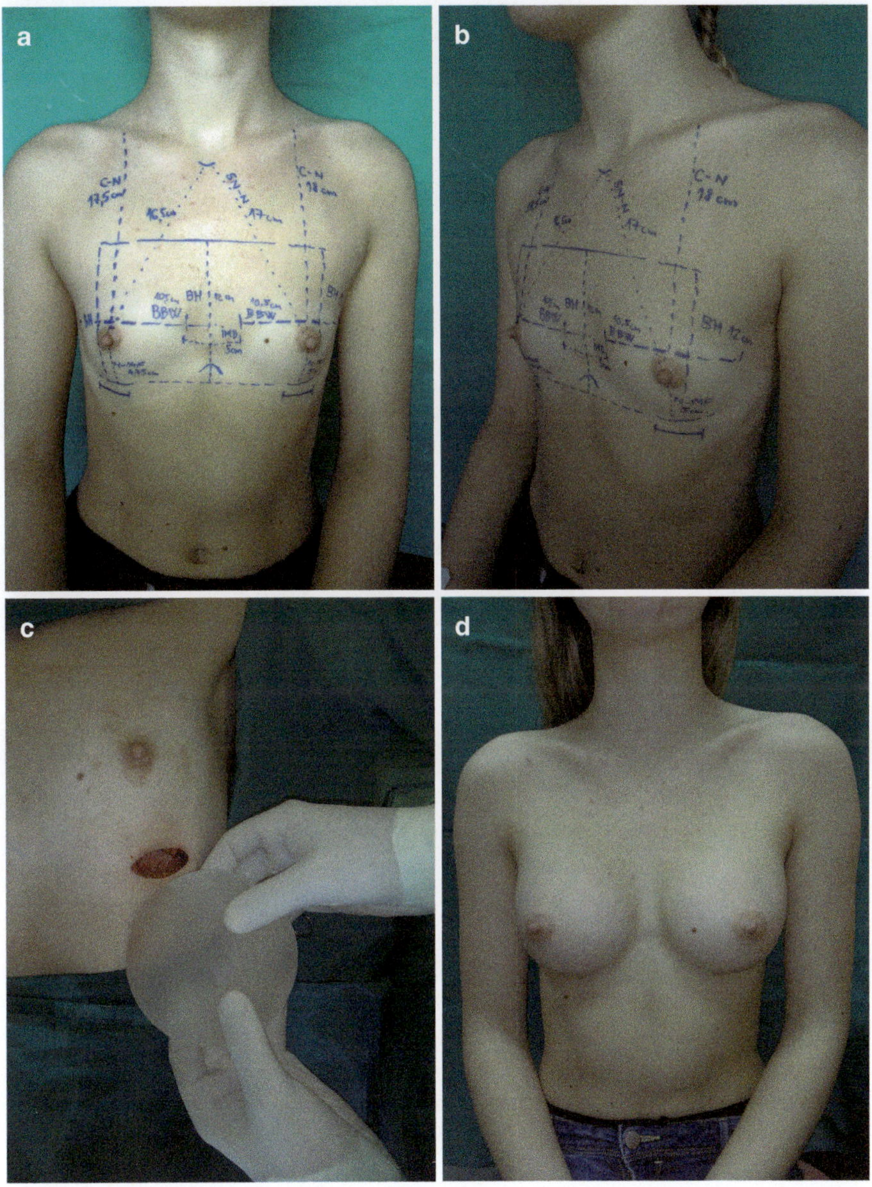

Fig. 4.1 Bilateral augmentation of the breast: (**a**, **b**) preoperative markings; (**c**) implant placement; (**d**, **e**) postoperative result

Fig. 4.1 (continued)

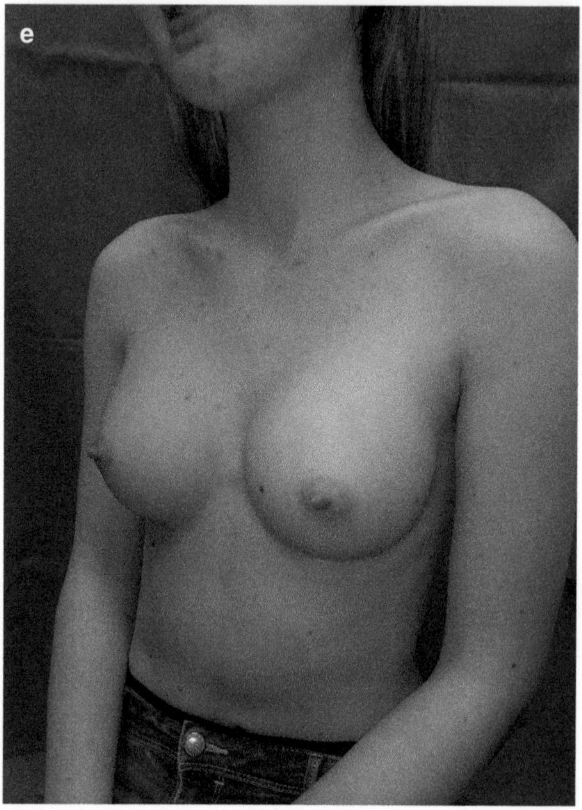

the breast midline [1, 2, 4]. For patients with significant hypoplasia, placement of the incision can be difficult (Fig. 4.2a–d) [4].

In periareolar approach, the incision is placed along the inferior portion of the areolar-cutaneous juncture [2, 4, 14]. The scar is well hidden, but there are disadvantages such as limited exposure of the surgical field, transaction of the parenchymal ducts, and potentially increased risk of nipple sensitivity changes [1–4, 14].

The transaxillary approach avoids scarring on the breast [2, 4, 5, 14]. The advantage of this approach is avoidance of injury of breast parenchyma, and disadvantages are difficulty to control hemorrhage (additional inframammary or periareolar incision is needed) and lack of control during surgery with high revision rate [1, 4, 14]. Transumbilical approach can be used only with saline implants, and this approach has not gained wider acceptance especially in pediatric population [1, 2, 4, 5, 11, 14].

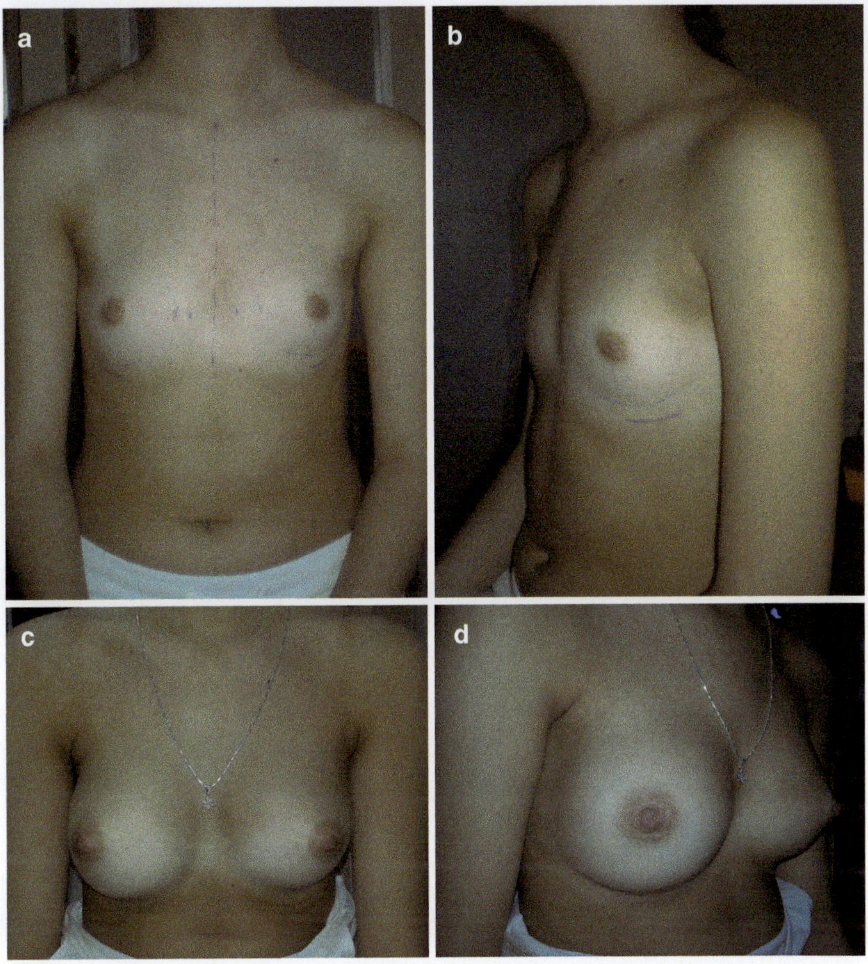

Fig. 4.2 Bilateral augmentation of the breast: (**a**, **b**) preoperatively; (**c**, **d**) postoperatively

4.7 Implant Type

There are two basic implant configurations—round and anatomical [2, 4, 5, 13]. The typical round-shaped breast implant has its greatest projection centrally, and anatomically shaped breast implants have the majority of the projection in the lower pole (Fig. 4.3a, b) [4, 5, 13]. Anatomical implants may be better for narrow breast width, small breast volume with minimal ptosis, noticeable asymmetry, and thoracic prominence, while round implants suit those with relative upper pole deficit, moderate pseudoptosis, and mild asymmetry [2, 4, 5, 13].

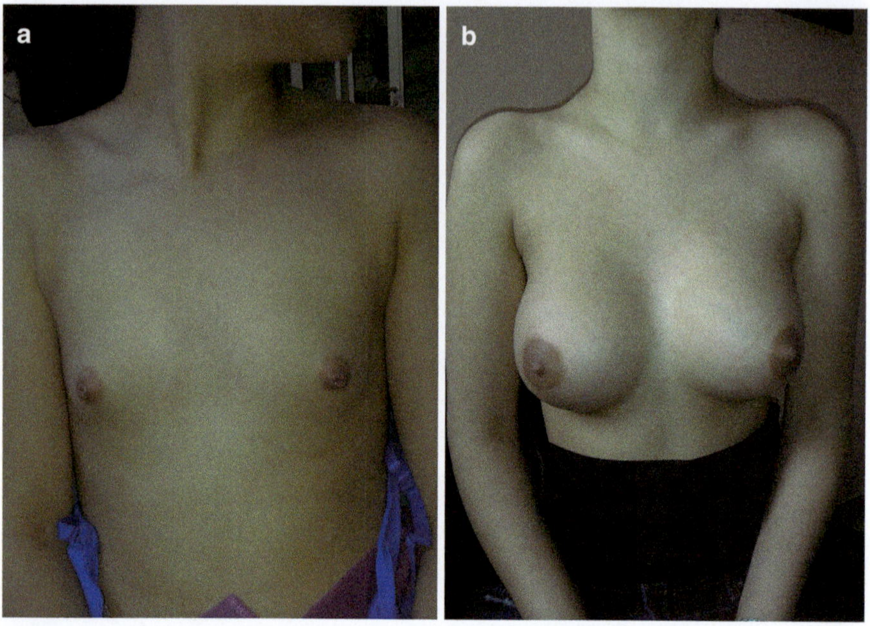

Fig. 4.3 Bilateral augmentation of the breast in a patient with Mayer-Rokitansky syndrome: (**a**) preoperative view; (**b**) postoperative view

4.8 Implant Placement

The implant placement sites are subglandular, submuscular, and subpectoral (dual plane) [1, 2, 4, 5, 14]. Placement of the implant in subglandular plane works best when there is adequate soft tissue coverage for the implant; however, there is a higher incidence of capsular contracture following this position of implant [3, 4]. When implant is placed in subpectoral pocket, it is covered by muscle in the upper pole and with glandular tissue in the lower pole [2–5]. The dual plane augmentation has developed as variation of the subpectoral plane augmentation [4, 5]. The origin of the pectoralis major muscle (PMM) is divided just above the inframammary fold, and the pectoralis muscle is retracted superiorly, which allowed better projection in the lower pole of the augmented breast [2, 4, 5, 14]. The difference between dual plane and subpectoral approach is that in dual plane approach, there is a possibility of subglandular dissection above the inferior border of PMM superiorly [2, 4, 5]. Exact implant "sizers" (gel or saline) are used when available to evaluate the pockets and resultant breast form, the pocket is irrigated with an antibiotic-containing solution, the implants are carefully placed, and multilayer closure is performed [1–3, 5]. Total submuscular and subfascial plane also exists, but they are not used as often as the previously described methods [4, 5]. Lipoaugmentation of the breast is new and also an effective method for breast reconstruction that can be also used in pediatric population [15–17].

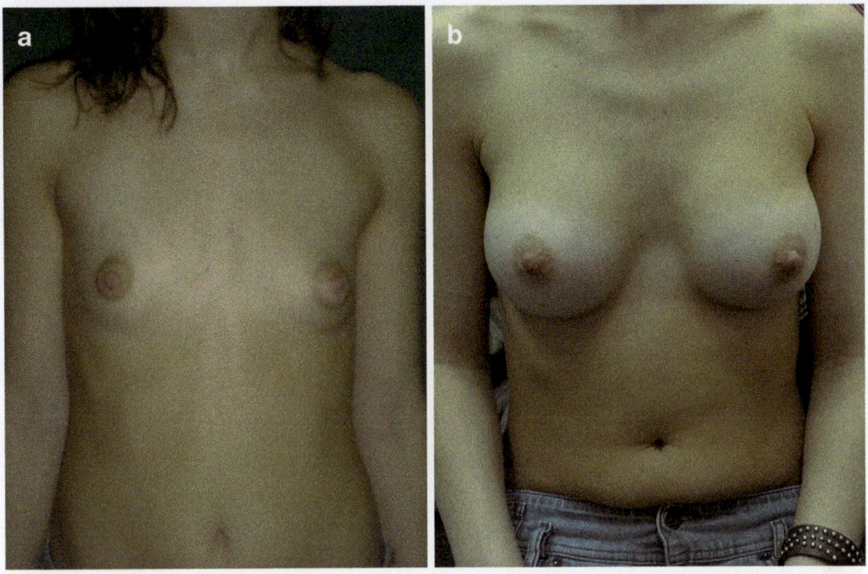

Fig. 4.4 Long-term follow-up of the breast augmentation: (**a**) preoperative view; (**b**) 8 years postoperatively

4.9 Postoperative Care

Pediatric patients are usually hospitalized, with analgetics and a 3-day course of prophylactic intravenous antibiotics followed by 5 days of peroral antibiotics [2]. Sports or surgical bra is recommended for 6 weeks after surgery, with early movement to allow stretching of PMM (to prevent contraction) [2, 10]. Breast massage is indicated twice daily for 10–15 min for 6 months [4, 5]. Rigorous exercise is not permitted for 6 weeks, and additional follow-up visits are scheduled at 1, 3, 6, and 12 months (Fig. 4.4a, b) [2, 4].

4.10 Complications

Besides capsular contracture as a complication of breast augmentation, hypertrophic scarring, infection, hematoma, and seroma may also occur [1, 5]. Capsular contracture is a common complication reported after breast enlargement (Fig. 4.5a, b) [1–3, 5, 15]. Baker's classification includes four degrees of capsular contracture, ranging from grade 1 contracture for near-normal breast to grade 4 for severely changed breast [1, 2, 18]. Women with Baker grade 3 or 4 capsular contracture often require treatment, including open capsulotomy or capsulectomy, and repositioning of the implant in a dual plane [1, 2]. Currently, there is no scientific evidence that silicone is a mutagen or teratogen, and implants do not interfere with lactation [1, 13].

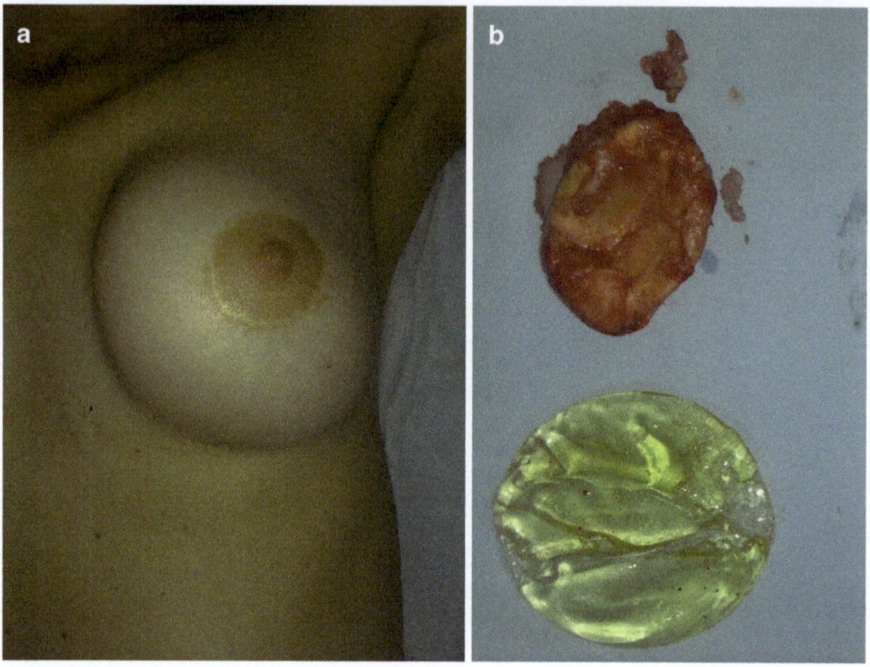

Fig. 4.5 Capsular contracture: (**a**) preoperative view; (**b**) excised capsule and prosthesis

Sensory changes occur in 10% of women (most often after subglandular placement of prosthesis), manifested as either anesthesia or hyperesthesia of nipple, and they are transitory in 85% of cases [2, 3]. *Hematoma* as complication is usually seen in the first 24 h after surgery, and in most cases, immediate evacuation of the hematoma and exploration of the pocket is recommended [1–3]. *Infection* occurs in 2–4% of cases (*Staphylococcus aureus* and *Staphylococcus epidermidis* are most common causes), and if the there is no response to oral or intravenous antibiotics, the implant should be removed [1–3].

Implant rupture may be intra- or extracapsular, and magnetic resonance imaging (MRI) of the breast is considered the state-of-the-art technique for evaluating breast implant integrity [2, 10, 13]. Any defect in the silicone elastomer shell of a saline-filled breast implant will ultimately result in *deflation* of the implant [2]. *Scars* are most visible with inframammary incision [1–3].

References

1. Slavin SA, Greene AK. Augmentation mammoplasty and its complications. In: Thorne CH, Beasley RW, Aston SJ, Bartlett SP, Gurtner GC, Spear SL, editors. Grabb and Smith's plastic surgery. Philadelphia: Lippincott Williams & Wilkins; 2007. p. 575–620.
2. Maxwell GP, Gabriel A. Breast augmentation. In: Neligen PC, Grotting JC, editors. Plastic surgery. Principles and practice, vol. 5. St Louis: Elsevier; 2013. p. 15–38.

3. Bostwick III J. Breast augmentation, reduction, and mastopexy. In: Jurkiewitz MJ, Krizek TJ, Mathes SJ, Ariyan S, editors. Plastic surgery. Principles and practice. St Louis: Mosby; 1990. p. 1063–93.
4. Spear SL, Bulan EJ, Venturi ML. Breast augmentation. Plast Reconstr Surg. 2006;118(7 Suppl):188S–96S.
5. Adams Jr WP, Mallucci P. Breast augmentation. Plast Reconstr Surg. 2012;130(4):597e–611e.
6. Larson K, Gosain AK. Cosmetic surgery in adolescent patient. Plast Reconstr Surg. 2011;129(1):135e–41e.
7. Rohrich RJ, Cunningham BL, Jewell ML, Spear SL. Teenage breast augmentation: validating outcome data and statistics in plastic surgery. Plast Reconstr Surg. 2005;115(3):943–4.
8. van Aalst JA, Phillips JD, Sadove AM. Pediatric chest wall and breast deformities. Plast Reconstr Surg. 2009;124(1 Suppl):38e–49e.
9. Latham K, Fernandez S, Iteld L, Panthaki Z, Armstrong MB, Thaller S. Pediatric breast deformity. J Craniofac Surg. 2006;17(3):454–67.
10. De la Torre J, Davis M. Anatomy for plastic surgery of the breast. In: Neligen PC, Grotting JC, editors. Plastic surgery. Principles and practice, vol. 5. St Louis: Elsevier; 2013. p. 44–56.
11. Ribas JMM. Breast problems and diseases in puberty. Best Pract Res Clin Obstet Gynaecol. 2010;24:223–42.
12. Sadove AM, van Aalst JA. Congenital and acquired pediatric breast anomalies: a review of 20 years' experience. Plast Reconstr Surg. 2005;115(4):1039–50.
13. Berry MG, Davies DM. Breast augmentation: part I—a review of the silicone prosthesis. J Plast Reconstr Aesthet Surg. 2010;63:1761–8.
14. Berry MG, Cucchiara V, Davies DM. Breast augmentation: part III—preoperative considerations and planning. J Plast Reconstr Aesthet Surg. 2011;64:1401–9.
15. Rosing JH, Wong G, Wong MS, Sahar D, Stevenson TR, Pu LL. Autologous fat grafting for primary breast augmentation: a systematic review. Aesthet Plast Surg. 2011;35(5):882–90.
16. Wilson H, Spear SL. Fat grafting to breast. In: Neligen PC, Grotting JC, editors. Plastic surgery. Principles and practice. St Louis: Elsevier; 2013. p. 581–604e2.
17. Spear SL, Pittman T. A prospective study on lipoaugmentation of the breast. Aesthet Surg J. 2014;34(3):400–8.
18. Berry MG, Cucchiara V, Davies DM. Breast augmentation: part II—adverse capsular contracture. J Plast Reconstr Aesthet Surg. 2010;63:2098–107.

Breast Reconstruction in Congenital Deformities

5

5.1 Introduction

Breast anomalies in pediatric population are common and they can have a significant psychological effect on teenage and adolescent girls (especially during breast development) [1–5]. Mammary pathology is very often a reason for consultation in medical practice [3]. The spectrum of breast disorders in pediatric population is different from that in adults, with significant physiological impact on patients and parents [1, 3–5]. Even most of pediatric breast lesions are benign, we have to think about malignancies [1, 2, 5, 6]. There is lack of comprehensive categorization of these abnormalities [1, 2].

5.2 Embryology

Breast development begins during the sixth week of gestation [1, 5, 7]. The breast originates from the ectoderm, along the milk line from the primitive axilla to the primitive groin [1, 5, 7–9]. By the tenth week, the upper and lower part of ridge disappears and the normal breast develops on the anterolateral chest wall [1, 7, 9]. The areola develops at the fifth month of gestation [7]. The average age of female thelarche (when the breast growth begins) is approximately 11 years of age (range from 8 to 15 years) [5, 8, 9]. Typically, breast growth is complete between 16 and 18 years [7, 9].

5.3 Anatomy

The glandular tissue of the breast (with significant amount of adipose tissue) is fixed in place by the superficial fascial system [10, 11]. The Cooper's ligaments provide interconnections between the deep and superficial fascial layers [4, 10, 11]. The breast overlies the anterolateral thorax principally the second through sixth ribs, with the nipple areola complex as the primary landmark of the breast [1, 4, 10, 11].

A.M. Vlahovic, E.Q. Haxhija, *Pediatric and Adolescent Plastic Surgery for the Clinician*, DOI 10.1007/978-3-319-56004-5_5

5.4 Diagnosis

Evaluation of breast-related symptoms in children begins with a thorough history (regarding menstrual history for adolescent and family history of similar problems, and other breast diseases) and physical examination [12, 13]. During physical examination (which is performed with maximal care) besides the breast evaluation, any pre-existing asymmetries, spinal curvature, or chest wall deformities should be recognized and noted [10, 12, 13]. Breast sonography is generally the primary imaging modality used in pediatric population [1, 5, 6, 12]. Magnetic resonance imaging (MRI) of the breast is rarely used in children, likewise open biopsy and fine needle aspiration biopsy (FNAB), while mammography has practically no use in pediatric patients [5, 6, 12, 13].

5.5 Classification

There is no adequate categorization of breast abnormalities in pediatric population [1, 2]. Breast anomalies can be roughly classified into four groups: hyperplasia, hypoplasia, asymmetry, and deformation [1, 2, 7, 9].

5.5.1 Breast Hyperplasia

There are several possible causes of breast hyperplasia in pediatric population such as premature thelarche, juvenile hypertrophy-macromasty, polythelia, polymasty, benign tumors (fibroadenoma, vascular anomalies), malignant tumors (breast carcinoma, phyllodes tumor, metastatic disease), non-tumorous masses (cysts, galactocele), and gynecomasty (Figs. 5.1, 5.2, 5.3) [2, 6, 13].

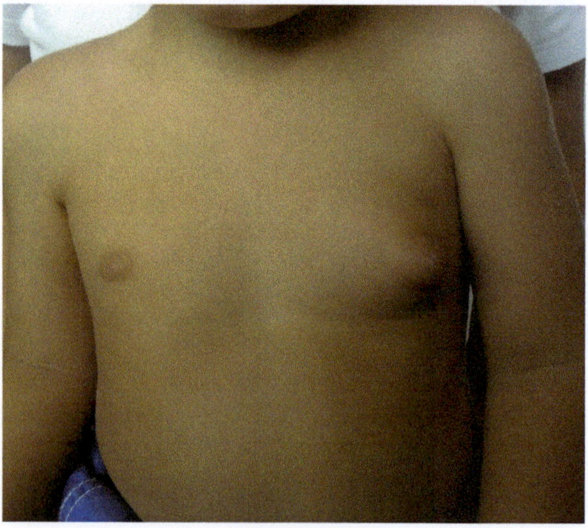

Fig. 5.1 Galactocele of the left breast

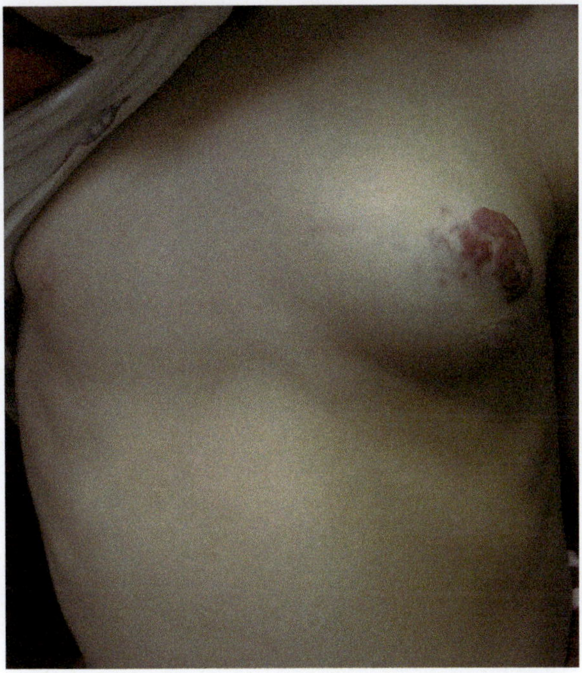

Fig. 5.2 Hemangioma of the left breast

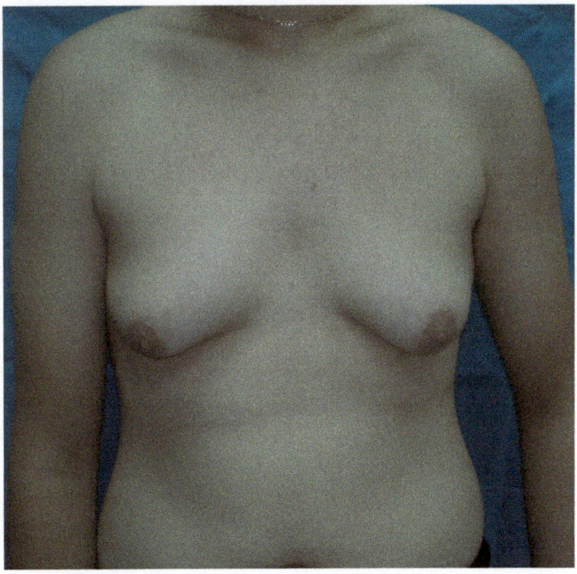

Fig. 5.3 Clinical appearance of bilateral gynecomastia

5.5.1.1 Premature Thelarche and Precocious Puberty

Premature thelarche presents as enlargement of one or both breasts from 6 months to 9 years of age and it occurs without other evidence of precocious puberty [4, 6]. Precocious puberty implies premature breast development in association with other secondary sex characteristics (only 18% of girls with premature thelarche develops precocious puberty) [4, 6, 14]. For premature thelarche, biopsy is contraindicated since it is a benign and self-limited condition, and reevaluation is indicated every 6–12 months [6, 14].

5.5.1.2 Gigantomastia (Virginal Hypertrophy)

Virginal hypertrophy is massive enlargement of breast with patients generally aged 11–16 years when the growth begins [1–4]. It is an uncommon primary condition with high sensitivity to estrogens as possible etiological factor [1]. Excessively large breast in a teenager can cause physical problem, such as pain and skin maceration, along with a psychological problem [15, 16]. Treatment of virginal hypertrophy is surgical (in most cases breast reduction with free nipple grafts, or mastectomy), with adjunct medical therapy (medroxyprogesterone, dydrogesterone, tamoxifen) to prevent regrowth after reduction mammoplasty [1, 3, 4, 13]. Psychologist and psychiatrist consultations are also needed [1]. Reduction mammaplasty is rarely performed in pediatric population (with similar indication as in adults) [10, 13, 15–21]. Surgery should be delayed, whenever it is possible, until the end of puberty because of continued breast growth [1, 2, 4, 7, 15, 21]. There are two important decisions in breast reduction surgery: choice of incision and choice of pedicle type, and breast amputation with free nipple graft remains as an alternative to breast reduction with nipple-bearing pedicle [15–21].

Mammary ptosis is a rare entity in pediatric population. The Regnault classification system for mammary ptosis describes mild, moderate, severe, and pseudoptosis according to the relative positions of the nipple and the inframammary fold [10, 16, 18, 22]. Mastopexy is a procedure designed to elevate breast tissue and the nipple areola complex to correct breast ptosis with several techniques involved (inverted-T mastopexy, concentric mastopexy procedures, periareolar "round-block" mastopexy, and vertical-incision mastopexy) used with different success and frequently combined with breast augmentation [16, 18, 22].

5.5.1.3 Polymastia

Polymastia is the presence of the supernumerary breast, usually manifested at puberty when hormonal influence started with an incidence of 1–2% of all live births [1–4, 9]. It is typically located along the primitive milk line (most commonly in the axilla) (Fig. 5.4a–d) [1, 4, 7]. When it is located outside of the mammary line, it is called ectopic mamma (Fig. 5.5a–c) [1, 3]. Since it is a subject to the same pathology as normally located breast tissue, complete resection is recommended [1–4].

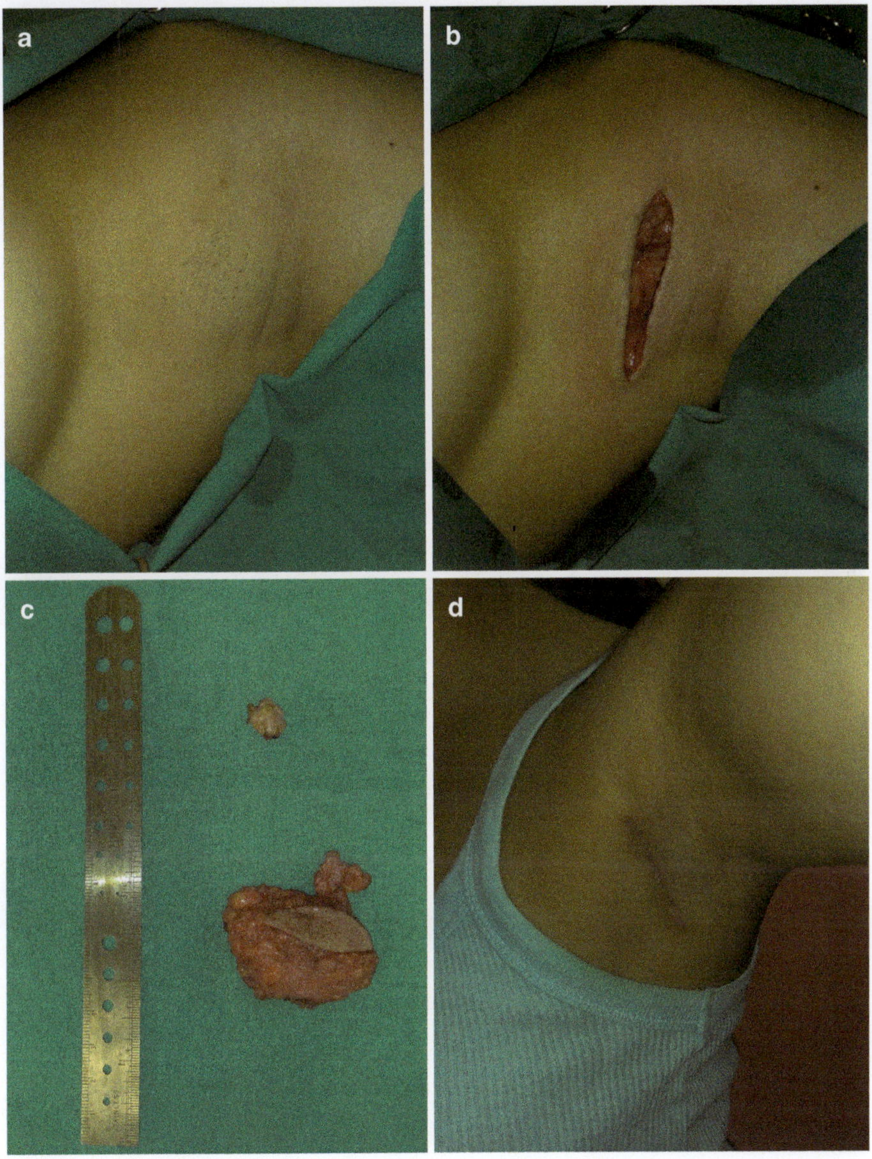

Fig. 5.4 Polymastia: (**a**) lesion in the left axillary region; (**b**) intraoperative view; (**c**) excised lesion; (**d**) 1 month after excision

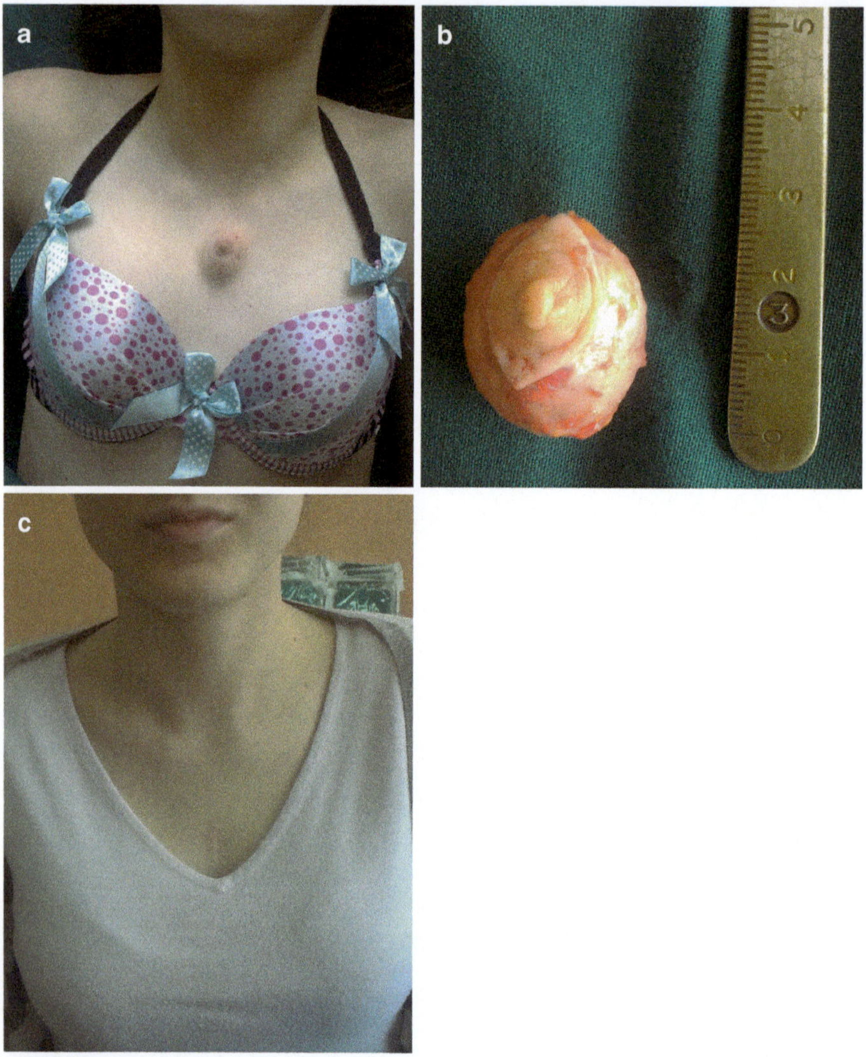

Fig. 5.5 Ectopic breast at sternal region: (**a**) preoperative appearance; (**b**) excised lesion; (**c**) post-operative hypertrophic scar at sternal region

5.5.1.4 Polythelia

Polythelia (supernumerary nipple) is a benign, most commonly encountered pediatric breast anomaly [1, 2, 4, 7, 9]. The incidence is 1–3%, and there is a male predominance [1, 7, 9]. It results from the failure of mammary ridge to regress in utero, but it can be located out of the mammary ridge also [1, 13]. If it is associated with polymastia, it is generally recognized at birth, and as a sole entity, polythelia is often unrecognized until the puberty (often misdiagnosis for nevi) [1]. Associated renal anomalies should be evaluated (physical exam, urinalysis, and renal ultrasound (US)) [1, 2, 4]. Excision is mostly because of surgery (Fig. 5.6a, b) [1, 2, 4, 7].

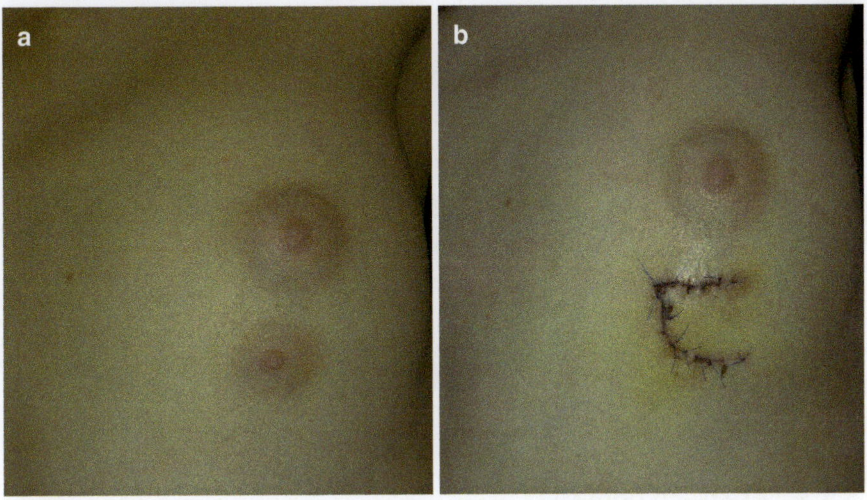

Fig. 5.6 Polythelia: (**a**) left female breast polythelia; (**b**) excision and reconstruction with local flap

5.5.2 Breast Masses

In neonatal and prepubertal period, there is often a palpable breast mass, in one or both breasts, in either sex, that typically resolves spontaneously in a few months [4]. Benign breast masses include fibroadenoma, phyllodes tumors, and fibrocystic disease (non-tumorous mass) [4, 13]. Adolescent breasts are typically fibrous with small lumps and cysts present through the breast [3, 13]. Biopsy of the prepubertal breasts is rarely indicated [4]. Firm support, analgesics, and reassurance are treatment options [3, 13]. Simple fibroadenoma is the most common breast lesion in adolescent females (91% of solid breast masses in girls under 19 years) (Fig. 5.7a, b) [4, 6, 13]. It is benign, nontender mass that grows as the result of tissue hypersensitivity to normal levels of gonadal hormones [1, 7, 9]. In 75% common fibroadenoma is presented as single lesion, the diagnosis is made by physical examination and ultrasound (US), and most of them can be observed safely [4, 13]. For patients with giant fibroadenoma (greater than 5 cm in size), complex fibroadenomas, positive family history, or associated proliferative disease, excision is recommended (increased risk of breast Ca) [2, 3, 6, 7, 9, 13]. Vascular anomalies, if located in the breast, can cause breast hypertrophy (they can be ruled out with US and MRI) [4, 6].

Cystosarcoma phyllodes represents 0.4% of all adolescent breast masses; it occurs de novo from lobular connective tissue, and in most cases it exhibits a benign behavior [4, 6, 12, 13]. Treatment is total excision of the tumor mass or mastectomy [12, 13]. *Primary breast cancer* is extremely rare, and it accounts for less than 1% of all childhood cancers and less than 0.1% of all reported breast cancers [6, 12]. Radiation-induced breast carcinoma is most frequently seen in young girls with Hodgkin disease, and there are also rhabdomyosarcomas, sarcomas, and non-Hodgkin lymphoma reported as primary malignancies in the breast, with surgical treatment as a primary option [6, 12, 13].

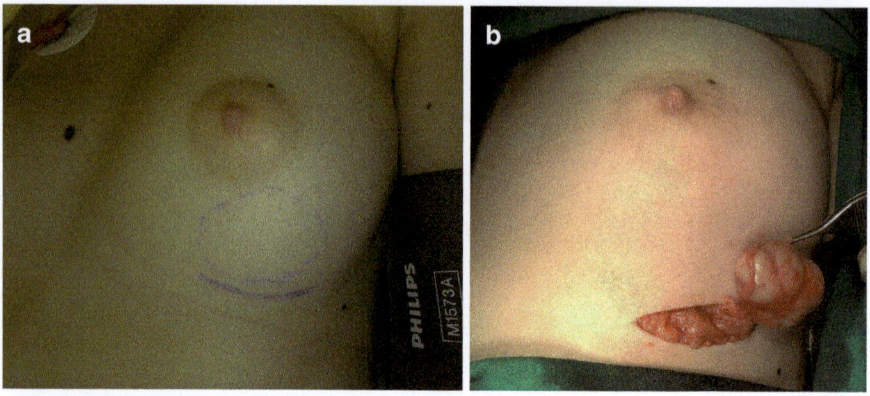

Fig. 5.7 Left breast fibroadenoma: (**a**) preoperative view; (**b**) complete excision of the tumor

5.5.3 Breast Hypoplasia

Breast hypoplasia includes the following conditions: athelia, amazia, amastia, and hypoplasia in Poland's syndrome.

5.5.3.1 Athelia

Athelia is an extremely rare condition, defined as congenital absence of the nipple areola complex (NAC) [1, 2, 4, 7, 9, 13]. It should be differentiated from amazia and amastia [1, 2, 7]. Incidence and etiology are not known, and it is usually associated with syndromes [1, 7]. In males, reconstruction is performed after puberty, and in females, if there is associated amastia, reconstruction is performed along with breast reconstruction [1].

5.5.3.2 Hypomasty

Hypomasty (breast hypotrophy) is the condition when the breast and NAC are present but underdeveloped and reconstruction is performed by augmentation with implants (Fig. 5.8) [2, 3].

5.5.3.3 Amastia

Amastia presents a very rare condition with complete absence of breast tissue and NAC that occurs in males and females, unilateral or bilateral, sole or as a part of syndrome (Sy Mayer-Rokitansky-Kuster-Hauser) (Fig. 5.9) [1, 2, 4, 9]. Breast reconstruction in amastia is usually performed with tissue expansion and subsequent implant placement, or with autologous tissue (transverse rectus abdominis or latissimus dorsi flap) [1, 2, 7]. Amazia presents complete absence of breast tissue (Fig. 5.10) [1, 2, 7, 9].

5.5.3.4 Poland's Syndrome

Alfred Poland had described a chest and hand deformity in 1841 at an executed convict, with only chest wall presented in picture [1, 23]. Patrick Clarkson

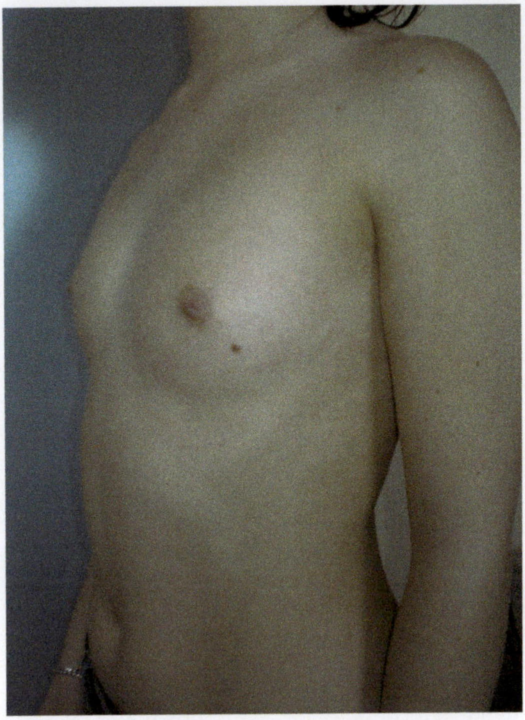

Fig. 5.8 Clinical appearance of bilateral hypomastia

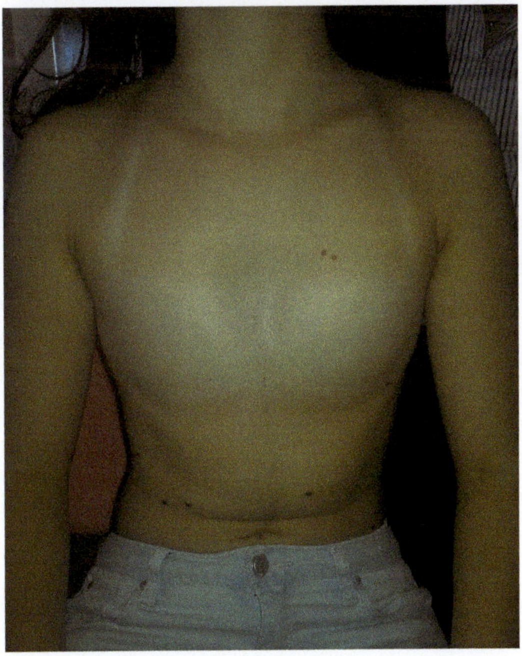

Fig. 5.9 Bilateral amastia: complete absence of the breast tissue and nipple-areola complex

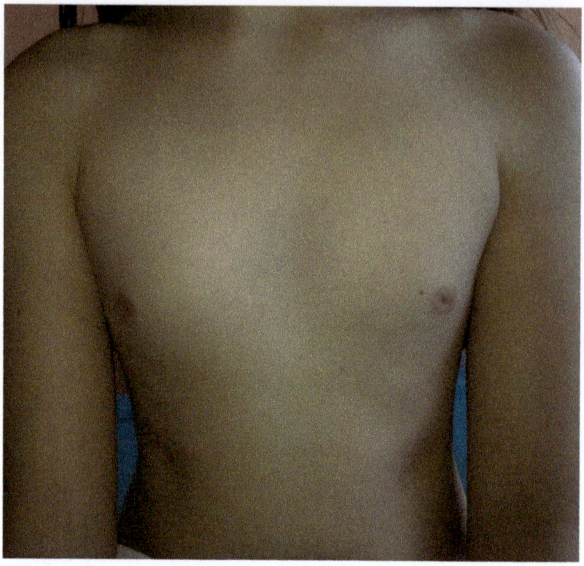

Fig. 5.10 Amazia: breast tissue absence

named it Poland's syndrome in 1962 describing three patients with chest and hand deformity at the same hospital [23, 24]. The incidence of Poland's syndrome varies from 1:7000 to 1:10,000; it is mostly sporadic, but it can be familial also [1, 2, 4, 7, 23–27]. There is male predominance in sporadic form (3:1), with right side more involved, and in familial form both sides and sexes are equally affected [1, 7, 27]. Poland's syndrome is characterized in most cases by partial or complete underdevelopment or absence of sternocostal head of pectoralis major muscle [1, 4, 23–27]. It rarely involves full spectrum of following anomalies: hypoplasia of the breast and nipple, scarcity of subcutaneous tissue over pectoral region, absence of the pectoralis minor, deficiency of additional chest wall muscles, aplasia of costal cartilages or ribs II–V, alopecia of axillary and mammary regions, and unilateral brachysyndactyly [1]. Interruption of the embryonic blood supply to the upper limb in the six embryonic weeks is the most probable etiological factor [1, 4, 23–27]. Renal anomalies should be excluded [1]. Surgical management of Poland's syndrome depends on the extent of the anomaly [1, 27]. The operation can be performed from 11 to 12 years, but when it is possible, repair should be delayed until after puberty (Fig. 5.11a–d) [1]. Corrective procedures include subcutaneous breast implants with or without tissue expanders, lipofilling, nipple areola reconstruction, and complete chest wall reconstruction with free muscle flap transfers [1, 2, 4, 7, 23, 25–27]. Contralateral procedures are used to achieve symmetry [1, 24].

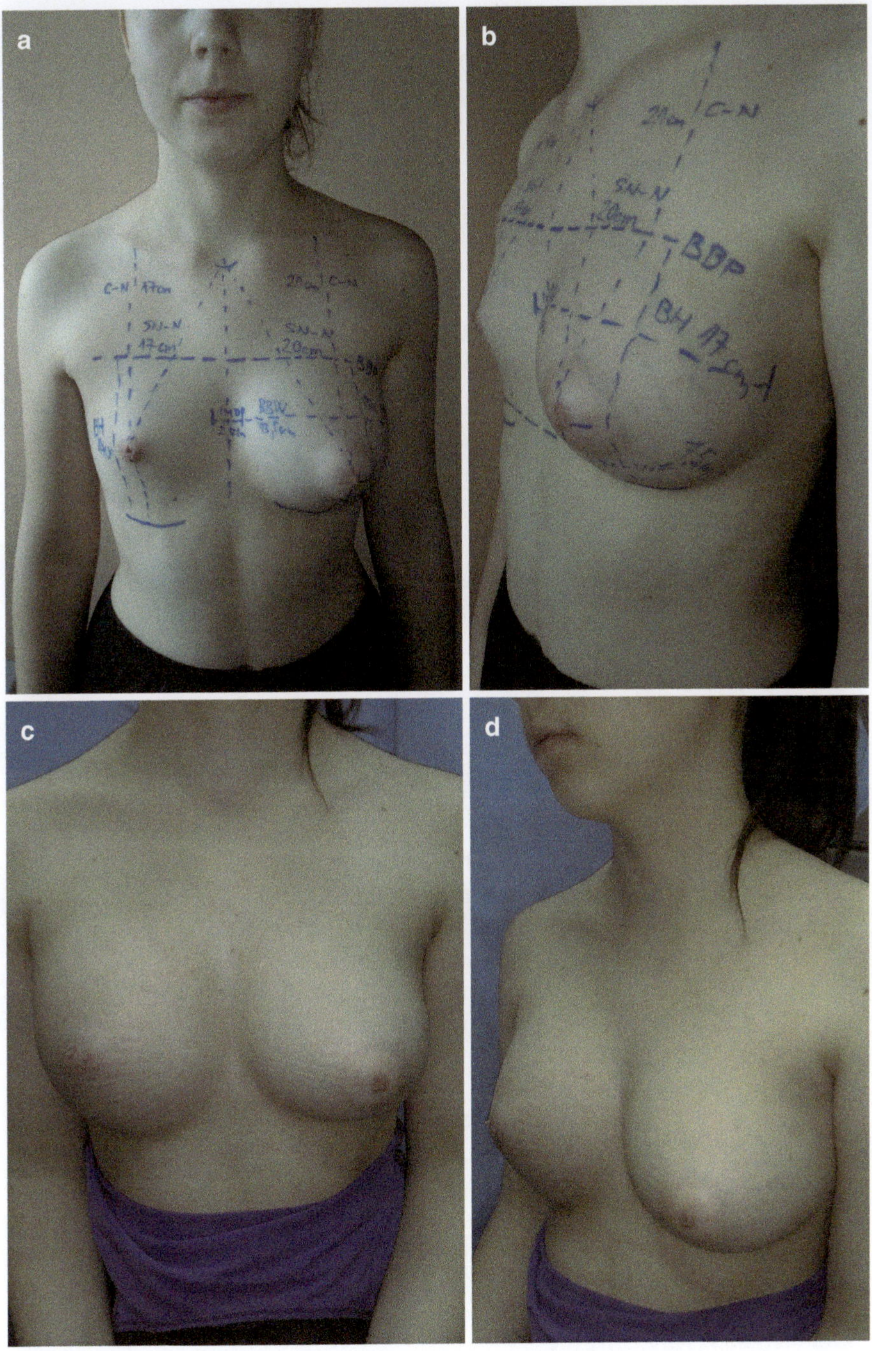

Fig. 5.11 Poland's syndrome breast deformity: (**a**, **b**) preoperative view; (**c**, **d**) reconstruction with silicone gel implants

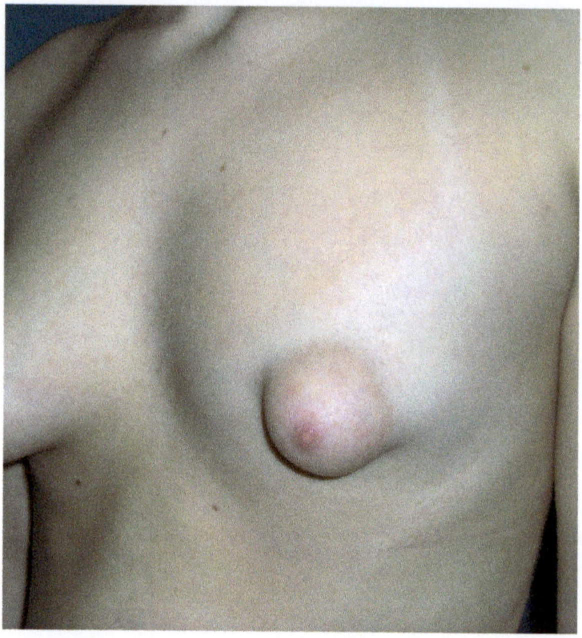

Fig. 5.12 Unilateral tuberous breast

5.5.4 Tuberous Breasts

This is a congenital anomaly with herniation of breast tissue through constrictive fascial ring (snoopy nose deformity) [2, 4, 7, 9, 13]. There is narrow mammary base, elevation of inframammary crease, and hypoplasia of one or more breast quadrants (Fig. 5.12) [1, 4]. Tuberous breasts most probably occur because of abnormal adherence of superficial fascia to dermis [1, 28]. It is a rare anomaly, in most cases bilateral and asymmetric, usually diagnosed at 12–13 years of life, with functionally normal breasts [1, 2, 4, 24, 28]. The diagnosis is made by physical examination of the breasts [28]. There are several different classification systems proposed by Heimburg et al., Meara et al., and Muti [1, 7, 9, 28, 29]. Surgical repair of tuberous breast is challenging and it should be postponed until the breast development is complete [1, 4, 7, 9, 28].

For mild and moderate deformities with adequate breast volume, breast parenchyma may simply be scored or divided, allowing for redraping, and if additional volume is needed, augmentation mammaplasty should be performed [4, 24]. In severe cases more than one procedure is needed (with tissue expansion and skin flaps employed) [1, 4, 7, 9]. Muti describes four types of glandular flaps that are used for reconstruction of tubular breasts along with mammary prosthesis [28].

5.5.5 Breast Asymmetry

Breast asymmetry occurs in more than half of the female population defined as asymmetric morphology of the shape, volume, or position of the breast, NAC, or both [3, 4, 12, 14]. They are roughly classified as congenital or acquired [14, 29–33]. Breast asymmetry may cause physical discomfort and early surgical correction may be warranted [4]. There are several classification systems for breast asymmetry, and one of them includes six categories of breast asymmetry: (1) bilateral asymmetric hypertrophy, (2) unilateral hypertrophy/contralateral normal, (3) unilateral hypertrophy/contralateral amastia or hypoplasia, (4) unilateral amastia or hypoplasia/contralateral normal, (5) asymmetric bilateral hypoplasia, and (6) unilateral mammary ptosis (Fig. 5.13a–f) [4, 14]. Only in extreme cases the surgery is needed, and the correction is performed

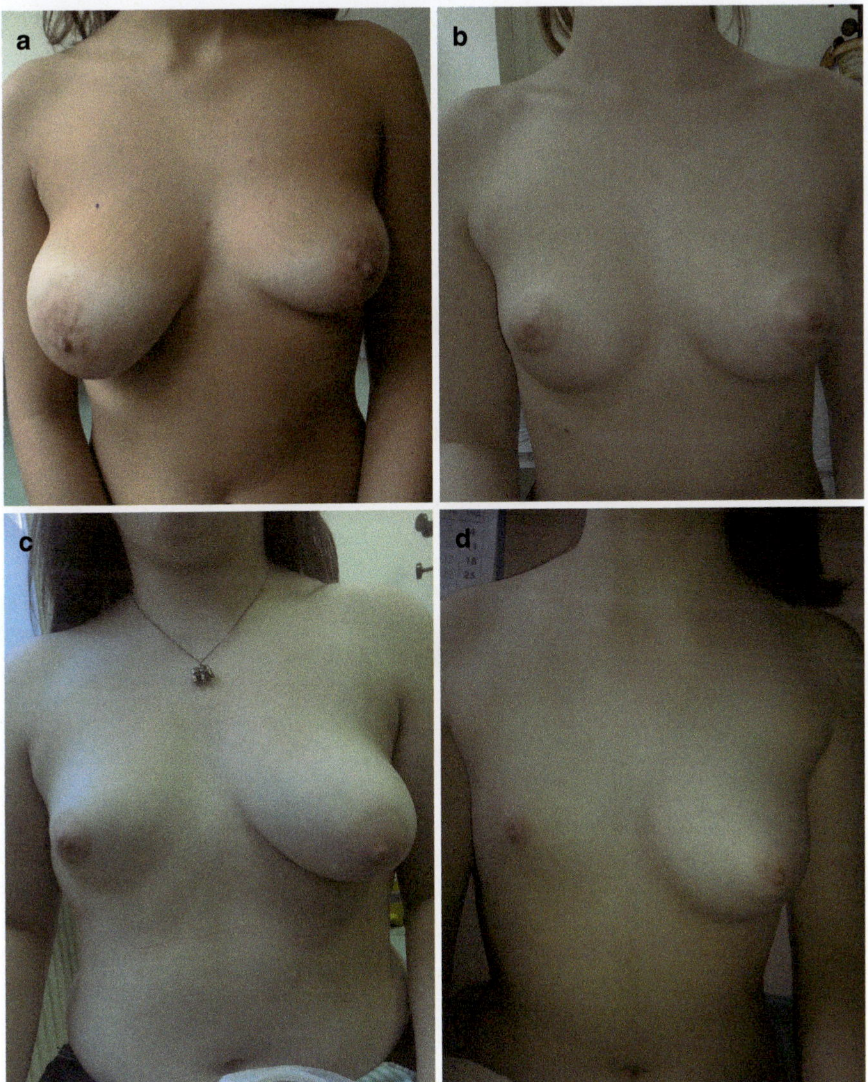

Fig. 5.13 Breast asymmetry: (**a**) bilateral asymmetric hypertrophy; (**b**) unilateral hypertrophy/contralateral normal; (**c**) unilateral hypertrophy/contralateral amastia or hypoplasia; (**d**) unilateral amastia or hypoplasia/contralateral normal; (**e**) asymmetric bilateral hypoplasia; and (**f**) unilateral mammary ptosis

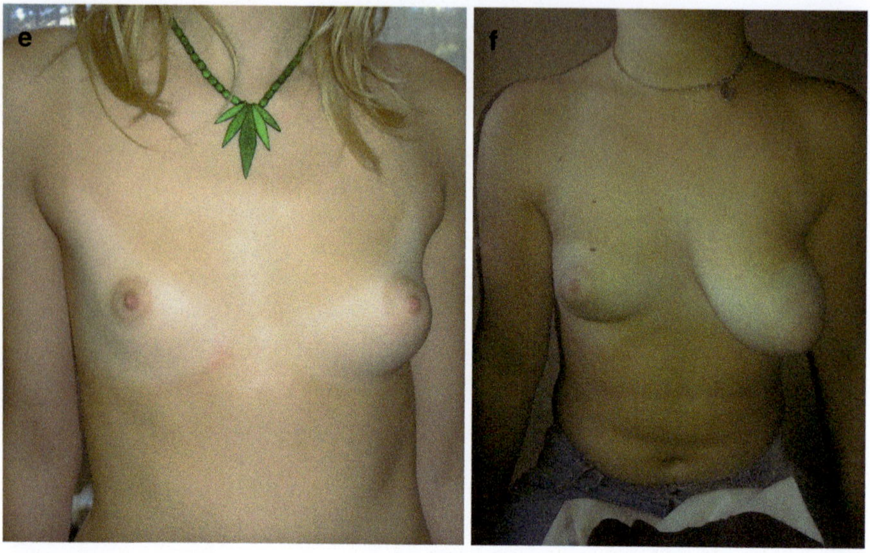

Fig. 5.13 (continued)

after the breast development is finished (Fig. 5.14a–d) [3, 14]. In case of hypertrophy, reduction is performed in group I and II, reduction and augmentation on opposite side in group III, muscular flap techniques in group IV, augmentation mammaplasty in group V, and mastopexy and augmentation mammaplasty in group VI [4, 14]. Tissue expansion is performed until the breast volume of the reconstructed breast is symmetric with the contralateral breast [3, 4, 30].

5.5.6 Traumatic and Iatrogenic Breast Disease

Burns, traumatic lacerations, dog bites, and surgical procedures can lead to damage of skin, subcutaneous, or deeper tissue of the breast as well (Fig. 5.15a–c) [1, 2, 4, 7, 9, 28, 30]. Inadequate tissue volume can be managed with tissue expansion and augmentation mammaplasty, and for nipple areola complex, cosmetic reconstruction can be performed using nipple sharing, full-thickness skin graft (FTSG) with a tattoo, and cartilage or toe pulp for reconstruction of nipple [1, 2, 7, 9].

5.5.7 Breast Infection

In neonates (2–3 weeks) and prepubertal children, mastitis usually involves the entire breast complex and is caused most often by gram-positive bacteria (*Staphylococcus aureus*) (Fig. 5.16) [6, 12, 13]. Antibiotics are required (systemic or perorally), and in the presence of breast abscess, incision and drainage may be necessary (with maximal care) [3, 12, 13].

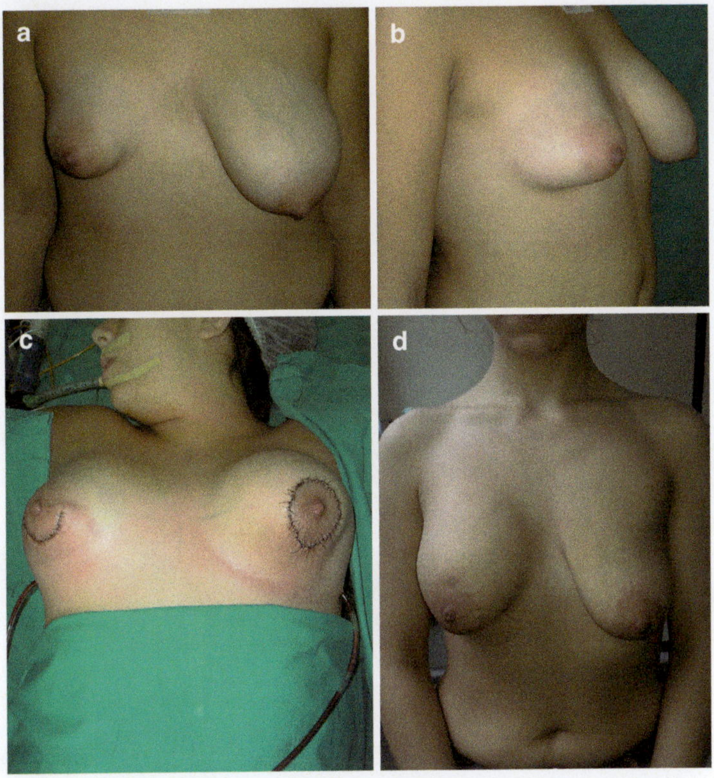

Fig. 5.14 Mammary ptosis of the left breast and hypoplasia of the right breast: (**a**, **b**) preoperative view; (**c**) mastopexy of the left breast and augmentation mammoplasty of the right breast; (**d**) the same patient as adult, 8 years after surgery and significant weight loss (reoperation is indicated)

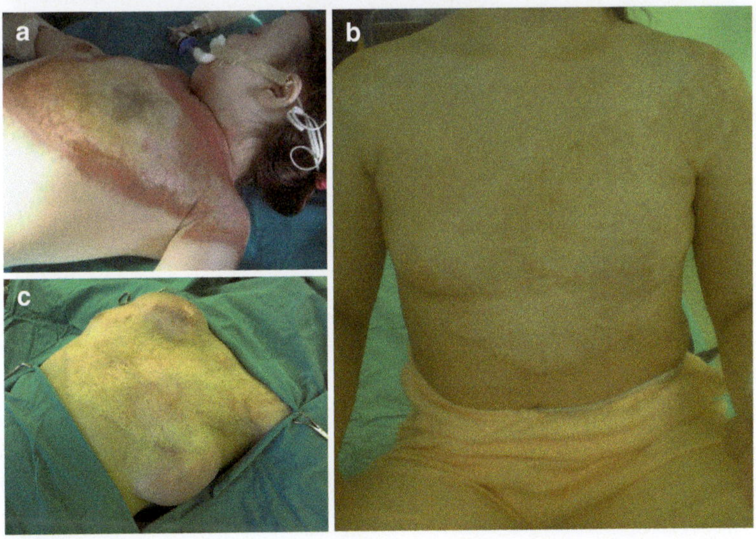

Fig. 5.15 Breast deformity caused by burn scar: (**a**) chemical burn; (**b**) result after necrectomy and skin grafting; (**c**) scar reconstruction with tissue expanders

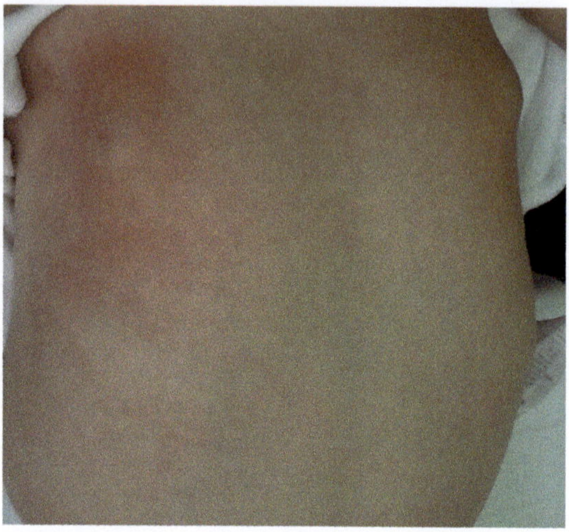

Fig. 5.16 Mastitis of the right breast

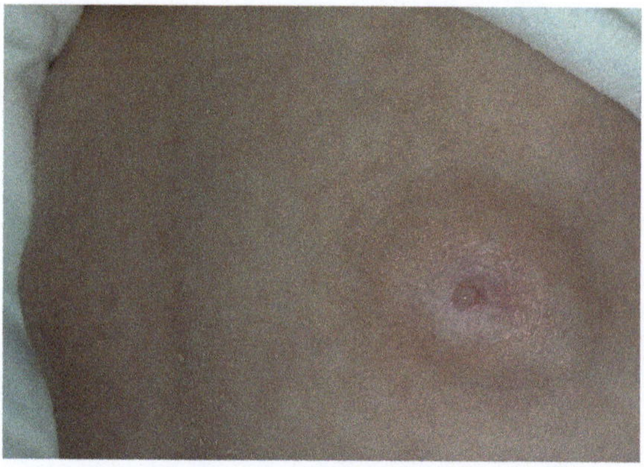

Fig. 5.17 Serous nipple discharge

5.5.8 Nipple Discharge

Nipple discharge is rare in pediatric population [3]. The characteristics of fluid provide clues to the underlying pathology [12, 13]. Serous discharge is not important, and bloody nipple discharge in prepubertal patients is sometimes associated with infantile mammary duct ectasia, intraductal papilloma or cyst (extremely rare in adolescents), or chronic cystic mastitis (Fig. 5.17) [3, 12, 13]. Treatment is surgical excision of the entire involved duct. Purulent discharge is associated with infection of the breast, and galactorrhea may be caused in adolescents by increase in prolactin, endocrine abnormalities, and drugs [3, 13, 34].

References

1. Latham K, Fernandez S, Iteld L, Panthaki Z, Armstrong MB, Thaller S. Pediatric breast deformity. J Cran Surg. 2006;17(3):4564–7.
2. Sadove AM, van Aalst JA. Congenital and acquired pediatric breast anomalies: a review of 20 years' experience. Plast Reconstr Surg. 2005;115(4):1039–50.
3. Ribas JMM. Breast problems and diseases in puberty. Best Prac Res Clin Obst Gyn. 2010;24:223–42.
4. Schermak MA. Congenital and developmental abnormalities of the breast. In: Jatoi I, Kaufmann M, editors. Management of breast diseases. Berlin: Springer; 2010. p. 37–51.
5. Bock K, Duda VF, Hadji P, Ramaswamy A, Schulz-Wendtland R, Klose KJ, Wagner U. Pathologic breast conditions in childhood and adolescence: evaluation by sonographic diagnosis. J Ultrasound Med. 2005;24(10):1347–54. Quiz 1356–7.
6. Kaneda HJ, Mack J, Kasales CJ, Schetter S. Pediatric and adolescent breast masses: a review of pathophysiology, imaging, diagnosis, and treatment. AJR Am J Roentgenol. 2013;200(2):W204–12.
7. van Aalst JA, Phillips JD, Sadove AM. Pediatric chest wall and breast deformities. Plast Reconstr Surg. 2009;124(1 Suppl):38e–49e.
8. Larson K, Gosain AK. Cosmetic surgery in the adolescent patient. Plast Reconstr Surg. 2012;129(1):135e–41e.
9. van Aalst JA, Sadove AM. Treatment of pediatric breast problems. Clin Plast Surg. 2005;32(1):65–78.
10. Higdon KK, Grotting JC. Mastopexy. In: Neligen PC, Gurtner GC, editors. Plastic surgery. Principles and practice. St Louis: Elsevier; 2013. p. 119–151e2.
11. De la Torre J, Davis M. Anatomy for plastic surgery of the breast. In: Neligen PC, Grotting JC, editors. Plastic surgery. Principles and practice. St Louis: Elsevier; 2013. p. 44–56.
12. Lam VT, Bambini DA. Breast lesions. In: Arensman RM, Bambini DA, Almond PS, editors. Pediatric surgery. Texas: Landes Bioscience; 2000. p. 206–10.
13. Arca MJ, Caniano DA. Breast disorders in the adolescent patient. Adolesc Med Clin. 2004;15(3):473–85.
14. Araco A, Gravante G, Araco F, Gentile P, Castrì F, Delogu D, Filingeri V, Cervelli V. Breast asymmetries: a brief review and our experience. Aesthet Plast Surg. 2006;30(3):309–19.
15. Soleimani T, Evans TA, Sood R, Hadad I, Socas J. Pediatric reduction mammaplasty: a retrospective analysis of the kids' inpatient database (KID). Surgery. 2015;158(3):793–801.
16. Cerrato F, Webb ML, Rosen H, Nuzzi L, McCarty ER, DiVasta AD, Greene AK, Labow BI. The impact of macromastia on adolescents: a cross-sectional study. Pediatrics. 2012;130(2):e339–46.
17. Spear SL. Breast reduction: inverted-T technique. In: Thorne CH, Beasley RW, Aston SJ, Bartlett SP, Gurtner GC, Spear SL, editors. Grabb and Smith's plastic surgery. Philadelphia: Lippincott Williams & Wilkins; 2007. p. 593–603.
18. Bostwick III J. Breast augmentation, reduction, and mastopexy. In: Jurkiewitz MJ, Krizek TJ, Mathes SJ, Ariyan S, editors. Plastic surgery. Principles and practice. St Louis: Mosby; 1990. p. 1063–93.
19. McMahan JD, Wolfe JA, Cromer BA, Ruberg RL. Lasting success in teenage reduction mammaplasty. Ann Plast Surg. 1995;35(3):227–31.
20. Evans GR, Ryan JJ. Reduction mammaplasty for the teenage patient: a critical analysis. Aesthet Plast Surg. 1994;18(3):291–7.
21. Xue AS, Wolfswinkel EM, Weathers WM, Chike-Obi C, Heller L. Breast reduction in adolescents: indication, timing, and a review of the literature. J Pediatr Adolesc Gynecol. 2013;26(4):228–33.
22. Karp NS. Mastopexy and mastopexy augmentation. In: Thorne CH, Beasley RW, Aston SJ, Bartlett SP, Gurtner GC, Spear SL, editors. Grabb and Smith's plastic surgery. Philadelphia: Lippincott Williams & Wilkins; 2007. p. 585–92.

23. Clarkson JH, Harley OJ, Kirkpatrick JJ. Alfred Poland's syndrome: a tidy little controversy. J Plast Reconstr Aesthet Surg. 2006;59(9):1006–8.
24. Kulkarni D, Dixon JM. Congenital abnormalities of the breast. Womens Health. 2012;8(1):75–86.
25. Dolas SC, Poovamma CU, Prema M, Khandelwal R, Pais AV, Kaul A. Poland's syndrome: a case report with review of literature regarding management. Breast Dis. 2014;34(3):121–5.
26. Freitas RS, Tolazzi ARD, Martins VD, Knop BA, Graf RM, Cruz GA. Poland's syndrome: different clinical presentations and surgical reconstructions in 18 cases. Aesthet Plast Surg. 2007;31(2):140–6.
27. Cingel V, Bohac M, Mestanova V, Zabojnikova L, Varga I. Poland syndrome: from embryological basis to plastic surgery. Surg Radiol Anat. 2013;35(8):639–46.
28. Muti E. Congenital anomalies of the breast. In: Neligen PC, Gurtner GC, editors. Plastic surgery. Principles and practice. St Louis: Elsevier; 2013. p. 521–47e2.
29. Heimburg DV, Exner K, Kruft S, Lemperle G. The tuberous breast deformity: classification and treatment. Br J Plast Surg. 1996;49:339–45.
30. Oakes MB, Quint EH, Smith YR, Cederna PS. Early, staged reconstruction in young women with severe breast asymmetry. J Pediatr Adolesc Gynecol. 2009;22(4):223–8.
31. Chan W, Mathur B, Slade-Sharman D, Ramakrishnan V. Developmental breast asymmetry. Breast J. 2011;17(4):391–8.
32. Eidlitz-Markus T, Mukamel M, Haimi-Cohen Y, Amir J, Zeharia A. Breast asymmetry during adolescence: physiologic and non-physiologic causes. Isr Med Assoc J. 2010;12(4):203–6.
33. Nuzzi LC, Cerrato FE, Webb ML, Faulkner HR, Walsh EM, DiVasta AD, Greene AK, Labow BI. Psychological impact of breast asymmetry on adolescents: a prospective cohort study. Plast Reconstr Surg. 2014;134(6):1116–23.
34. Kelly VM, Arif K, Ralston S, Greger N, Scott S. Bloody nipple discharge in an infant and a proposed diagnostic approach. Pediatrics. 2006;117(4):e814–6.

Male Breast Reduction

6

6.1 Introduction

Gynecomastia is defined as benign proliferation of male breast (ductal tissue, stroma, and/or fat) [1–4]. The term gynecomastia is derived from Greek words *gyne*, women, and *mastos*, breast [5]. Reported incidence of gynecomastia is different, and it ranges from 32 to 36% and up to 65% [1, 5–8]. Gynecomastia can be confused with pseudogynecomastia (accumulation of subareolar fat without real proliferation of glandular tissue, usually in the presence of general obesity) [3, 5, 7, 9].

6.2 Embryology

The breast originates from the ectoderm, and the connective tissue is derived from the mesoderm [2, 5–8]. By the tenth week of gestation, the upper and lower part of milk line (from the primitive axilla to the primitive groin) disappears, and the limited portion at the level of the fourth intercostal space of embryo remains and forms the basis for development of the neonatal breast [5–8]. By birth, neonatal mammary tissue becomes functional; it grows proportionally with the child during childhood [8]. Until the puberty, the growth of breast is identical for males and females [2, 5, 6].

6.3 Anatomy

In adults, breasts are in position between the second and third and seventh and eighth rib; medially, there are sternal edge and laterally midaxillary line [5, 8]. Besides the skin and subcutaneous tissue, the breast is made up of parenchymatous

A.M. Vlahovic, E.Q. Haxhija, *Pediatric and Adolescent Plastic Surgery for the Clinician*, DOI 10.1007/978-3-319-56004-5_6

and stromal tissue [5, 7, 8]. The breast is supplied by a vascular network consisting of the internal mammary, lateral thoracic, and intercostal arteries [5, 8]. Sensory supply of the breast is provided by T3–T5 nerve roots; the superior portion of the breast is supplied by supraclavicular nerve, and the nipple receives sensory innervation from T4 [7].

6.4 Pathophysiology

The etiology of gynecomastia is not completely understood [2]. It is thought to be the result of an imbalance of estrogen action relative to androgen action at the breast tissue level [3, 5, 10–12].

Gynecomastia can be classified as asymptomatic (with high incidence) and symptomatic (it is rare) [3, 5, 7]. Bailey et al. categorized gynecomastia in four groups: physiologic, pathologic, pharmacologic, and idiopathic [13].

Most commonly, gynecomastia is *idiopathic* [3, 10].

Physiologic (asymptomatic) gynecomastia is very common; it is related to hormonal changes; and it has three peaks of occurrence in neonatal, pubertal (in almost 66% of adolescent boys), and old age period (older than 65 years) [1–3, 5, 7, 8, 10, 11]. Leptin may play role in the development of physiologic gynecomastia [2].

Pathologic (symptomatic) gynecomastia is very rare, and it can be caused by increase in estrogen, a decrease in testosterone, medication, or drug use, or it may be idiopathic [2, 10].

Elevated serum estrogen levels may be a result of estrogen-secreting neoplasms or their precursors or with increase extragonadal conversion of androgens to estrogens by tissue aromatase [2, 5]. Increase aromatization of the precursors of the estrogen can result in the elevation of the estrogens (testicular germ cell tumors, liver disease, hyperthyroidism, Klinefelter syndrome) [2, 3, 12]. Levels of free serum testosterone are decreased in patients with gonadal failure [1–3, 9]. Serum levels of sex hormone-binding globulin (SHBG) can affect the estrogen/androgen balance in hyperthyroidism and chronic liver disease [1, 3, 9, 10].

Drugs may be associated with gynecomastia *(pharmacologic gynecomastia)* [1–3, 5–7, 10]. The use of medications such as hormones (antiandrogens, anabolic steroids, estrogen), antibiotics (metronidazole, ketoconazole, isoniazid), antiulcer medications (cimetidine, omeprazole, ranitidine), chemotherapeutic agents (methotrexate), cardiovascular drugs (digoxin, nifedipine, verapamil, spironolactone), psychoactive agents (diazepam, haloperidol), and marihuana is believed to cause gynecomastia [3, 9, 10, 12].

There is no increased risk of breast cancer in patients with gynecomastia when compared to the unaffected male population (with the exception of patients with Klinefelter syndrome) [1, 2, 9].

6.5 Pathology

Three types of gynecomastia have been described: florid, fibrous, and intermediate [1, 5, 9]. The florid type is characterized by an increase in ductal tissue and vascularity with a variable amount of fat, the fibrous type has more stromal fibrosis and few ducts, and the intermediate type is a mixture of the two [7, 11]. Florid gynecomastia is usually seen when the duration is 4 months or less, the fibrous type is usually present after duration of 1 year, and the intermediate type is usually seen between 4 and 12 months [8, 11].

6.6 Classification

Various classification schemes have been proposed for gynecomastia [11, 14–16]. There are two classifications of gynecomastia mostly used in practice presented by Simon and Rohrich [11, 16]. Simon et al. proposed a qualitative classification of volume and skin redundancy dictating treatment: grade I, small enlargement, no skin excess; grade IIA, moderate enlargement, no skin excess; grade IIB, moderate enlargement with extra skin; and grade III, marked enlargement with extra skin (Fig. 6.1a–d) [7, 11, 17].

Rohrich's classification is based on the amount of tissue mass requiring excision (adipose versus fibrous tissue predominance): grade I, minimal hypertrophy (<250 g of breast tissue) without ptosis, (IA primarily glandular, IB primarily fibrous); grade II, moderate hypertrophy (250–500 g of breast tissue) without ptosis (IIA primarily glandular, IIB primarily fibrous); grade III, severe hypertrophy (>500 g of breast tissue) with grade I ptosis (glandular or fibrous); and grade IV, severe hypertrophy with grade II or III ptosis (glandular or fibrous) [11, 16].

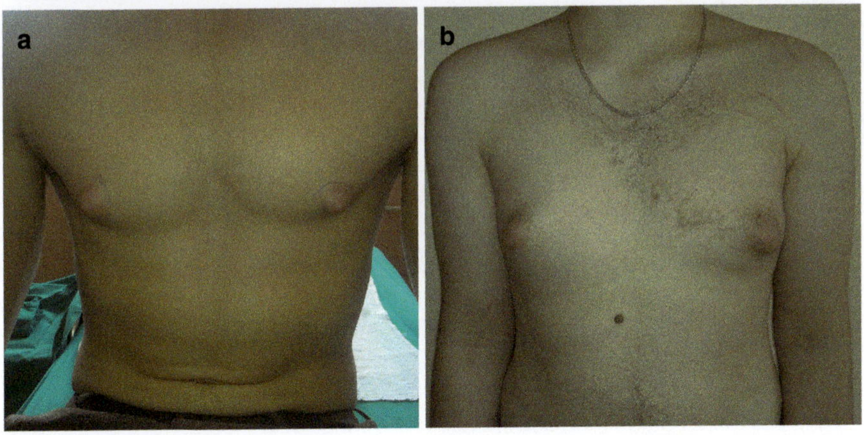

Fig. 6.1 Different types of gynecomastia (according to Simon classification): (**a**) grade 1; (**b**) grade 2a; (**c**) grade 2b; (**d**) grade 3

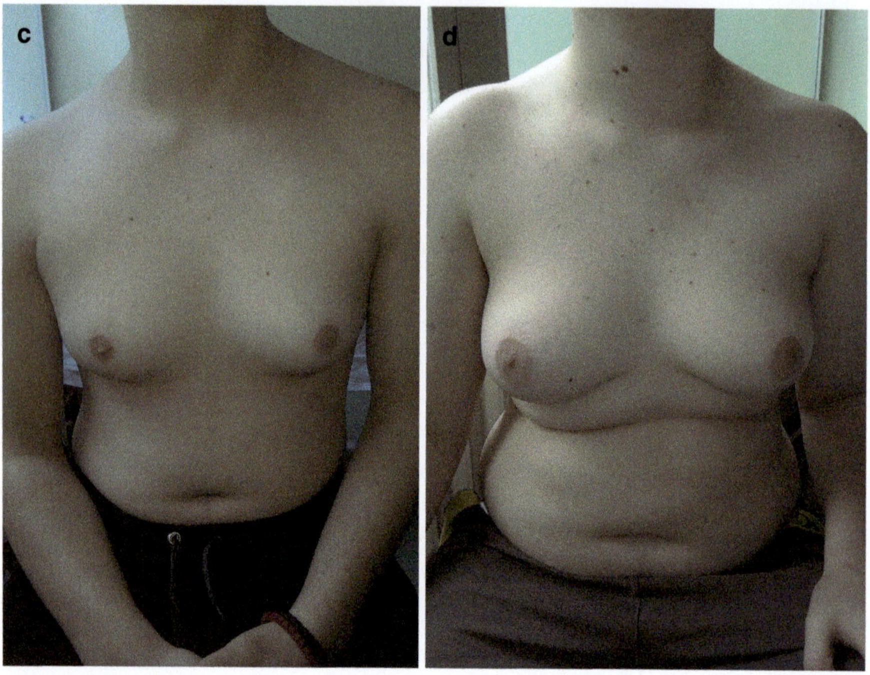

Fig. 6.1 (continued)

6.7 Clinical Manifestation

Gynecomastia is usually bilateral (it may also appear as asymmetrical or unilateral) [1, 3, 10]. On examination, gynecomastia presents as palpable, firm, tender, mobile, mound of tissue [1, 3, 9, 10].

There is positive family history in more than half of patients with persistent pubertal gynecomastia [3]. The testicular exam should be included in physical examination since it may reveal presence of malignancy or varicoceles [1, 3, 7, 8].

6.8 Diagnosis

A careful history (time of onset, associated symptoms, drug use, careful review of organ systems) and physical examination is the most important part of any workup for gynecomastia [1–3, 9]. Patients with pseudogynecomastia have diffuse breast enlargement without a subareolar palpable nodule (Fig. 6.2) [2, 3, 9, 10]. These patients do not require additional workup and only require reassurance [2, 3, 9].

Physical examination should include assessment of the breast gland (nature of the tissue, isolated masses, and tenderness), thyroid gland, and the testis [3, 9, 10]. Any other new positive findings on physical examination should be evaluated [1, 3, 9, 10]. Patients with pseudogynecomastia do not need further workup [3].

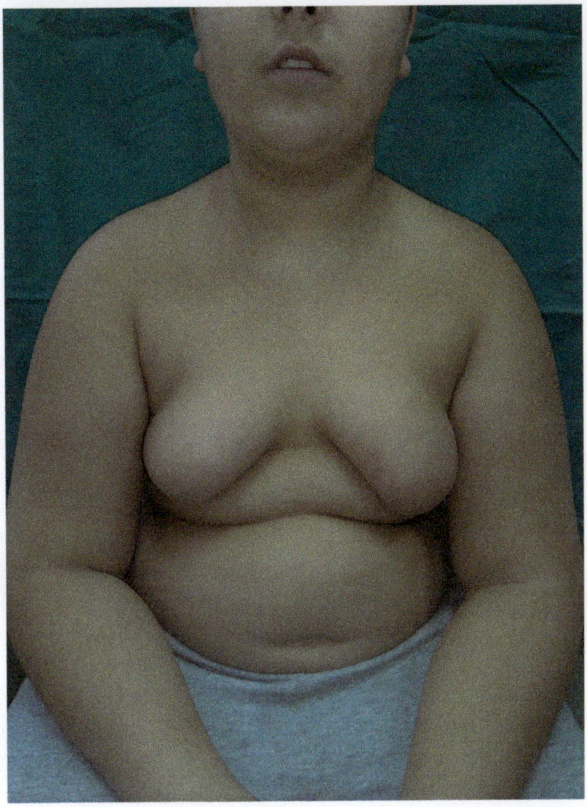

Fig. 6.2 Bilateral pseudogynecomastia

If the history and physical examination revealed a painful gynecomastia, without known cause, laboratory evaluation is indicated; liver, kidney, and thyroid tests should be performed, and estradiol, testosterone, prolactin, luteinizing hormone, serum DHEA-sulfate, and hCG should be measured [3, 6, 9, 10]. If all endocrine testing in patient with feminizing characteristics is negative, idiopathic gynecomastia is diagnosed [3]. Imaging studies or biopsy are rarely used [10].

Differential diagnosis of gynecomastia includes pseudogynecomastia, dermoid cyst, sebaceous cyst, ductal ectasias, hematoma, fat necrosis, galactocele, and breast carcinoma (extremely rare in children) [1–3, 7, 9, 10, 18].

6.9 Treatment Option

Treatment of gynecomastia depends on underlying cause, and it can be conservative or surgical [1, 4, 5, 9, 10].

6.9.1 Conservative Treatment

Conservative treatment is possible until there is no fibrosis with antiestrogens (tamoxifen), androgens (danazol), and aromatase inhibitors [3, 4, 6, 9, 10, 12, 13]. In some cases (drug-induced gynecomastia, chemotherapy, hypothyroidism, tumors) by eliminating the cause, one can resolve gynecomastia [1, 6, 9–11, 15]. In near 25% of gynecomastia, the cause is not identified, and for these patients, the treatment is recommended only if there is pain, psychological discomfort, or embarrassment [3, 4, 10]. These patients can be initially treated with drug therapy [3, 10].

6.9.2 Surgical Treatment

Surgery is treatment of choice for gynecomastia, and it is usually performed under general anesthesia [3, 4, 14, 19]. Surgery is performed if gynecomastia persists beyond 1 year despite of treatment, and it can be performed in any stage of gynecomastia [4, 9, 11, 13]. A wide range of surgical techniques has been described for appropriate gynecomastia stage [1, 3, 4, 7, 11, 13, 15–17, 19–21]. There is a shift from open approach to minimally invasive techniques [3, 4, 15, 19]. The surgical procedures used to treat gynecomastia include excision, conventional liposuction with or without excision, power-assisted liposuction (PAL), ultrasound-assisted liposuction (UAL), and vibration amplification of sound energy at resonance (VASER)-assisted liposuction (newer form of UAL) [4, 11, 14, 15, 19].

The traditional reduction mammoplasty is still required for a selected group of patients with well-localized fibrous gynecomastia under the nipple or with significant amount of excess skin and ptosis (Fig. 6.3a, b) [11, 15].

Current literature supports the use of ultrasound-assisted liposuction or liposuction alone, and combination of these procedures with direct excision of the residual breast tissue [13, 19]. UAL has several advantages in the treatment of gynecomastia

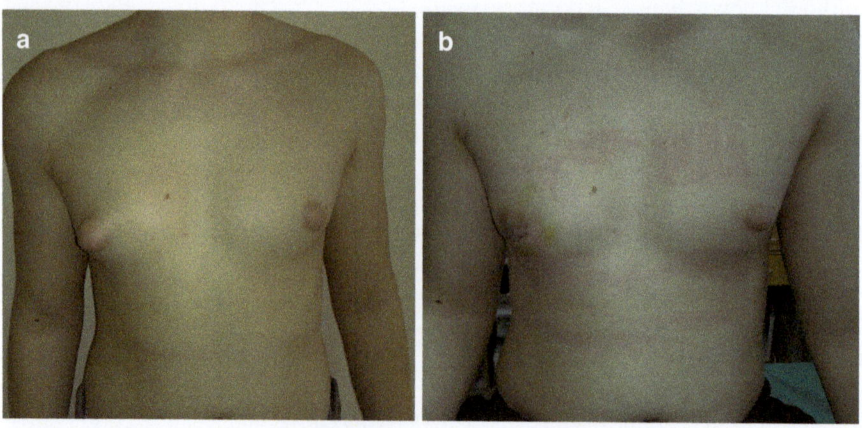

Fig. 6.3 Surgical treatment of unilateral gynecomastia: (**a**) preoperative view; (**b**) postoperative result

(better emulsification of the fat and efficient removal; it promotes skin retraction) [4, 13, 15, 19].

Most fibrous or solid lesions (Simon grade I or IIA - Rochrich grade I and II) are usually treated with surgical excision or, in some cases, with UAL [11, 16]. The skin incision is placed at the junction of the areola and skin; a cuff of tissue 1–1.5 cm in thickness is left directly under the NAC to prevent postoperative nipple areola depression [11].

If the patient has a lesion that is glandular, fatty, or mixed in nature and is Simon grade I or IIA, the area could be treated with liposuction, and if liposuction is unsuccessful, there are several additional options ("pull-through" technique, periareolar incision, arthroscopic shavers insertion through small inframammary incisions) [11, 15].

In patients with Simon grade IIB and Rochrich grade III gynecomastia (fat, glandular, or mixed), the initial treatment is like in grade I or IIA gynecomastia followed by skin resection after 6–12 months [11, 14]. In solid or fibrous Simon grade IIB gynecomastia, UAL with pull-through or open approach with skin reduction should be performed [11].

There are numerous incisions and techniques described for severe gynecomastia (Simon grade III and Rochrich grade IV) similar to those used in female mastopexy and reduction mammaplasty, and liposuction with skin excision can also be used (Fig. 6.4a–e) [4, 11, 12, 17, 20, 21].

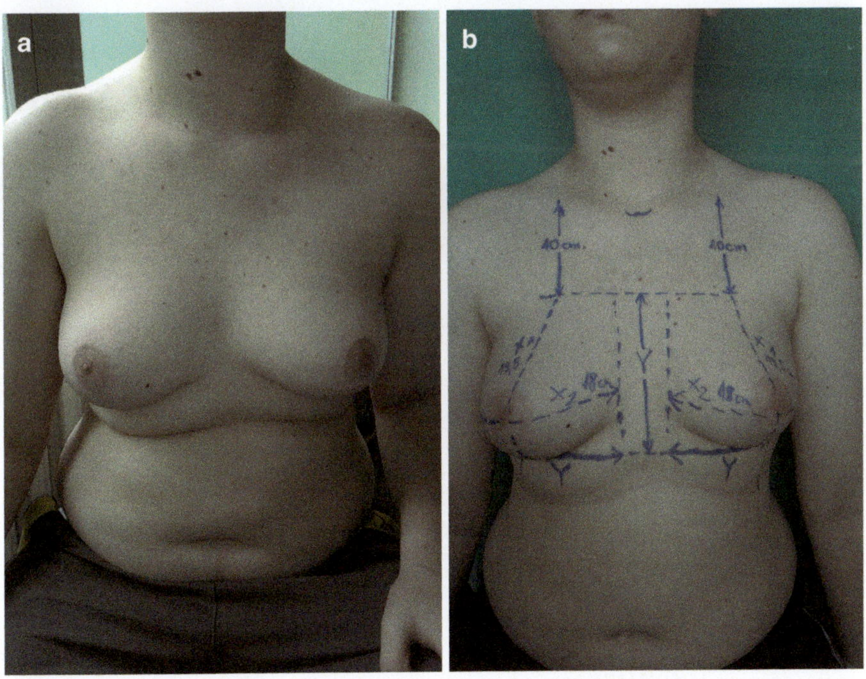

Fig. 6.4 Surgical treatment of grade 3 gynecomastia: (**a**) preoperative view; (**b**) preoperative markings; (**c**) right breast excision; (**d**) left breast excision; (**e**) early postoperative result

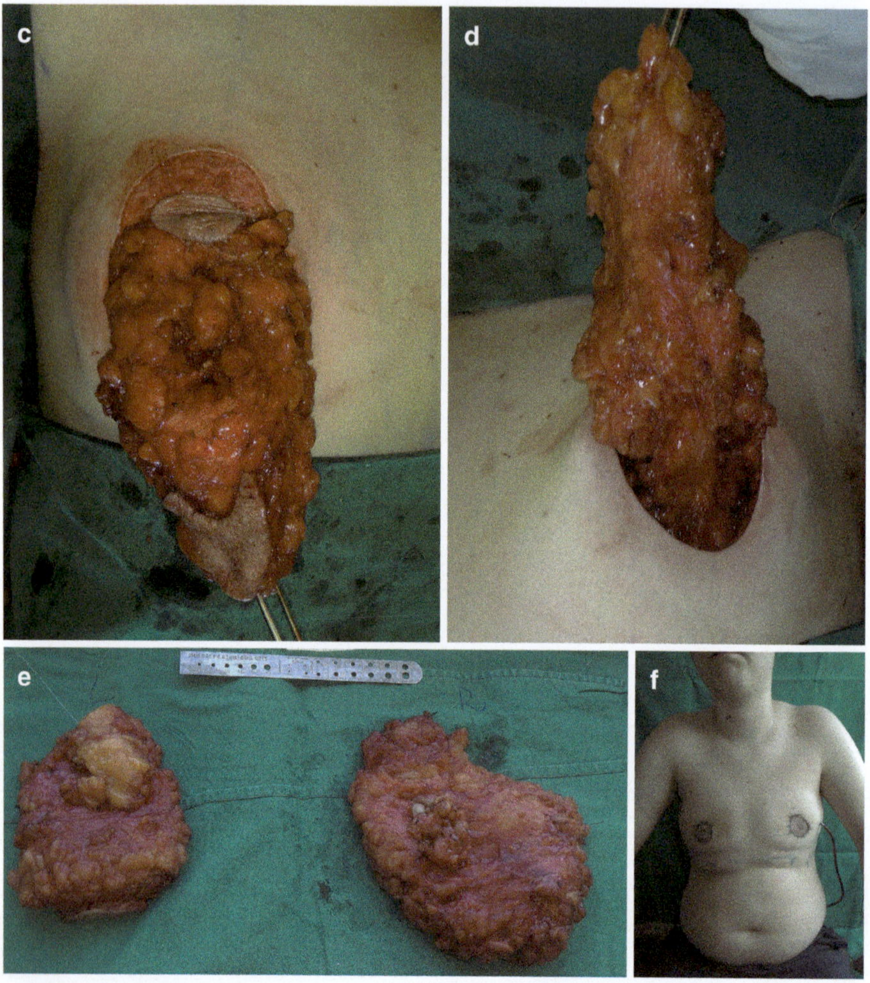

Fig. 6.4 (continued)

6.10 Complications

Complications of gynecomastia surgery has been reported up to 50% including hematoma, wound infection, scarring, contour deformity (underresection and overresection), breast asymmetry, pain, and sensory changes [1, 7, 15]. Hematoma is a common early complication after surgical treatment of gynecomastia (the incidence of hematoma decreases with postoperative closed suction drainage), and it should be evacuated to prevent complications [1, 7, 11, 15]. Postoperative wound infection is uncommon [15]. Underresection is the most common long-term complication, especially in liposuction cases, and overresection in the nipple areola can result in a saucer-type deformity (difficult to correct) [2, 15]. Loose skin is usually not considered a complication if it is part of the operative plan, and if it occurs as an unexpected manner, surgical excision is required [1, 2, 15].

6.11 Postoperative Care

Postoperative drainage may be used if the dead space is large, patients are placed in compression garments for 6–8 weeks, and sustaining of sport activities for several weeks is also advised [1, 15].

References

1. McGrath MH. Gynecomastia. In: Jurkiewitz MJ, Krizek TJ, Mathes SJ, Ariyan S, editors. Plastic surgery. Principles and practice. St Louis: Mosby; 1990. p. 1063–93.
2. Kaneda HJ, Mack J, Kasales CJ, Schetter S. Pediatric and adolescent breast masses: a review of pathophysiology, imaging, diagnosis, and treatment. AJR Am J Roentgenol. 2013;200(2):W204–12.
3. Johnson RE, Hassan MM. Gynecomastia: pathophysiology, evaluation, and management. Mayo Clin Proc. 2009;84(11):1010–5.
4. Fruhstorfer BH, Malata CM. A systematic approach to the surgical treatment of gynaecomastia. Br J Plast Surg. 2003;56(3):237–46.
5. Schermak MA. Congenital and developmental abnormalities of the breast. In: Jatoi I, Kaufmann M, editors. Management of breast diseases. Berlin: Springer; 2010. p. 37–51.
6. Baumann K, Pursche T. Congenital and developmental abnormalities of the breast. In: Jatoi I, Kaufmann M, editors. Management of breast diseases. Berlin: Springer; 2016. p. 41–55.
7. Latham K, Fernandez S, Iteld L, Panthaki Z, Armstrong MB, Thaller S. Pediatric breast deformity. J Cran Surg. 2006;17(3):454–67.
8. Arca MJ, Caniano DA. Breast disorders in the adolescent patient. Adoles med Clin. 2004;15(3):473–85.
9. Braunstein GD. Gynecomastia. N Engl J Med. 2007;357:1229–37.
10. Bembo SA, Carlson HE. Gynecomastia: its features, and when and how to treat it. Cleve Clin J Med. 2004;71(6):511–7.
11. Karp NS. Gynecomastia. In: Thorne CH, Beasley RW, Aston SJ, Bartlett SP, Gurtner GC, Spear SL, editors. Grabb and Smith's plastic surgery. Philadelphia: Lippincott Williams & Wilkins; 2007. p. 616–20.
12. Laituri CA, Garey CL, Ostlie DJ, St. Peter SD, Gittes GK, Snyder CL. Treatment of adolescent gynecomastia. J Ped Surg. 2010;45:650–4.
13. Bailey SH, Guenther D, Constantine F, Rohrich RJ. Gynecomastia Management: an evolution and refinement in technique at UT Southwestern Medical Center. Plast Reconstr Surg Glob Open. 2016;4(6):e734–41.
14. Cordova A, Moschella F. Algorithm for clinical evaluation and surgical treatment of gynaecomastia. J Plast Reconstr Aesthet Surg. 2008;61(1):41–9.
15. Brown RH, Chang DK, Siy R, Friedman J. Trends in the surgical correction of gynecomastia. Semin Plast Surg. 2015;29(2):122–30.
16. Rohrich RJ, Ha RY, Kenkel JM, Adams Jr WP. Classification and management of gynecomastia: defining the role of ultrasound-assisted liposuction. Plast Reconstr Surg. 2003;111(2):909–23. Discussion 924–5.

17. Cannistra C, Piedimonte A, Albonico F. Surgical Treatment of gynecomastia with severe ptosis: periareolar incision and dermal double areolar pedicle technique. Aesth Plast Surg. 2009;33:834–7.
18. Vlahovic A, Djuricic S, Todorovic S, Djukic M, Milanovic D, Vujanic GM. Galactocele in male infants: report of two cases and review of the literature. E J Ped Surg. 2012;22(3):246–50.
19. Petty PM, Solomon M, Buchel EW, Tran NV. Gynecomastia: evolving paradigm of management and comparison of techniques. Plast Reconstr Surg. 2010;125(5):1301–8.
20. Huang TT, Hidalgo JE, Lewis SR. A circumareolar approach in surgical management of gynecomastia. Plast Reconstr Surg. 1982;69(1):36–9.
21. Davidson BA. Concentric circle operation for massive gynecomastia to excise the redundant skin. Plast Reconstr Surg. 1979;63(3):350–4.

Cleft Lip and Palate

7

7.1 Introduction

Cleft lip and palate are the most common congenital craniofacial anomalies [1, 2]. Cleft lip (CL), cleft palate (CP), and cleft lip and palate (CLP) constitute a heterogenous group of birth defects with multifactorial origin [1]. Cleft care requires closely allied reconstructive and cosmetic principles, applied by a plastic surgeon as a member of a collaborative multidisciplinary team [3–8]. Major advances in the care of children born with CLP occurred in the last three decades, and there is a tendency for cleft care centralization [4].

7.2 Embryology

Primary palate develops from 4 to 8 gestational weeks (GW) and secondary palate develops from 5 to 12 GW [2, 9, 10]. Although they often occur together, they have different embryonic origins [2, 6, 7, 11]. Medial nasal, lateral nasal, and maxillary processes are involved in the formation of primary palate, and any failure of fusion will give a rise to the cleft of the lip, alveolus, and hard palate to the incisive foramen on one or both sides [6, 9–11]. The secondary palate develops from the paired lateral palatine processes [2, 10, 11]. This shelf-like mesodermal projections are fused together from anterior to posterior, after the tongue is moved inferiorly [7, 11]. If the shelves do not fuse (as a result of defective growth, failure to rise above the tongue, or there is a rupture after fusion), cleft palate occurs [2, 7].

7.3 Cleft Anatomy

Normal lip anatomy is a reconstructive goal [6]. The lip surface is divided into cutaneous, dry vermilion, and vet vermilion part, and superior to the upper lip in central position is the nose with philtrum lying between these two [6, 10, 12]. Deep to the

A.M. Vlahovic, E.Q. Haxhija, *Pediatric and Adolescent Plastic Surgery for the Clinician*, DOI 10.1007/978-3-319-56004-5_7

skin is the orbicularis oris muscle (OOM) which is striated and it encircles the mouth [6, 10]. The palate consists of anterior bony (hard) palate covered with mucoperiosteal lining, and posterior muscular (soft) palate, with foramen incisivum that delimits primary from secondary palate [6, 11, 13]. Soft palate muscles (m. levator veli palatini and m. tensor veli palatini as most important) are involved in speech, swallowing, and hearing [6, 11, 13–15].

In unilateral CL, lip is short on medial side, philtral column is flattened, and vermilion is narrow [10, 12]. On lateral side vermilion border and red line converge as they approach to cleft, with the deficiency of OOM and misdirection to the alar base and columella [5, 6, 10, 12, 13]. The nasal floor, alveolus, and palate can also be involved [10, 12].

In bilateral CL, the prolabium and premaxilla remain entirely separated from the lateral lip and maxillary arch elements [1, 5, 6, 13]. The cutaneous roll of prolabium is of poor quality, the height of vermilion is inadequate, labial sulcus is shallow, there is lack of OOM, and the lateral elements are similar to lateral elements of unilateral cleft [1, 13].

Unilateral complete CLP is characterized by direct communication between the entire length of the nasal passage and oropharynx (there is a full thickeness palatal defect of nasal mucosa, bony palate, velar musculature, and oral mucosa), and the nasal septum is deviated and buckled toward the cleft side (in bilateral cleft palate vomer remains free of attachments to the palatal shelves) [1, 11, 13]. *Isolated cleft palate* can occur as an opening in the posterior soft palate to a cleft extending up to the incisive foramen, and *in submucous cleft palate*, there is underlying levator palatine muscle discontinuity with triad of symptoms midline clear zone (zona pellucida), bifid uvula, and a palpable notch in the posterior hard palate [1, 11].

7.4 Epidemiology

The overall incidence of CLP is 1/700 [2, 4, 6, 8, 15]. Isolated cleft palate has an overall incidence of 0.4–0.5 per 1000 live births [1, 2, 4, 16]. The most common diagnosis is CL/P, followed by isolated cleft palate and then isolated cleft lip [2, 6]. Unilateral clefts are nine times as common as bilateral clefts, the left side is more often involved than right side, and the majority of bilateral and unilateral cleft lips are associated with a cleft palate [1, 2, 6]. Males are predominant in the CL/P population and females in isolated CP [2, 6].

7.5 Etiology

Both environmental (phenytoin, thalidomide, retinoic acid, maternal cigarette smoking, alcohol use) and genetic factors are involved in the genesis of cleft lip and palate [1, 2, 6, 15]. Gender differences (palate develops 1 week later in males), low socioeconomic status, parents' age, as well as maternal obesity play a role in clefting [1, 2, 6].

Clefts are classified as non-syndromic (without other physical or developmental anomalies, and known teratogenic exposures) and syndromic [2, 15, 16]. Isolated CP is most commonly a part of the syndromes compared to all cleft types (in 50% of all cases) [1, 2, 6].

There are more than 350 Mendelian disorders associated with CLP (Van der Woude, Treacher-Collins, Waardenburg, Apert's, Stickler's, Carey-Fineman-Ziter, velocardiofacial syndrome, Pierre Robin sequence, etc.) (Fig. 7.1) [1, 2, 6, 10, 11].

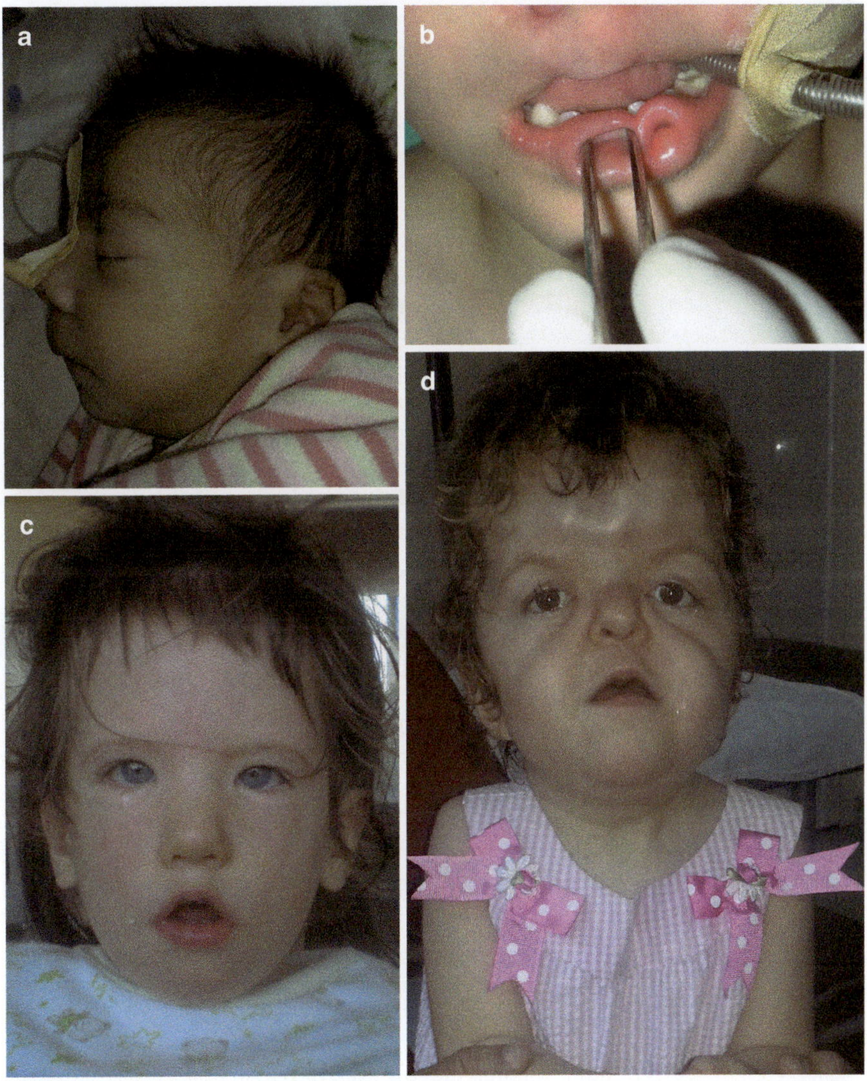

Fig. 7.1 Syndromic cleft palate: (**a**) Pierre Robin syndrome; (**b**) Van der Woude syndrome (lower lip pits); (**c**) Möbius syndrome; (**d**) Apert's syndrome

7.6 Diagnosis

Prenatal diagnosis of CL by ultrasound (US) is possible in more than 70% of cases [17, 18]. This is very important to establish because the birth of a child with cleft is a very large stress for unprepared parents, and it allows early preparation of the family [4, 8, 16–18]. The mean gestational age at detection of CL reported by some authors is 25.5 weeks [6].

Neonatologist or pediatrician has to be available at the time of the delivery (patients with clefts are in most cases already seen by pediatricians after the delivery and sent to the surgeon) [6, 8]. After cleft evaluation, complete examination of the oral cavity and entire body has to be performed (to exclude associated anomalies) [1, 8]. Instructions and assistance should be given to the parents regarding the feeding issues [8]. After birth, genetic counseling for the parents may be beneficial, and the child with CL and/or CP should be sent to regional cleft center [1, 3, 4, 8]. Parents are usually very upset and even angry with plethora of questions regarding etiology, care, and surgical treatment of their child [4, 6].

7.7 Surgical Evaluation and Classification

Clefts are typically divided into four groups: cleft of primary palate (unilateral, bilateral, total, or subtotal), cleft of secondary palate (total, subtotal, and submucosal), cleft of primary and secondary palate (unilateral, bilateral, total, or subtotal), and rare facial cleft [1, 6, 16].

Kernahan proposed a system to classify cleft lip and palate with the incisive foramen as central landmark and Y-shaped diagram (upper limbs represent primary palate and lower limb represent hard and soft palate) [1, 10, 16]. This classification is modified by adding numbers for more precise description [17]. Otto Kriens proposed a system that used letters to present components [1, 10]. The acronym LAHSHAL denotes the bilateral anatomy of the lip (L), alveolus (A), hard (H), and soft (S) palates, by convention from right to left [1, 10, 16]. Small letters represent incomplete clefts of the structure, and a period denotes no cleft [1, 10]. Clefts also can be recorded by letter codes (R, right; L, left; P, primary; S, secondary; C, complete, I, incomplete) [16].

There are several types of unilateral CL: *unilateral incomplete clefts* have in common an intact nasal sill, or Simonart band, and *unilateral complete clefts* are characterized by disruption of the lip, nostril sill, and alveolus (complete primary palate), and there is a group of unilateral CL named lesser-form clefts with three anatomical categories (*minor-form, microform, mini-microform clefts*) (Fig. 7.2a–e) [1, 10, 16, 19].

In *incomplete* bilateral primary clefts, there is a near-normal nose, a normally positioned premaxilla, and clefts involving only the lip, and in *complete bilateral primary cleft*, the protruding premaxilla with lateral palatal shelves is collapsed toward the midline (Fig. 7.3a–c) [1, 5].

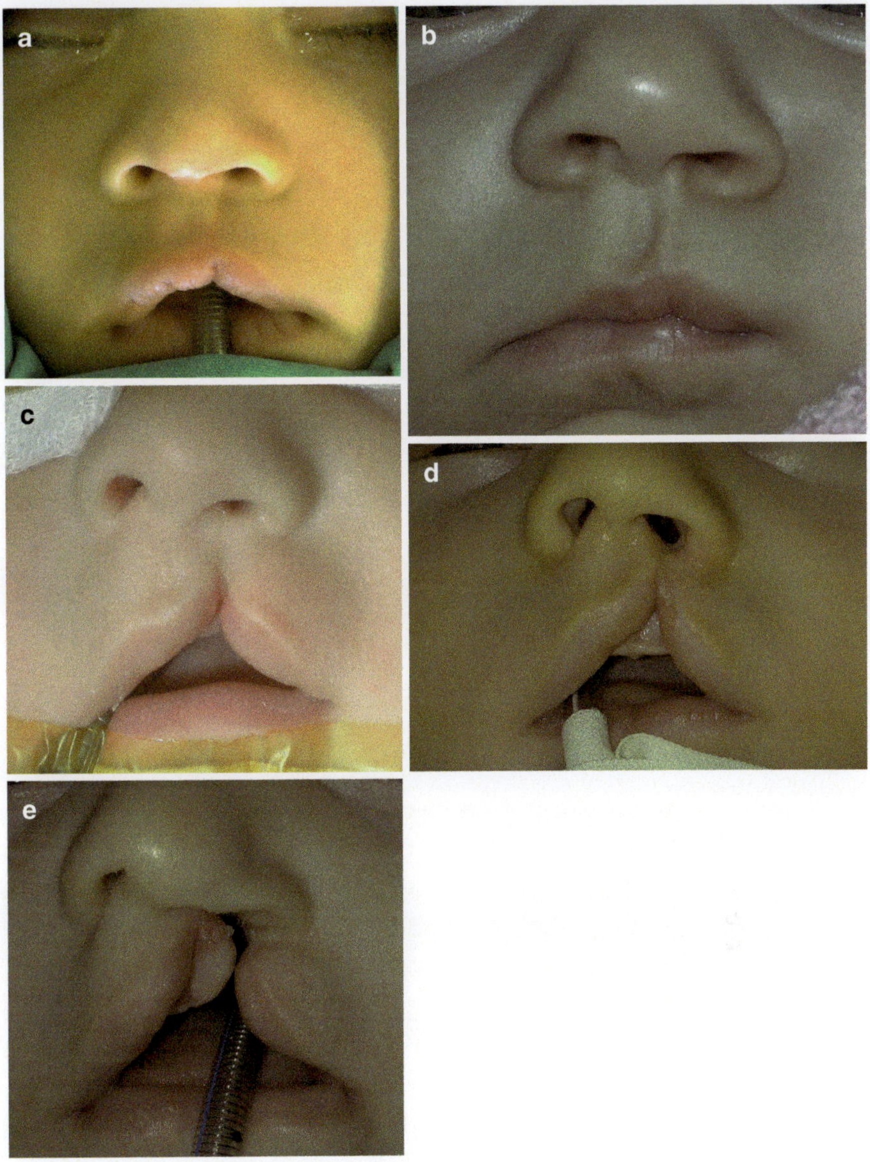

Fig. 7.2 Different types of unilateral cleft lip: (**a**) microform cleft lip; (**b**) mini-microform cleft lip; (**c**) minor form cleft lip; (**d**) unilateral incomplete cleft lip; (**e**) unilateral complete cleft lip

Unilateral complete clefts are characterized by disruption of the lip, nostril sill, and alveolus, hard and soft palates [1, 10]. Small group of patient with complete unilateral or bilateral CLP has nasolabiomaxillary hypoplasia and orbital hypertelorism, and they are named binderoid CLP [20].

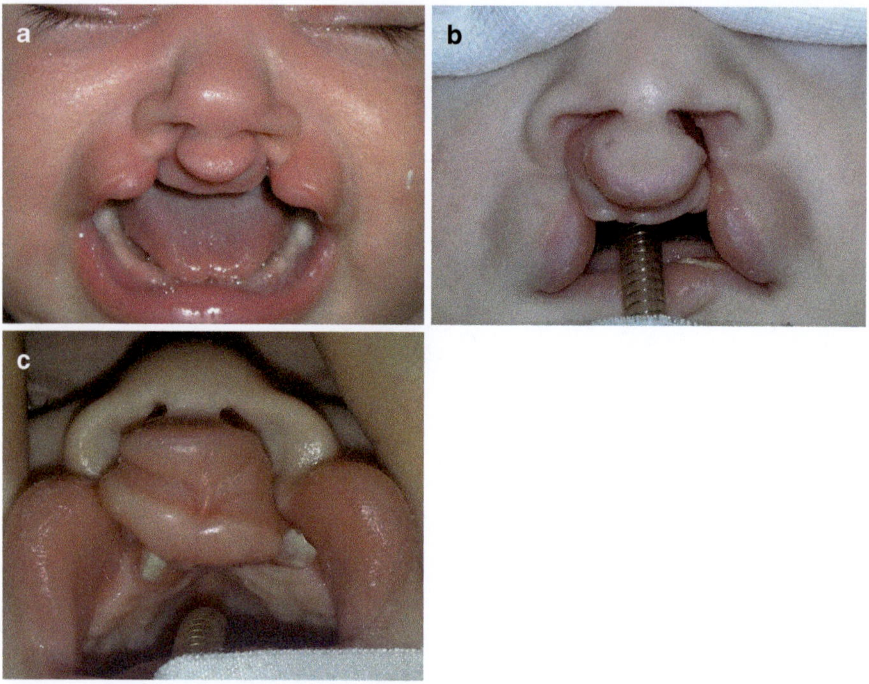

Fig. 7.3 Bilateral cleft lip: (**a**) incomplete bilateral cleft lip; (**b**) complete bilateral cleft lip; (**c**) complete isolated bilateral cleft of primary palate

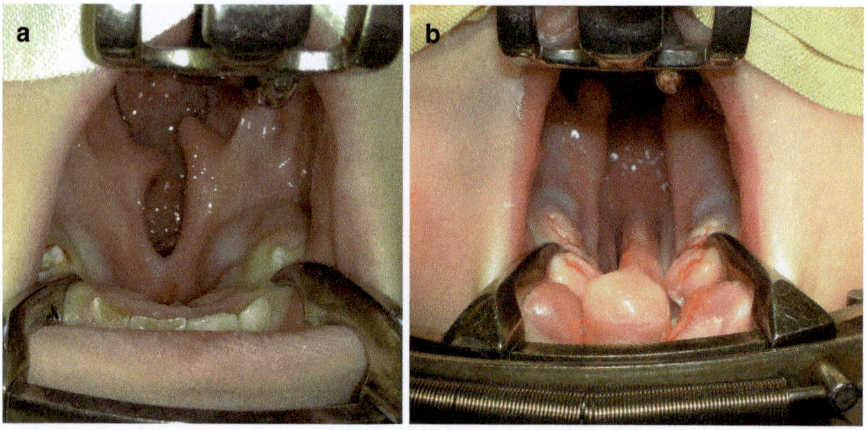

Fig. 7.4 Cleft palate types: (**a**) incomplete cleft palate; (**b**) complete cleft palate

Isolated cleft palate can be unilateral, bilateral, and medial (total or subtotal) (Fig. 7.4a, b) [1, 7, 11]. Pierre Robin sequence includes micrognathia, glossoptosis, and airway obstruction, typically associated with wide U-shaped cleft palate in up

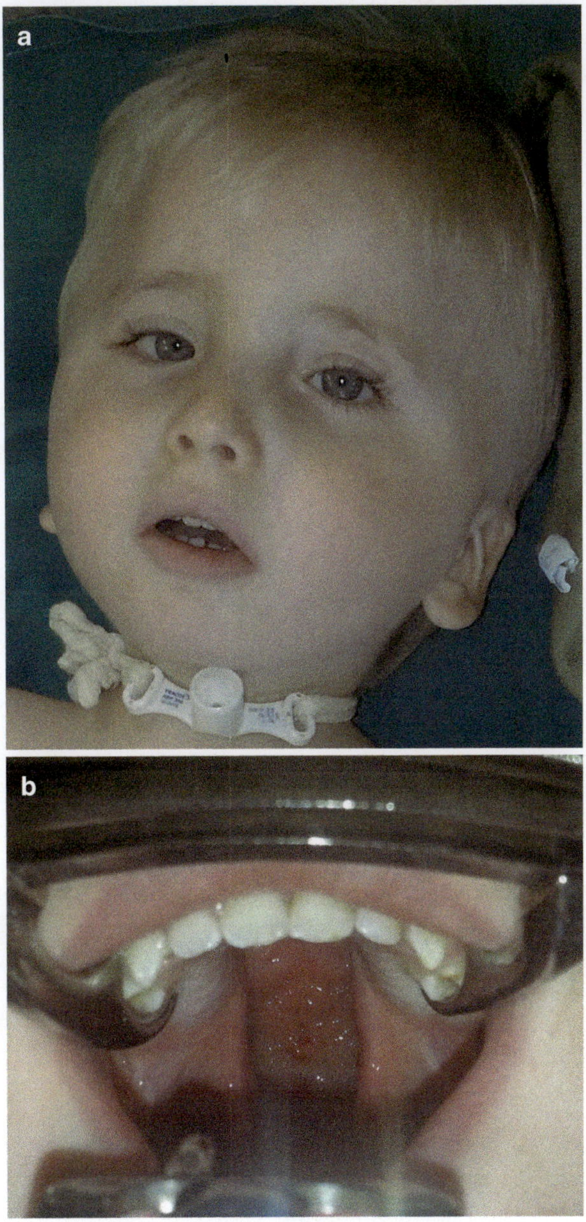

Fig. 7.5 Pierre Robin syndrome: (**a**) tracheostomy performed because of airway problems; (**b**) cleft palate of the same child

to 73–90% of cases (Fig. 7.5) [11, 21]. Patients with submucous cleft palate are in generally asymptomatic, although approximately 15% will develop velopharyngeal insufficiency (VPI) (Fig. 7.6) [1, 6, 11].

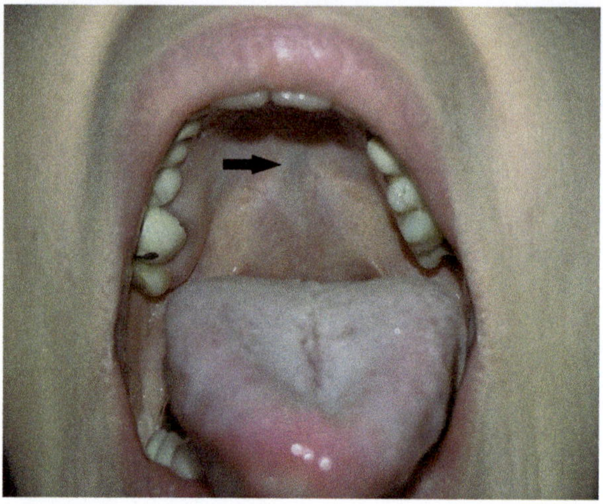

Fig. 7.6 Submucosal cleft palate (zona pellucida)

7.8 Treatment of Cleft Patients

Goals of treatment for patients with clefts include generally: feeding counseling, surgical treatment, hearing and speech evaluation, orthodontic treatment, and additional surgical treatment [1, 8, 11, 13, 18].

7.8.1 Feeding

Most infants with CP are unable to breast feed because they cannot generate intraoral vacuum, and food may reflux into the nasal passage (Fig. 7.7) [7, 8, 11]. There are proper feeding techniques with the upright position (30°–45°) with special devices, bottles, and nipples (with enlarged hole) made to make low resistance to flow [7, 11]. When surgery on palate is performed and the palate is closed, there is no need for special feeding methods [11].

7.8.2 Presurgical Nasoalveolar Molding

Presurgical infant orthopedics (PSIO) is classified as passive which include using of alveolar molding plate (Liu's and Grayson's method) and active (Latham pinned coaxial screw appliance) which requires a surgical procedure to introduce the device and to remove it [1, 6, 7, 10, 13, 16, 22]. Gingivoperiosteoplasty (GPP)

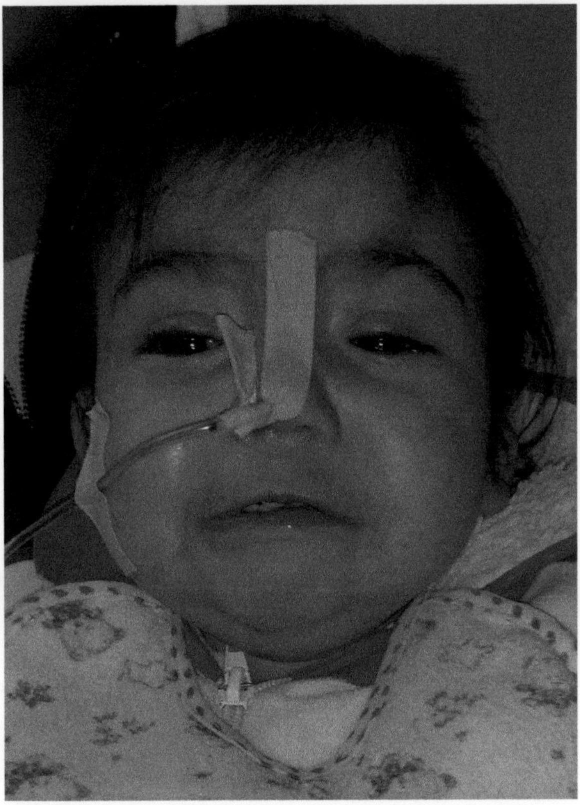

Fig. 7.7 Nasogastric feeding tube left in place by child's mother for 10 months without any visit to a hospital or outpatient clinic (low socioeconomic status)

is a procedure used for correction of the cleft alveolar segments at the time of cleft lip repair [5, 13]. There are concerns about influences of PSIO and GPP on maxillary growth [1, 10, 22]. Lip adhesion can also reduce the gap of alveolar segments by 60% [6, 10, 16, 22].

Objectives of presurgical nasal and alveolar molding (PNAM) are active molding and repositioning of the nasal cartilages and alveolar processes and lengthening of the deficient columella [1, 5, 10, 22]. PNAM is applied both to the patients with unilateral and bilateral clefts in most cases during 6 weeks after birth [1, 22].

The external taping is the simplest technique for presurgical molding used in combination with dental plate (Fig. 7.8a, b) [6]. Restoring the normal anatomy presurgically allows lip repair under less tension [1, 5].

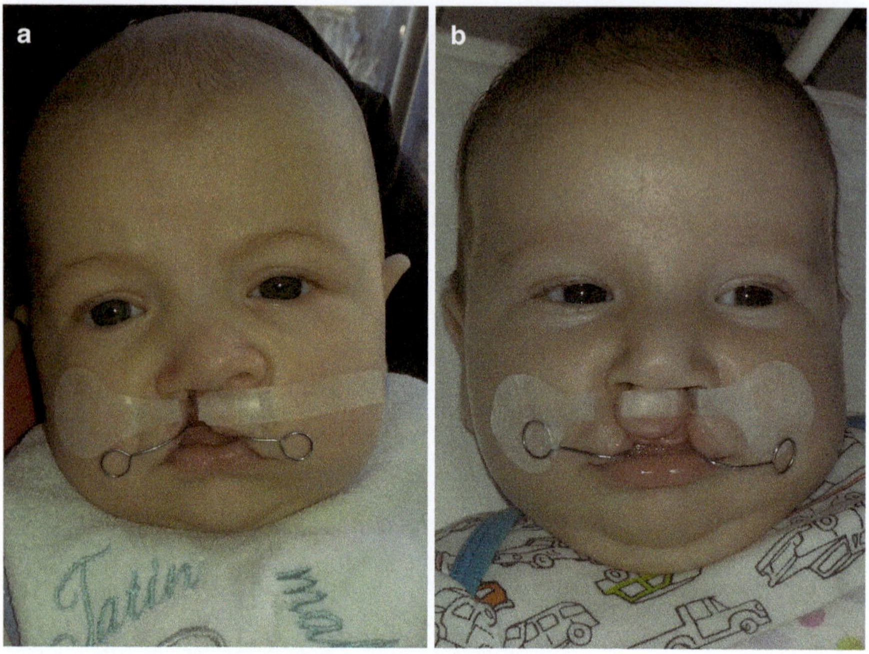

Fig. 7.8 Preoperative nasoalveolar molding (external taping in combination with dental plate): (**a**) unilateral cleft treatment; (**b**) bilateral cleft treatment

7.8.3 Cleft Lip Surgery

7.8.3.1 Primary Unilateral Cleft Lip Repair

Modern repairs of unilateral CL repair have in common the use of a lateral lip flap to fill a medial deficit [1, 6, 10, 13, 16, 23]. Most widely used techniques are those of Tennison and Millard and their modification [23]. Tennison repair employs a back-cut that extends from the Cupid's bow peak to the center of the philtrum that is filled by a lateral triangular flap (Fig. 7.9a–d) [6, 10, 23]. Millard described the concept of advancing a lateral flap into the upper portion of the lip combined with downward rotation of the medial segment (several modification of this technique has been described) (Fig. 7.10a–d) [1, 6, 10, 23]. Noordhoff (Chang Gung), Bardach, Mohler, and Fisher techniques for repair of the CL deformity have been most widely used (Fig. 7.11a–c) [6, 10, 13, 16, 23, 24].

The cleft lip repair is scheduled when the patient is approximately 12 weeks of age, and it is performed in general anesthesia [1, 6, 16]. If the alveolar segments are appropriately aligned and <2 mm apart, GPP can be performed at the time of the surgery (this is not possible if the collapse is present or the gap is too wide) [1, 13]. The goal of any operative technique for unilateral complete CL is to restore normal appearance including lip and nasal deformity [1, 16].

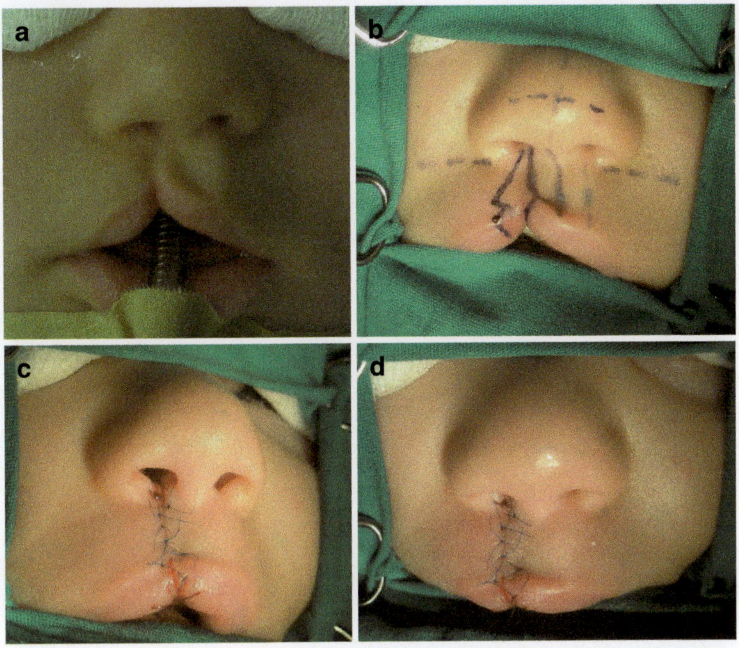

Fig. 7.9 Correction of incomplete unilateral cleft lip (Tennison technique): (**a**) preoperative view; (**b**) intraoperative markings; (**c**) triangular flap creation; (**d**) postoperative result

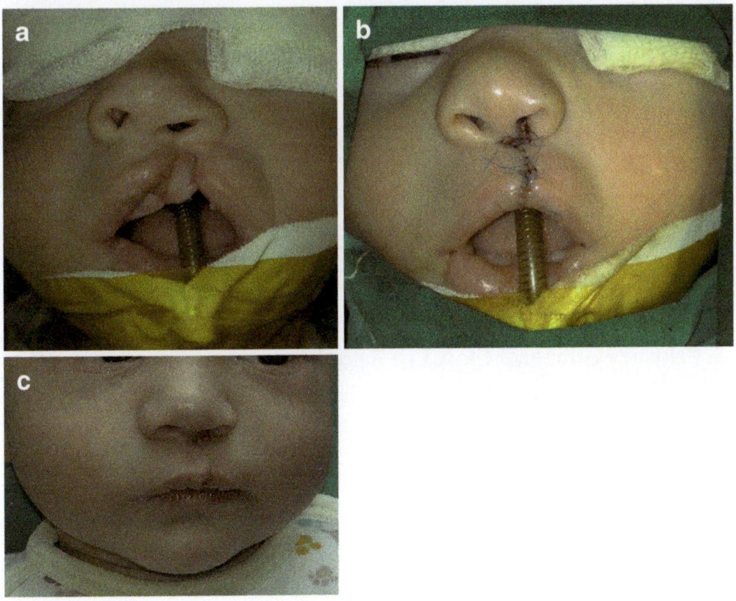

Fig. 7.10 Correction of unilateral cleft lip (Millard technique): (**a**) preoperative view; (**b**) intraoperative view; (**c**) early postoperative result; (**d**) 6 months after surgery

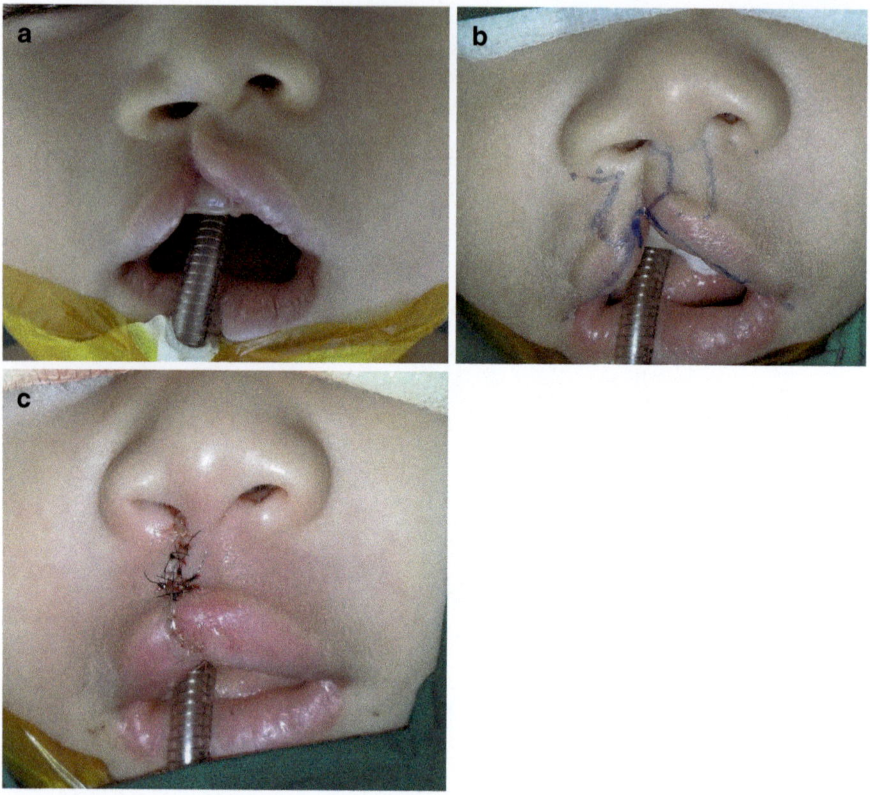

Fig. 7.11 Correction of unilateral cleft lip (Fisher technique): (**a**) preoperative view; (**b**) intraoperative markings; (**c**) postoperative result

7.8.3.2 Microform Cleft Operative Technique

An elliptical excision and a straight-line repair can be performed if the vertical height of the affected side approximates that of the normal side [1, 10, 16, 19]. When the vertical difference exceeds 1–2 mm, rotation-advancement repair is used [1, 19].

7.8.3.3 Primary Bilateral Cleft Lip Repair

Recently, because of positive NAM effects on labial elements, the results of one-stage primary bilateral cleft lip and nose repair are significantly improved [1, 6, 25]. Central lip vermilion is constructed with the vermilion tissue from the lateral lip segments [1, 13, 25].

There are numerous surgical techniques for bilateral cleft lip and nose repair, and most popular are those presented by Mulliken, McComb, Cutting, Trott, and Chen and Noordhoff (Fig. 7.12a–c) [1, 6, 13, 25, 26]. In cases with severe protrusion of premaxilla, two-stage procedure is performed [26] (Fig. 7.13a–c).

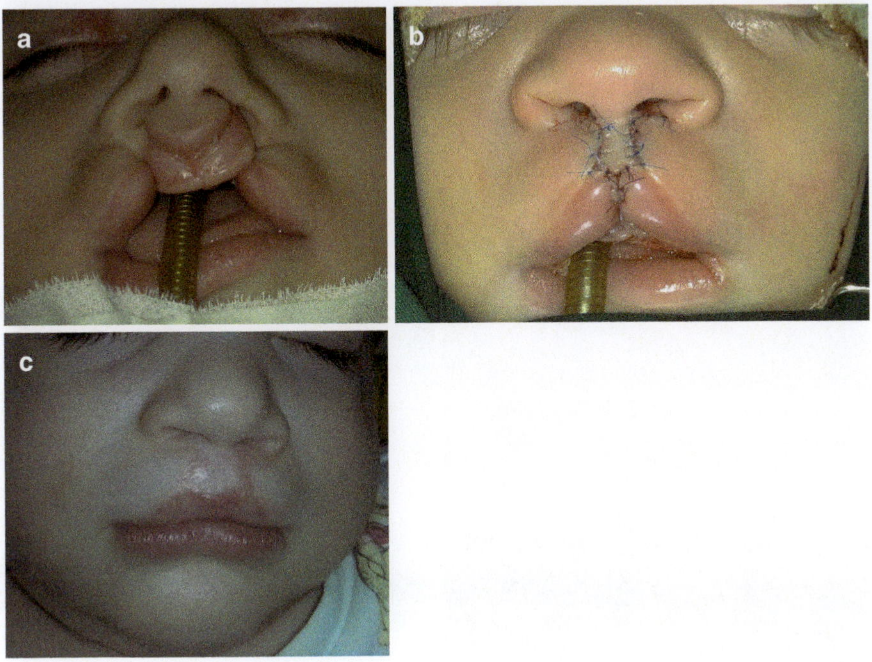

Fig. 7.12 Bilateral cleft lip repair (Mulliken technique): (**a**) preoperative view; (**b**) postoperative result; (**c**) 6 months after surgery

7.8.3.4 Postoperative Care

Postoperatively the airway maintaining is important, and infants are kept in soft arm restraints and feeded at the same postoperative day [1, 6]. Suture line care consists of regular cleansing and treatment with antibiotic ointment [1, 6, 16]. Sutures are removed on the fifth to seventh postoperative day; postsuture removal taping and silicone scar gel can be used along with massage of the lip scar [1, 16].

7.8.3.5 Cleft Palate Repair

The correct time for palatal repair is still unknown [7]. There are currently two common approaches to the timing of cleft palate repair: (a) single-stage repair around the age of 11–12 months and (b) two-stage repair, proposed by Schweckendiek and Doz, with the soft palate repair and veloplasty performed at the time of lip adhesion or primary lip repair (around 4–6 months), and the hard palate repaired at 18–24 months [1, 11, 27]. In children with airway issues (Pierre Robin sequence), the surgery can be delayed until age 14–18 months to allow further mandible growth and to decrease the chance of postoperative airway compromise [11, 21].

Oxford palatoplasty, described by Veau, Wardill, and Kilner with two bilateral mucoperiosteal flaps on major palatine arteries, is widely used (Fig. 7.14a–d) [1, 7, 11, 13]. In case of wide clefts, inferiorly based vomer flaps are used for closing nasal

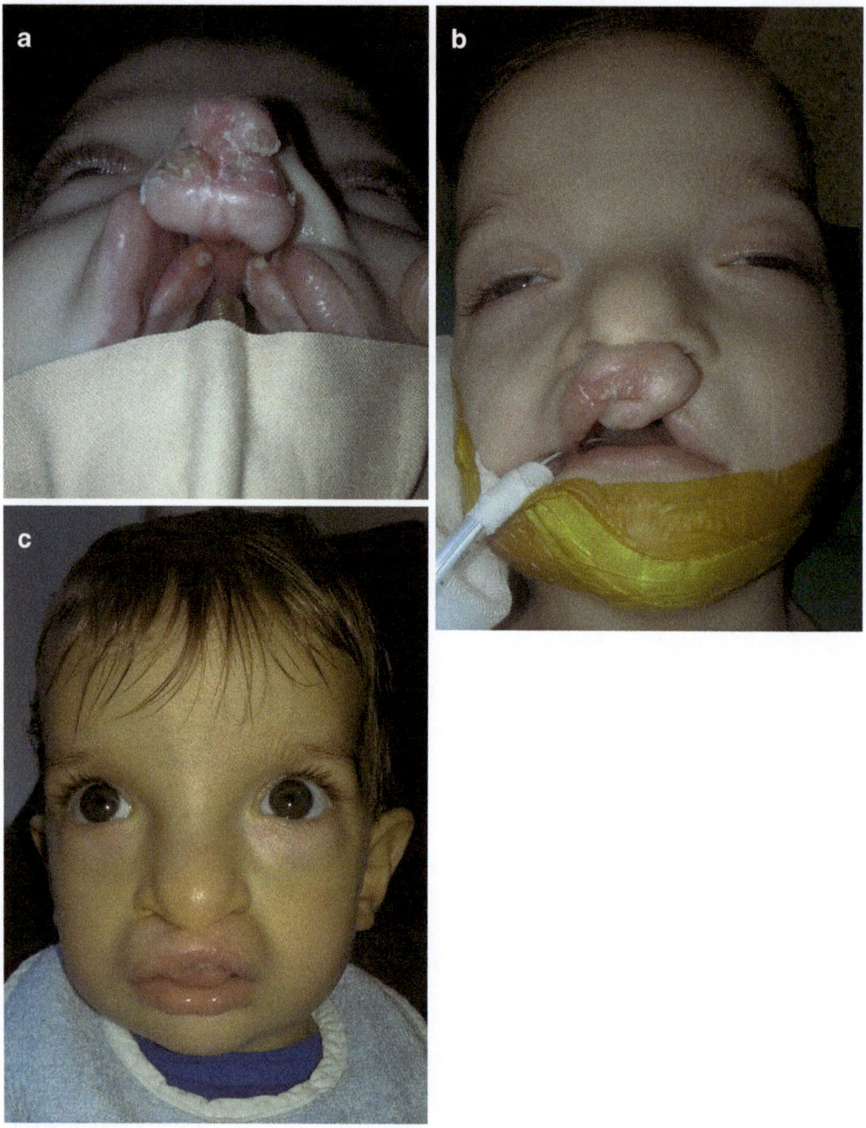

Fig. 7.13 Bilateral cleft lip (two-stage reconstruction): (**a**) preoperative view of bilateral cleft with severe protrusion of premaxilla; (**b**) right side reconstruction; (**c**) bilateral reconstruction completed

mucosa, and intravelar veloplasty encompasses dissection and freeing of muscles from the oral and nasal mucosa and from the posterior edge of the hard palate [11, 13].

Furlow describes his technique of double-opposing Z-palatoplasty on both the oral and the nasal surfaces (Fig. 7.15a, b) [1, 7, 11, 13, 14]. There are also modifications of this technique that are successfully used [28]. It can be used to treat velopharyngeal insufficiency [14, 28].

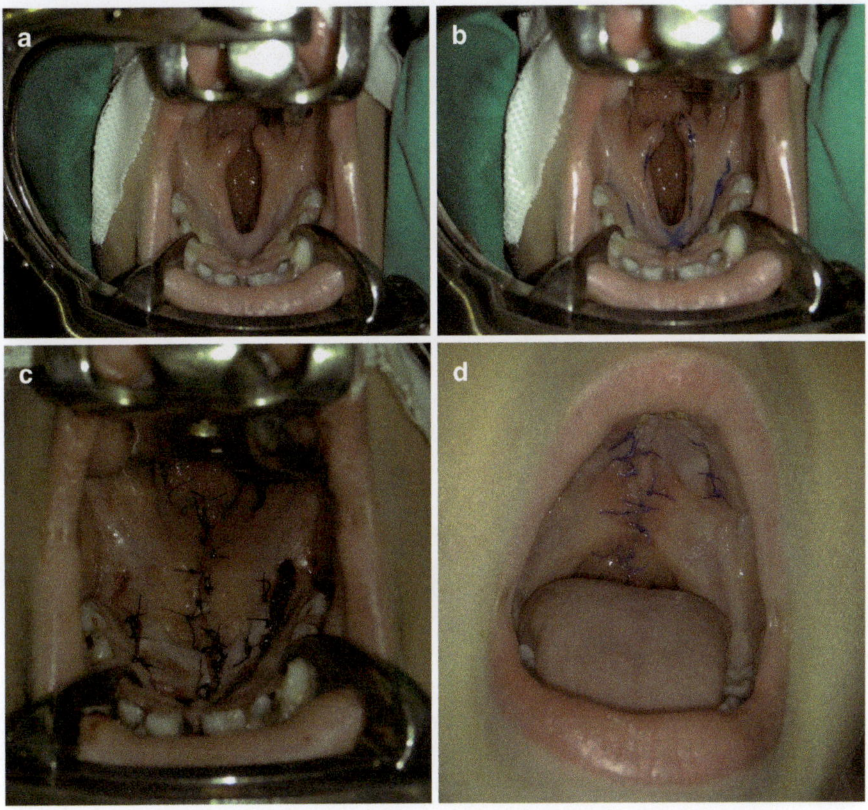

Fig. 7.14 Cleft palate repair by V-Y palatoplasty: (**a**) preoperative view; (**b**) intraoperative markings; (**c**) reconstruction of the cleft with mucoperiosteal flaps; (**d**) postoperative result

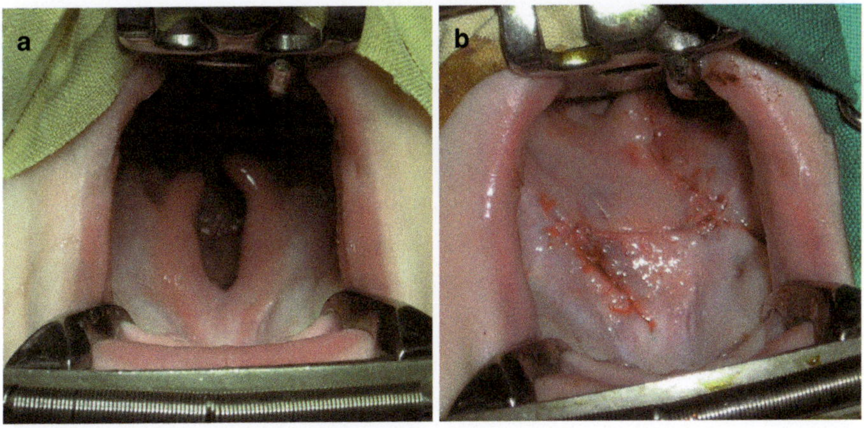

Fig. 7.15 Correction of subtotal cleft palate by Furlow technique: (**a**) preoperative view; (**b**) postoperative result

After the surgery the patient is placed in soft arm restraints [1, 7]. Hemostasis should be controlled, patient should be in a supine position, and liquid feeding may be postponed for 48 h [7, 11]. Liquid is taken for following 10 days and semisolid food for next 3–4 weeks [7, 11, 27].

Most common complications of palatoplasty include hemorrhage, suture line dehiscence, palatal scaring, and oronasal fistula formation [1, 7, 27]. The surgical intervention of cleft palate repair impairs future maxillary growth (there is a higher rate of maxillary hypoplasia following surgery of wider clefts, bilateral clefts, and syndromic patients) [1, 7, 11].

7.8.3.6 Speech, Hearing, and Dental Care

Normal speech is the primary goal of palatoplasty [7, 11]. Abnormal coupling of the nasal and oral cavities results in hypernasality, nasal emission, and imprecise consonant production [1, 29]. The diagnosis and work-up of language difficulties require involvement of the speech pathologist, audiologist, otolaryngologist, psychologist, and pediatrician [1].

Hearing loss is a well-known complication of cleft palate, and there is a 97% incidence of otitis media among the children with clefts younger than 24 months [7, 11, 30, 31]. These patients need ear, nose, and throat (ENT) specialist and audiological surveillance [7, 30].

The pathogenesis of middle ear problems in cleft patients is connected to mechanical, dynamic, infectious, and skeletal factors [30]. Tympanometry (objective test of the middle ear function) is used to test the condition of the middle ear and is classified as type A normal, As, B, and C [31]. Ventilation tube (grommet) insertion may be performed during or after the palatoplasty depending on the condition of the middle ear [30]. Cleft palate closure significantly reduces the prevalence of audiological problems [11, 30]. A child with CL/P should attend dentist (specialist pediatric dentist) regularly, and it is very important to keep the gingiva and teeth healthy because of the orthodontic treatment.

7.8.4 Additional Surgery

There are several surgical procedures that are, if needed, performed from 6 months to puberty: bone grafting, pharyngoplasty, fistuloraphy, rhinoplasty, and Le Fort osteotomies (middle face retraction) [29, 32–41]. It is very important that the indications are clear and to avoid over surgery.

Treatment of the alveolar cleft remains one of the most controversial topics in cleft care with functional and aesthetic significance [1, 18, 33]. Alveolar cleft is associated with variable anomalies in dental development [33]. If the alveolar anatomy and presurgical molding outcome are favorable, a GPP can be performed, and if the infant is not a candidate for GPP, alveolar bone grafting should be performed [1, 18, 33]. According to the age, treatment of alveolar cleft is divided into primary (during primary dentition), secondary (separate operation during mixed

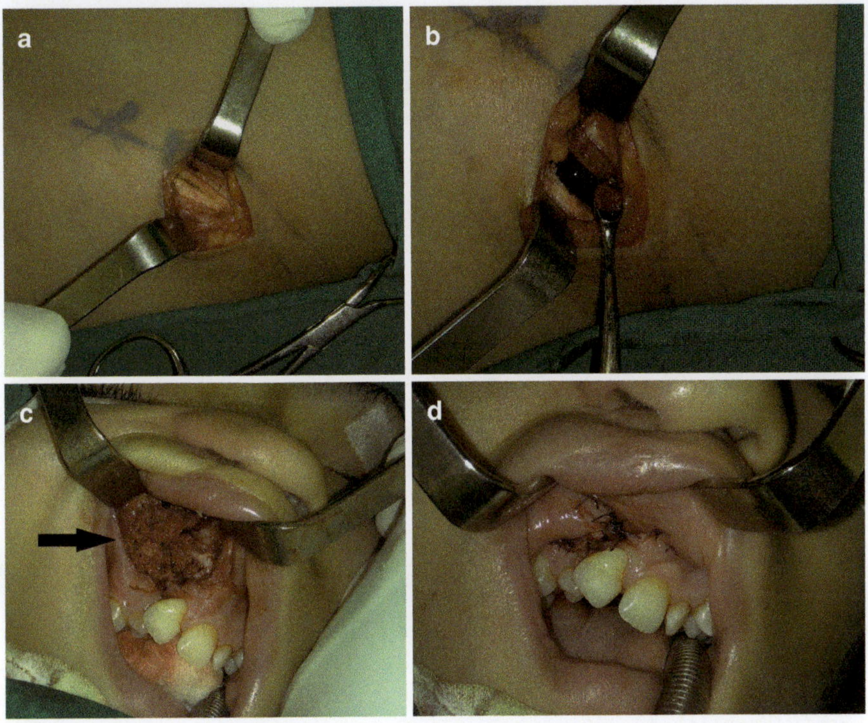

Fig. 7.16 Secondary alveolar bone grafting: (**a**, **b**) harvesting of autogenous cancellous bone from anterior iliac crest; (**c**) alveolar cleft reconstruction with cancellous bone graft; (**d**) postoperative view

dentition with autogenous iliac crest cancellous graft), and late (mostly abandoned) [18, 33, 37]. Secondary bone grafting at the time of mixed dentition remains by far the most common technique for the treatment of the alveolar cleft (Fig. 7.16a–d) [32, 33].

The velopharynx normally separates nasopharynx from the oropharynx [7, 11, 13, 29, 34–36]. Velopharyngeal insufficiency is characterized by hypernasality and nasal air emissions during speech production [29, 35]. Diagnosis of VPI is made by perceptual speech assessment (the presence of hypernasality on vowel production is a hallmark) and by instrumental assessment of VP function performed by nasoendoscopy and multiplanar videofluoroscopy [29, 34–36].

Treatment of VPI includes nonsurgical (speech therapy, prosthetic management with speech bulb, or palatal lift appliances) and surgical approach (palatal, palatopharyngeal, and pharyngeal procedures) [1, 7, 29, 35]. All surgical procedures for the management of VPI seek to reduce cross-sectional area of velopharyngeal port and/or improve the dynamic function of the velopharyngeal valve [29, 35]. Furlow double-opposing Z-palatoplasty is an ideal procedure for selected patient with VPI [14, 35].

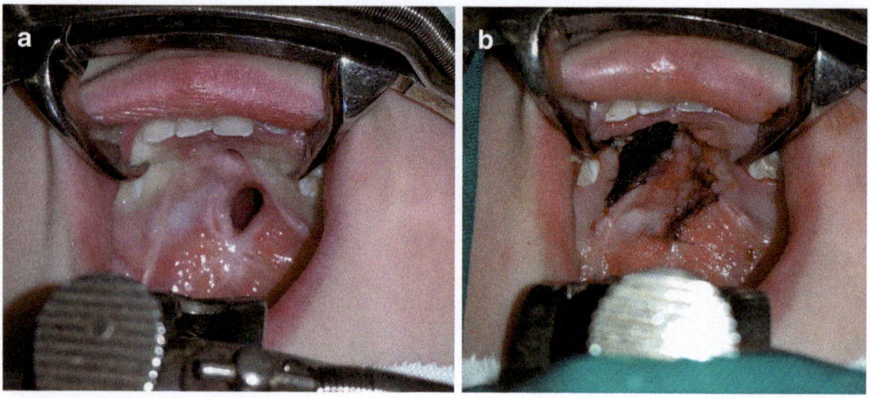

Fig. 7.17 Hard palate fistula reconstruction: (**a**) two fistulous opening at the anterior part of the hard palate; (**b**) two-layer reconstruction with local transposition flap

Palatal fistula occurs as a result of nonrepair cleft or as a result of a breakdown palate, it may occur in any anatomic site of the original cleft, and it may be asymptomatic or symptomatic including speech problems and nasal regurgitation [1, 12, 37–39]. Reconstruction of fistulas is complicated, and it may involve local, palatal, intraoral (buccal, tongue, and pharyngeal flap), and distant (microvascular) flaps (Fig. 7.17a, b) [12, 37–39].

It should be performed in a two-layered fashion with minimal tension and with avoiding of overlapping of oral and nasal suture lines [39]. Recently biomaterials such as acellular dermal to augment palatal fistula repair are used [12].

7.8.5 Secondary Surgery

Secondary deformities mostly depend on the severity of primary defect, effectiveness of orthodontic treatment, and the method of repair (Fig. 7.18a–e) [12, 40].

Lip deformities after unilateral cleft lip repair include short, long, wide, or tight lip, philtral column, and Cupid's bow distortion, and vermilion deformities include thin lip, thick lip, vermilion mismatch, and whistle deformity [6, 12, 40].

The secondary deformities after bilateral cleft lip repair may involve the lip, the nose, and the skeleton (alveolus, premaxilla), but they are recently minimized by using adequate surgical approach [1, 25, 40].

Repair of secondary nasal deformities is a challenge and is still best treated by preventive surgery at the time of the primary repair [1, 25, 40, 41]. The nasal defects are different after unilateral and bilateral cleft lip repair, and prior to the definitive secondary rhinoplasty, the position of the premaxilla must be assessed [1, 12, 40]. Timing of cleft nasal surgery can be divided into primary (at the time of cleft surgery), intermediate (before the patient enters the school), and secondary repairs (when the facial growth is finished) [41].

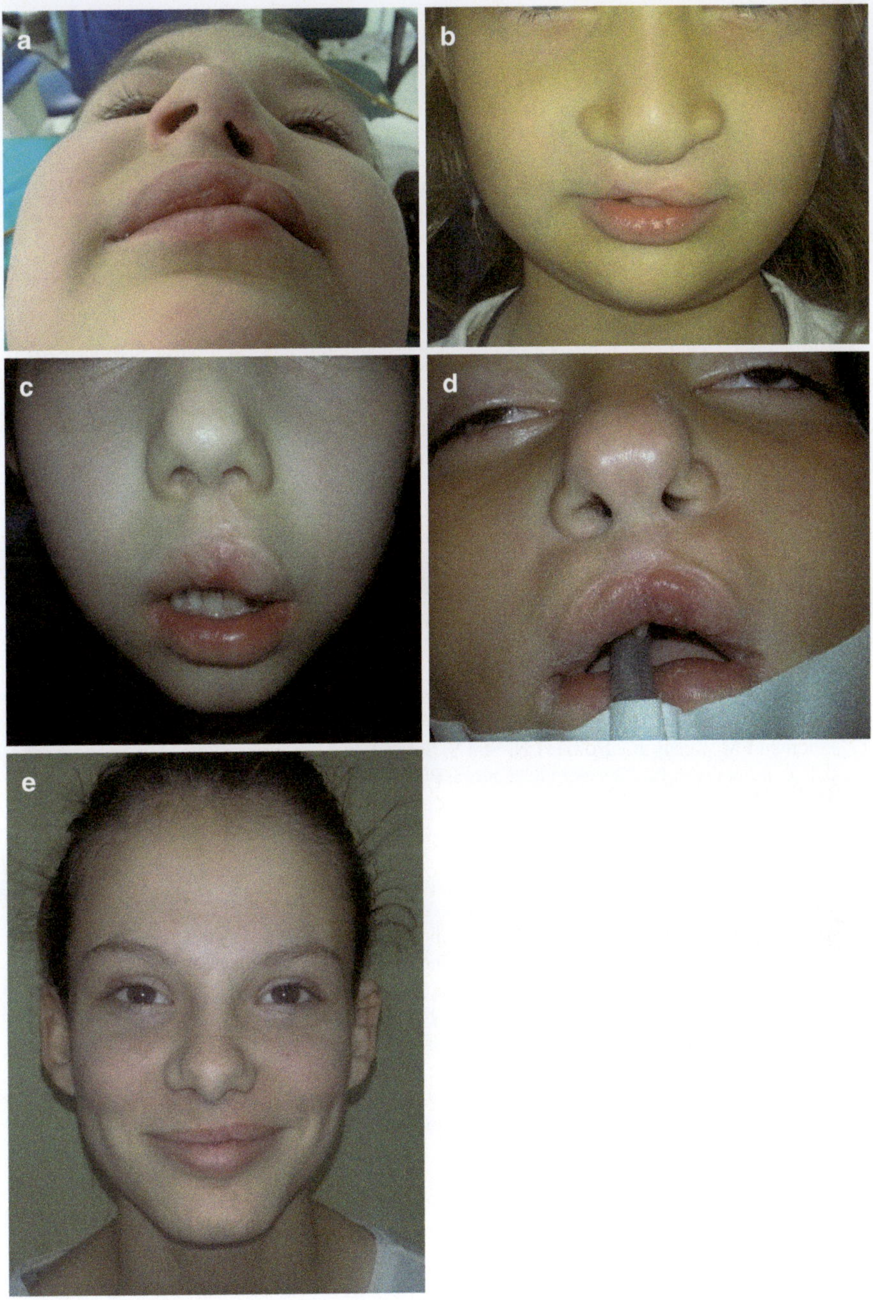

Fig. 7.18 Secondary deformities after cleft lip surgery: (**a**) left side nasal deformity; (**b**) whistle deformity after bilateral cleft lip surgery; (**c**) hypertrophic lateral side of the reconstructed lip; (**d**) wide nasal tip after bilateral cleft lip reconstruction; (**e**) patient with minimal scar after surgery of unilateral cleft lip admitted for otoplasty

References

1. Hopper RA, Cutting C, Grayson B. Cleft lip and palate. In: Thorne CH, Beasley RW, Aston SJ, Bartlett SP, Gurtner GC, Spear SL, editors. Grabb and Smith's plastic surgery. Philadelphia: Lippincott Williams & Wilkins; 2007. p. 201–25.
2. Bernheim N, Georges M, Malevez C, De Mey A, Mansbach A. Embryology and epidemiology of cleft lip and palate. B-ENT. 2006; 2 Suppl 4:11–9.
3. Capone RB, Sykes JM. The cleft and craniofacial team: the whole is greater than the sum of its parts. Facial Plast Surg. 2007;23(2):83–6.
4. Mulliken JB. The changing faces of children with cleft lip and palate. N Engl J Med. 2004;351(8):745–7.
5. Figueroa AA, Polley JW. Orthodontics in cleft lip and palate management. In: Neligen PC, Gurtner GC, editors. Plastic surgery. Principles and practice. St Louis: Elsevier; 2013. p. 595–613e3.
6. Sando WC, Jurkiewicz MJ. Cleft lip. In: Jurkiewicz MJ, Krizek TJ, Mathes SJ, Ariyan S, editors. Plastic surgery. Principles and practice. St Louis: Mosby; 1990. p. 59–79.
7. Sando WC, Jurkiewicz MJ. Cleft palate. In: Jurkiewicz MJ, Krizek TJ, Mathes SJ, Ariyan S, editors. Plastic surgery. Principles and practice. St Louis: Mosby; 1990. p. 81–97.
8. Kasten EF, Schmidt SP, Zickler CF, Berner E, Damian LA, Christian GM, Workman H, et al. Team care of the patient with cleft lip and palate. Curr Probl Pediatr Adolesc Health Care. 2008;38(5):138–58.
9. Senders CW, Peterson EC, Hendrickx AG, Cukierski MA. Development of the upper lip. Arch Facial Plast Surg. 2003;5(1):16–25.
10. Tse R. Unilateral cleft lip: principles and practice of surgical management. Semin Plast Surg. 2012;26(4):145–55.
11. Hoffman WY. Cleft palate In: Neligen PC, Gartner GC, editors. Plastic surgery. Principles and Practice. St Louis Missouri: Elsevier; 2013. p 569-83e4.
12. Feldman EM, Koshy JC, Hollier LH, Stal S. Secondary deformities of the cleft lip, nose, and palate. In: Neligen PC, Gurtner GC, editors. Plastic surgery. Principles and practice. St Louis: Mosby; 2013. p. 630–54e2.
13. Fisher DM, Sommerlad BC. Cleft lip, cleft palate, and velopharyngeal insufficiency. Plast Reconstr Surg. 2011;128(4):342e–60e.
14. Furlow LT. Cleft palate repair by double opposing Z plasty. Op Tech Plast Reconstr Surg. 1995;2(4):223–32.
15. Yu W, Serrano M, Miguel SS, Ruest LB, Svoboda KK. Cleft lip and palate genetics and application in early embryological development. Indian J Plast Surg. 2009;42(Suppl):S35–50.
16. Chen PKT, Noordhoff MS, Kane A. Repair of unilateral cleft lip. In: Neligen PC, Gurtenr GC, editors. Plastic surgery. Principles and practice, vol. 3. St Louis: Elsevier; 2013. p. 517–49e3.
17. Mulliken JB, Benacerraf BR. Prenatal diagnosis of cleft lip: what the sonologist needs to tell the surgeon. J Ultrasound Med. 2001;20(11):1159–64.
18. Robinson JN, McElrath TF, Benson CB, Doubilet PM, Westgate MN, Holmes L, Lieberman ES, Norwitz ER. Prenatal ultrasonography and the diagnosis of fetal cleft lip. J Ultrasound Med. 2001;20(11):1165–70.
19. Yuzuriha S, Mulliken JB. Minor-form, microform, and mini-microform cleft lip: anatomical features, operative techniques, and revisions. Plast Reconstr Surg. 2008;122(5):1485–93.
20. Mulliken JB, Burvin R, Padwa BL. Binderoid complete cleft lip/palate. Plast Reconstr Surg. 2003;111(3):1000–10.
21. Côté A, Fanous A, Almajed A, Lacroix Y. Pierre Robin sequence: review of diagnostic and treatment challenges. Int J Pediatr Otorhinolaryngol. 2015;79(4):451–64.
22. Grayson BH, Shetye PR. Presurgical nasoalveolar moulding treatment in cleft lip and palate patients. Indian J Plast Surg. 2009;42(Suppl):S56–61.
23. Millard Jr RD. Unilateral cleft lip deformity. In: McCarthy JG, May JW, Littler JW, editors. Plastic surgery. Philadelphia: W.B. Saunders Company; 1990. p. 2627–52.

24. Demke JC, Tatum SA. Analysis and evolution of rotation principles in unilateral cleft lip repair. J Plast Reconstr Aesthet Surg. 2011;64(3):313–8.
25. Mulliken JB. Repair of bilateral cleft lip. In: Neligen PC, Gurtner GC, editors. Plastic surgery. Principles and practice. St Louis: Elsevier; 2013. p. 550–68e3.
26. Cronin TD, Cronin ED, Roper P, Millard Jr RD, McComb H. Bilateral clefts. In: McCarthy JG, May JW, Littler JW, editors. Plastic surgery. Philadelphia: W.B. Saunders Company; 1990. p. 2653–722.
27. Randal P, LaRossa D. Cleft palate. In: McCarthy JG, May JW, Littler JW, editors. Plastic surgery. Philadelphia: W.B. Saunders Company; 1990. p. 2723–52.
28. Jackson OH, Stransky CA, Jawad AF, Basta M, Solot CB, et al. The Children's Hospital of Philadelphia modification of the Furlow double-opposing Z-palatoplasty: 30-year experience and long-term speech outcomes. Plast Reconstr Surg. 2013;132(3):613–22.
29. Sie KC, Chen EY. Management of velopharyngeal insufficiency: development of a protocol and modifications of sphincter pharyngoplasty. Facial Plast Surg. 2007;23(2):128–39.
30. Sharma RK, Nanda V. Problems of middle ear and hearing in cleft children. Indian J Plast Surg. 2009;42(Suppl):S144–8.
31. Narayanan DS, Pandian SS, Murugesan S, Kumar R. The incidence of secretory otitis media in cases of cleft palate. J Clin Diagn Res. 2013;7(7):1383–6.
32. Coots BK. Alveolar bone grafting: past, present, and new horizons. Semin Plast Surg. 2012;26(4):178–83.
33. Hopper RA. Alveolar clefts. In: Neligen PC, Gurtner GC, editors. Plastic surgery. Principles and practice, vol. 3. St Louis: Elsevier; 2013. p. 584–613e3.
34. Skirko JR, Weaver EM, Perkins JA, Kinter S, Eblen L, Martina J, Sie KC. Change in quality of life with velopharyngeal insufficiency surgery. Otolaryngol Head Neck Surg. 2015;153(5):857–64.
35. Kirschner RE, Baylis AL. Velopharyngeal dysfunction. In: Neligen PC, Gurtner GC, editors. Plastic surgery. Principles and practice. St Louis: Elsevier; 2013. p. 615–630e4.
36. David D, Bagnall AD. Velopharyngeal incompetence. In: McCarthy JG, May JW, Littler JW, editors. Plastic surgery. Philadelphia: W.B. Saunders Company; 1990. p. 2903–21.
37. Honnebier MB, Johnson DS, Parsa AA, Dorian A, Parsa FD. Closure of palatal fistula with a local mucoperiosteal flap lined with buccal mucosal graft. Cleft Palate Craniofac J. 2000;37(2):127–9.
38. Murthy J. Descriptive study of management of palatal fistula in one hundred and ninety-four cleft individuals. Indian J Plast Surg. 2011;44(1):41–6.
39. Lehman JA. Closure of palatal fistulas. Oper Tech Plast Reconstr Surg. 1995;2(4):255–62.
40. Jackson IT, Fasching MC. Secondary deformities of cleft lip, nose and cleft palate. In: McCarthy JG, May JW, Littler JW, editors. Plastic surgery. Philadelphia: W.B. Saunders Company; 1990. p. 2772–877.
41. Kaufman Y, Buchanan EP, Wolfswinkel EM, Weathers WM, Stal S. Cleft nasal deformity and rhinoplasty. Semin Plast Surg. 2012;26(4):184–90.

Polydactyly

8

8.1 Introduction

Congenital anomalies of the upper extremity vary from a barely noticeable to an absent extremity [1–3]. They are noted in approximately 2 per 1000 live births, with boys affected more commonly than girls (3:2) [2]. The diagnosis is in most cases made by physical and radiological exam, and vascular studies are rarely indicated [1–3]. Patients with hand anomalies can have associated malformations, most often involving the heart, kidneys, or tracheoesophageal complex [2]. Treatment of patients with congenital hand anomalies is multidisciplinary with the primary surgical goals to improve hand function and aesthetic appearance [2, 3].

8.2 Embryology

Around 4 weeks after fertilization, the upper limb bud appears as an oblong ventrolateral bulge on the body wall [1–6]. The emerging limb bud is composed of somatic lateral plate mesoderm covered by the ectoderm [2, 4]. Subsequent limb bud growth and differentiation are controlled by distinctive region-signaling centers: apical ectodermal ridge (AER) (proximodistal growth), Wnt (Wingless type) (dorsoventral growth), and zone of polarizing activity (ZPA) (anteroposterior-radioulnar growth) [1, 3–5]. Signaling pathways critical to limb formation include several other factors such as Sonic Hedgehog (Shh) protein and fibroblast growth factors (FGF) [2, 5, 7, 8]. Digits are recognizable at 41–43 days and fully separate at 53 days of gestation [5].

A.M. Vlahovic, E.Q. Haxhija, *Pediatric and Adolescent Plastic Surgery for the Clinician*, DOI 10.1007/978-3-319-56004-5_8

8.3 Classification

Oberg and colleagues proposed a modified Swanson classification of hand anomalies, and by this classification all hand anomalies are placed within one of three groups: *malformations* (abnormal cell formation), *deformations* (insult to cells which have formed normally), and *dysplasias* (lack of normal cell organization) [2, 3, 8].

1. *Malformations*
   (a) Failure in axis formation and differentiation—entire upper limb
   - Proximal-distal outgrowth (symbrachydactyly, transverse deficiency, intersegmental deficiency)
   - Radial-ulnar (anteroposterior) axis (radial longitudinal deficiency, ulnar longitudinal deficiency, ulnar dimelia, radioulnar synostosis, humeroradial synostosis)
   - Dorsal-ventral axis (nail-patella syndrome)

   (b) Failure in axis formation and differentiation—hand plate
   - Radial-ulnar (anteroposterior) axis (radial polydactyly, triphalangeal thumb, ulnar polydactyly)
   - Dorsal-ventral axis (dorsal dimelia, hypoplastic/aplastic nail)

   (c) Failure in hand plate formation and differentiation—unspecified axis
   - Soft tissue (syndactyly, camptodactyly, trigger digits)
   - Skeletal deficiency (brachydactyly, clinodactyly, Kirner's deformity, metacarpal and carpal synostosis)
   - Complex (cleft hand, synpolydactyly, Apert's hand)
2. *Deformations* (constriction ring syndrome)
3. *Dysplasias* (macrodactyly, limb hypertrophy, tumorous condition)

8.4 Polydactyly

Polydactyly is the presence of extra digits or duplication of digital parts [1, 2, 4–6, 9–11]. The pathogenesis of polydactyly is not known [11, 12]. It is easily detected, most frequently observed congenital hand anomaly that causes cosmetic and functional impairment ranging from minor cutaneous protuberance to complete duplication of a limb [1, 5, 10, 11, 13]. Polydactyly can be detected by ultrasound (US) as early as 14 weeks of gestational age [9].

The true incidence of polydactyly is not known, it depends on the studied population, and it varies from 0.3–3.6/1000 and 1.6–10.7/1000 in general population [7, 9, 10]. The incidence of radial polydactyly varies from 0.08:1000 to 1.4:1000 live births, and it represents 90% of all polydactyly cases [1, 2, 5, 8]. Polydactyly affects Blacks more commonly than Whites [2, 9, 13]. Upper limbs are more involved than lower limbs and right hand more than the left [9]. Preaxial polydactyly is the most common (mostly isolated), followed by postaxial (mostly syndromic and bilateral), and meso-axial (central) [7, 10]. Polydactyly has been associated with more than 300 diseases and syndromes (patient with atypical presentation (syndromes) should be referred to genetics) [7, 9, 10].

8.4.1 Classification

Classification of polydactyly proposed by Temtamy-McKusick as *preaxial polydactyly*, *postaxial polydactyly*, *complex polydactyly*, *central polydactyly*, and *mixed polydactyly* (syndromic or nonsyndromic) is most widely used (Figs. 8.1a–c, 8.2a, b, and 8.3) [5, 7, 9–12].

There are also several classification systems of radial, central, and postaxial polydactyly: Wassel-Flatt classification of thumb duplication, Wood and Miura modification of Wassel-Flatt classification, Stelling and Turek classification of central polydactyly, and Ryan classification of postaxial polydactyly [2, 5, 9, 10, 12].

Wassel-Flatt classification of radial polydactyly is based on the radiological findings, including seven types of splitting of the thumb at different levels [1, 3, 5, 7, 9, 14]. Recently, the classification of thumb polydactyly is named Flatt classification (Harry Wassel was a hand surgery fellow of Adrian Flatt) [4]. Wassel-Flatt types of thumb duplication include type I (distal phalanx), type II (interphalangeal joint, IPJ),

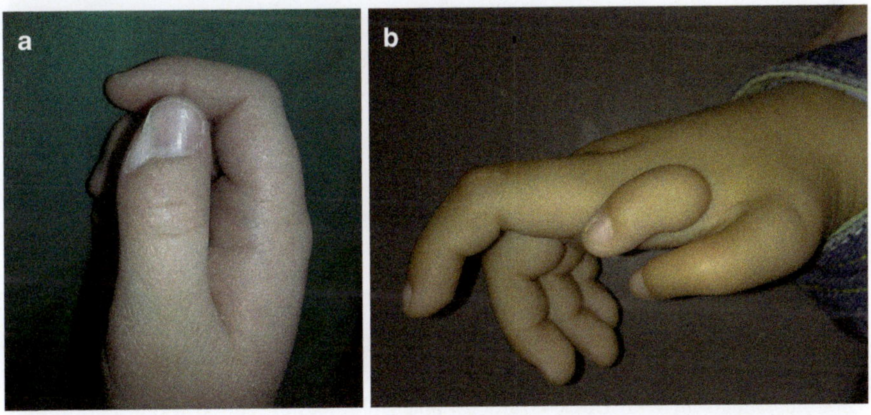

Fig. 8.1 Preaxial polydactyly: (**a**) barely noticeable deformity; (**b**) complex radial polydactyly including floating thumb and hypoplastic thumb

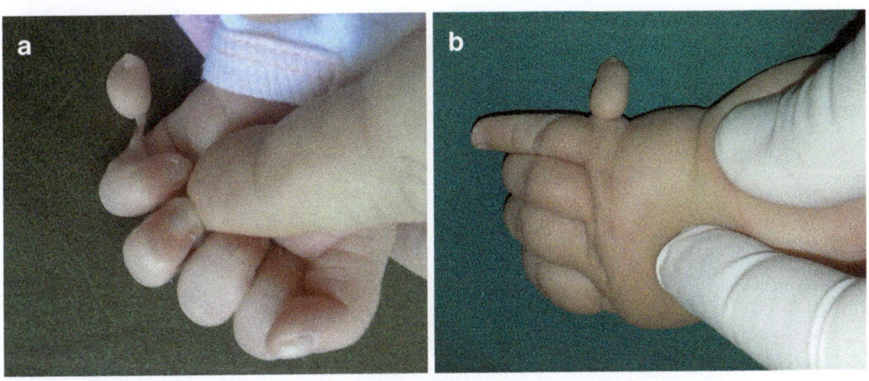

Fig. 8.2 Postaxial polydactyly: (**a**) rudimentary digit; (**b**) fully developed digit

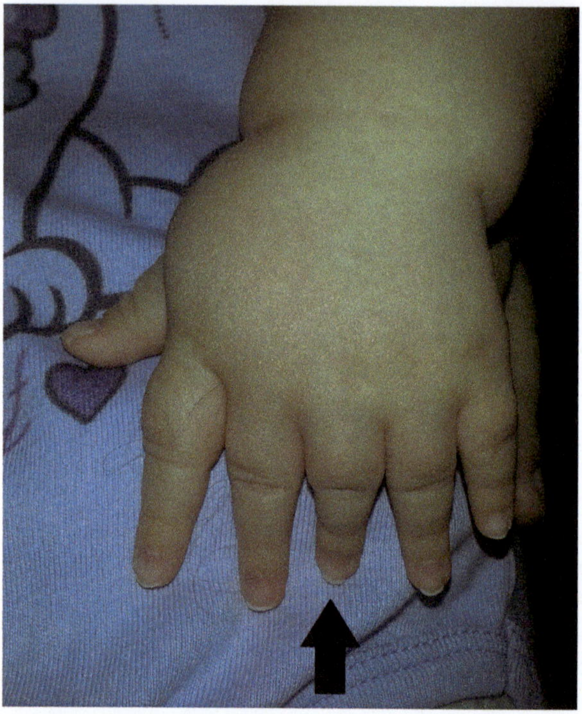

Fig. 8.3 Central polydactyly

type III (proximal phalanx), type IV (metacarpophalangeal joint, MCPJ), type V (metacarpal, MC), type VI (carpometacarpal joint, CMCJ), and type VII (at least on thumb is triphalangeal) [5, 7, 8, 11].

Wood and Miura presented a modification of Wassel-Flatt classification dividing type IV thumbs into three subtypes and type VII into four subtypes [5, 8]. Zuidam et al. proposed the Rotterdam classification system in 2008 that includes Wassel-Flatt classification, with Buck-Gramcko and Behrens intercarpal modification and suffixes to indicate different complex deformities (Tph, triphalangism; T, triplication; S, symphalangism; D, duplication; H, hypoplasia) [4, 8].

8.4.2 Patient Evaluation

A thorough medical history and general physical examination has to be obtain, and both upper limbs have to be examined from proximal to distal [3, 7].

8.4.3 Treatment Option

Surgical treatment of polydactyly seeks to remove the least functional component, to reconstruct normal parts, and to allow normal hand function [2, 3, 5, 9, 11]. Anatomic level of duplication, musculoskeletal components involved, stability, developmental stage, and cosmetic outcome have to be considered carefully [1, 2, 5,

7, 9, 11–16]. Floating little fingers with narrow soft tissue stalk <2 mm can be removed early in the newborn nursery by ligation, and simple excision is possible when there is no bone connection and joints are stable [3, 5, 9]. Surgical treatment ideally occurs before the supernumerary elements displace the normal elements and before fine motor skills have developed with the abnormal anatomy (from 6 to 9 months of life, at the end of the first year of life, or during second year of life) [5, 9, 11, 14]. Radiological examination is usually adequate in obtaining additional preoperative information [3].

8.4.3.1 Radial Polydactyly

Regarding radial polydactyly, Wassel-Flatt type II and type IV are the most frequent [1, 7, 8, 14]. In Wassel-Flatt type II, there is a broad proximal phalanx with two (partial) distal phalanges [2, 7, 8]. If there is an unequal duplication, the smaller thumb has to be excised along with the part of articular surface of the proximal phalanx, preserving the collateral ligament [2, 5, 7]. If necessary, tendon augmentation with smaller finger tendons is performed [6]. In case of symmetrical duplication, Bilhaut-Cloquet procedure is performed [5, 9, 14–16].

In Wassel-Flatt type IV, there is often a hypoplastic extra thumb on the radial side [1, 5, 7, 9]. The radial thumb has to be excised similar to the technique for Wassel type II, and the broad MC is partially excised in distal part (with asymmetric tendons realigned in the "ulnar" thumb) (Fig. 8.4a–c) [5, 7, 9]. Deviation at the IPJ should be corrected with a transverse wedge osteotomy [2, 7, 9].

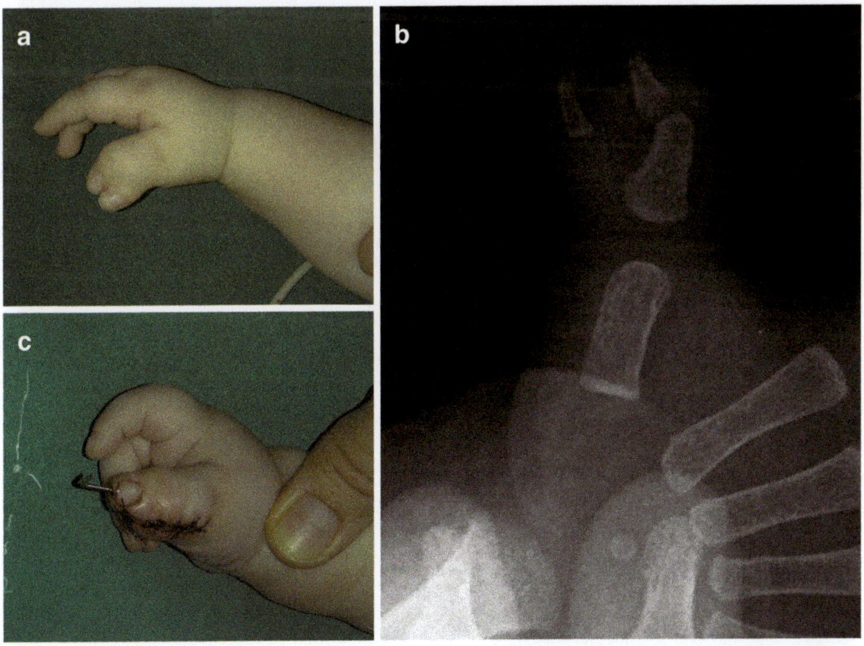

Fig. 8.4 Reconstruction of thumb duplication by excision of the radial part of the thumb: (**a**) preoperative view; (**b**) radiography of the thumb; (**c**) postoperative view

When there is minimal size mismatch between the two thumbs (Wassel-Flatt type I, II, III and occasionally IV), the two outer halves can be joined after excising the two inner halves longitudinally, in the Bilhaut-Cloquet operation (Fig. 8.5a–c)

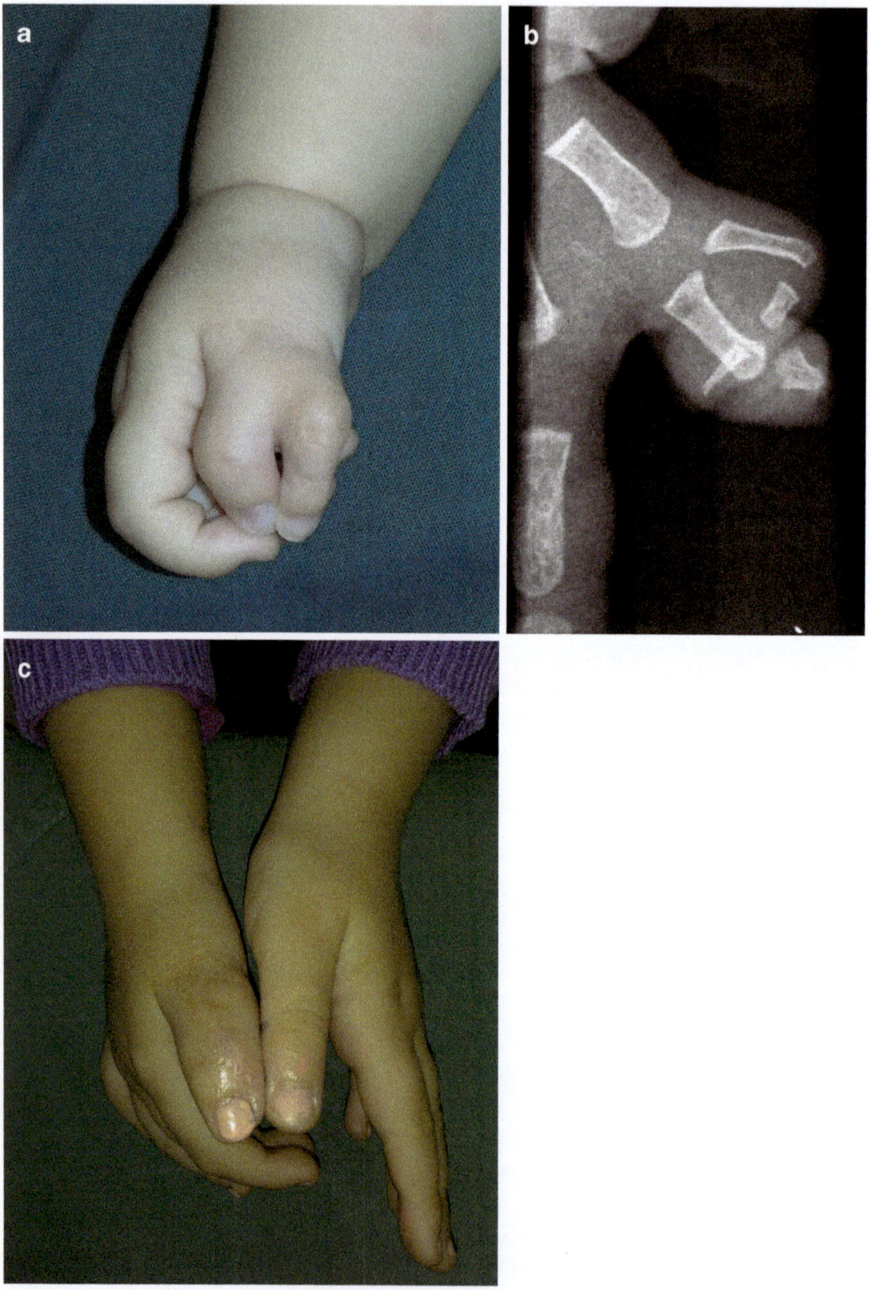

Fig. 8.5 Reconstruction of the thumb duplication (Bilhaut-Cloquet procedure): (**a**) preoperative finding; (**b**) radiography of the thumb; (**c**) postoperative view

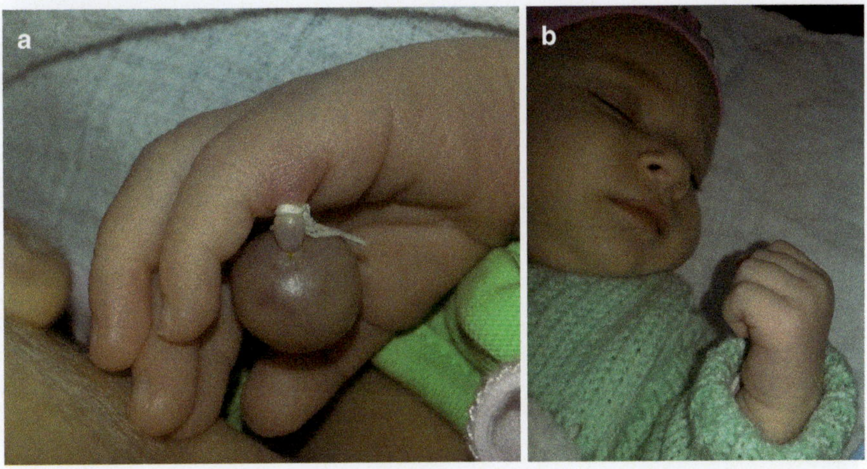

Fig. 8.6 Postaxial polydactyly: (**a**) unsuccessful ligature of the postaxial polydactylous finger performed by pediatrician; (**b**) result after excision was performed

[2, 5, 11, 14, 16]. This procedure can be complicated by joint stiffness, growth arrest, asymmetric growth, and longitudinal nail bed deformities (this can be avoided by Baek modification) [2, 11, 16].

8.4.3.2 Postaxial Polydactyly

Postaxial polydactyly includes duplication of small finger of the hand [2, 5]. It has high incidence in African and African-American population [1, 5, 6]. There are two most common used classifications of postaxial syndactyly proposed by Stelling Turek and Temtamy-McKusick [1, 2, 5, 7]. According to Stelling and Turek classification, there are three types of postaxial polydactyly (type I soft tissue, type II partial duplication, and type III complete duplication), and according to Temtamy-McKusick, there are two types of postaxial polydactyly (A, fully developed finger; B, a rudimentary digit) [1, 2, 5, 9, 10]. Postaxial type B digits with narrow stalk can be ligated (revisions may be necessary later in life) (Fig. 8.6a, b) [2, 5, 7, 9]. For more developed extra little finger, surgical excision is recommended [1, 5, 7]. Postaxial type A digits are excised through large ulnar-sided flap with zigzag incisions, spearing ulnar collateral ligament, and with trimming of articular surface of the MC [2, 5].

8.4.3.3 Central Polydactyly

Central polydactyly is duplication of nonborder digits, and it is less prevalent than radial or ulnar polydactyly [1, 5, 7, 12]. Stelling and Turek proposed classification of central polydactyly into three types: *type I* with an extra soft tissue mass, *type II* that includes duplication of digit or part of the digit with normal components and bifid MC or phalanx, and *type III* presenting complete digit with its own MC [5, 12]. Tada et al. divided type II into type IIA with syndactyly and type IIB without syndactyly [5]. Involved fingers are insufficient or hypoplastic, and the joints are stiff (fully developed extra independent digits are rare) [5, 7]. Surgical treatment is complicated, and good results are difficult to achieve (Fig. 8.7a–e) [1, 5, 7]. Mirror hand

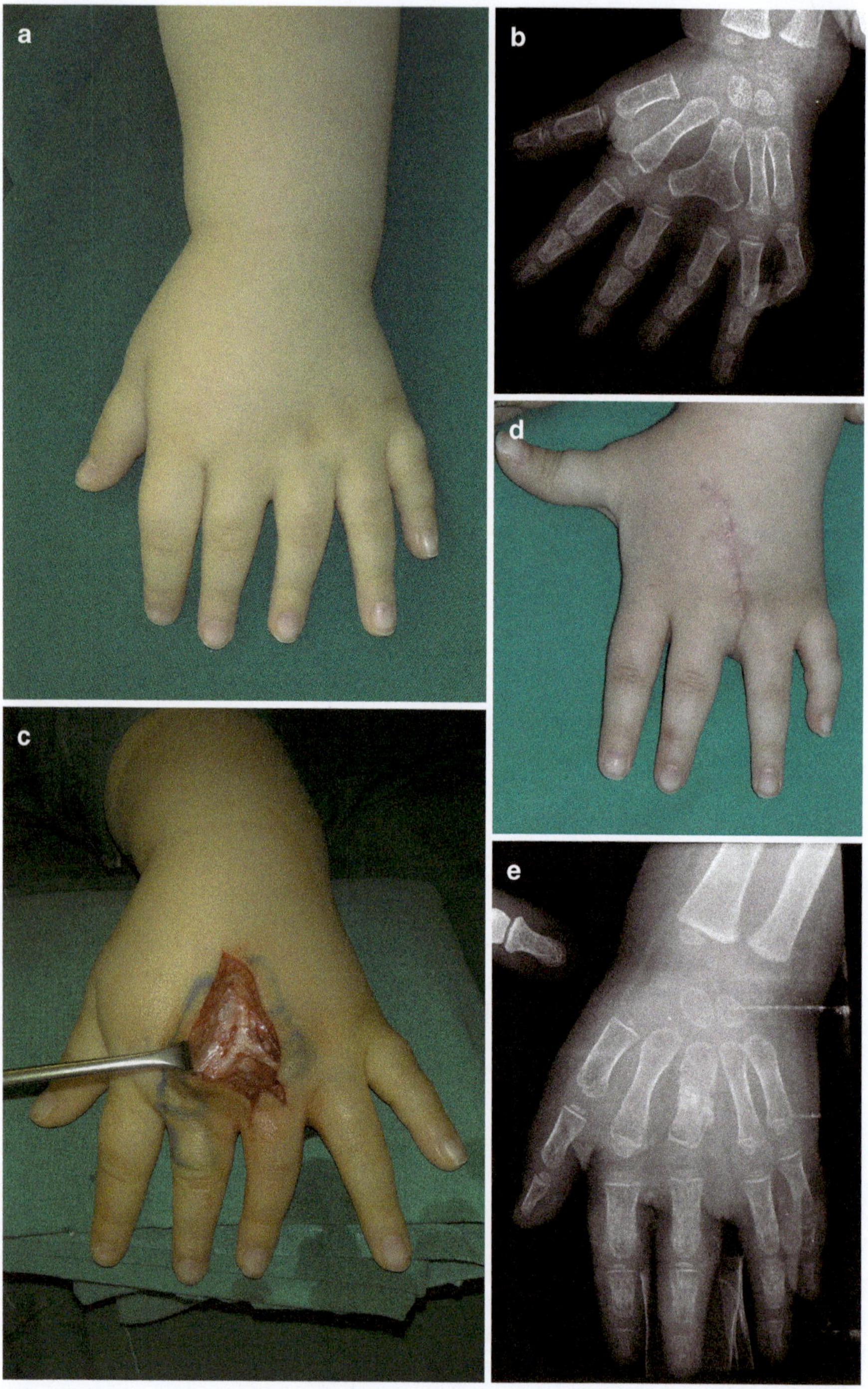

Fig. 8.7 Reconstruction of central polydactyly: (**a**) preoperative view; (**b**) preoperative radiography; (**c**) bifid III metacarpal bone and extensor tendons; (**d**) postoperative view; (**e**) postoperative radiography

is a very rare condition that requires hand reconstruction, making a thumb of the best finger and creating a sufficient first web [7].

8.4.3.4 Postoperative Care

In the simple polydactyly, a bandage is given as in regular wound care [7]. Cast or splint treatment is indicated when complex reconstruction is performed, and after splint removing, hand exercises are seldom necessary [2, 7]. In polydactyly, a reoperation rate of up to 25% has been reported, and in some cases definitive outcome can only be assessed after growth has been completed [7, 9]. Secondary procedures include procedures on ligaments, tendons, bones, nail deformity correction, and scar revision [7, 9].

8.5 Symphalangism (Synostosis)

This is a union of a two or more adjacent bones, and it can be classified as true symphalangism with normal length of digits, symbrachydactyly, and symphalangism with other anomalies (Poland's syndrome, Apert's syndrome) [6, 7]. In upper extremity, it can involve bones from distal phalanx to radius and ulna, but in most cases proximal IPJ is involved [7, 8]. If function is normal, there is no indication for surgery and the treatment is conservative [1, 7]. Surgical treatment depends of the type of the fusion [6, 7].

8.6 Triphalangeal Thumb

The extra middle phalange is constant finding in triphalangeal thumb (TPT), the incidence of TPT is 1:25,000 live births, and there is family history of thumb anomalies in two thirds of patients (Fig.8.8a–c) [7]. Surgical treatment includes excision of delta type extra phalanx and ligament reconstruction, different types of osteotomies, soft tissue reconstruction, and pollicization for five-fingered hand [7, 11].

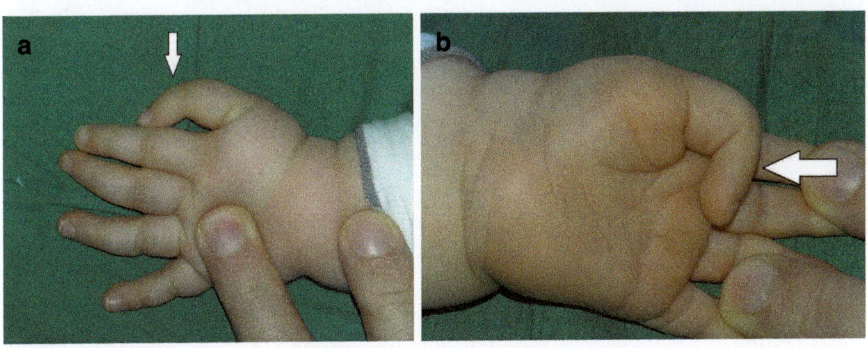

Fig. 8.8 Triphalangeal thumb: (**a**) clinical dorsal view; (**b**) clinical palmar view; (**c**) radiography of both thumbs revealing anomaly of the left thumb

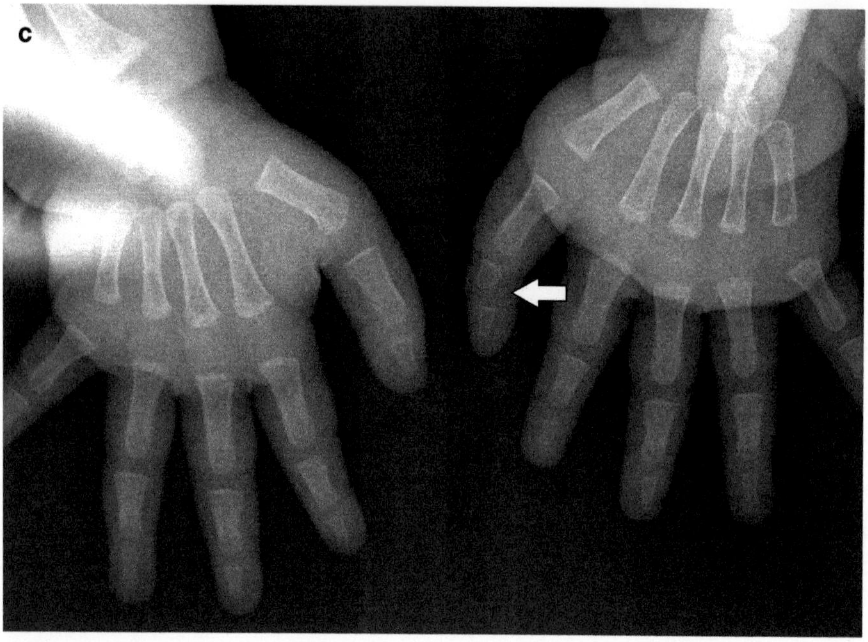

Fig. 8.8 (continued)

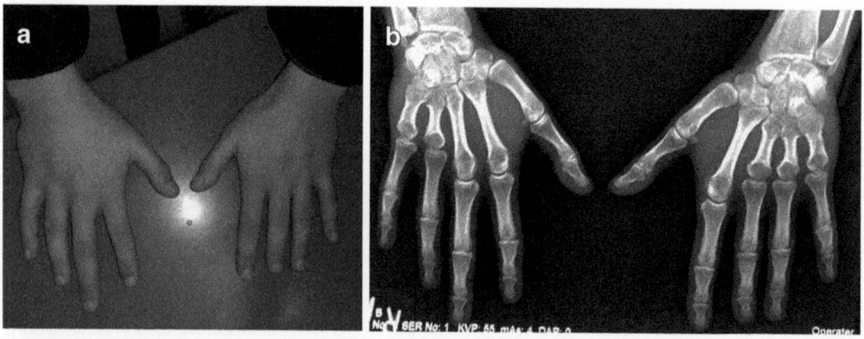

Fig. 8.9 Bilateral brachydactyly (short metacarpal bones): (**a**) clinical view of both hands; (**b**) radiography revealed bilaterally short metacarpal bones

8.7 Brachydactyly

Brachydactyly includes shortening of the digits due to abnormal development of phalanges, metacarpals, or both, and it can occur as isolated malformation or as a part of complex malformation syndrome (Fig. 8.9a, b) [8, 17, 18]. There are several classification of brachydactyly based on anatomic ground [17, 18]. Surgery is rarely indicated for minor deformities, and when it is indicated, surgery includes ligament reconstruction, osteotomies, bone distracting, removing of delta phalanx, syndactyly release, and bone transplantation [17, 18].

8.8 Kirner's Deformity

Kirner first described this deformity in 1927 [18–20]. It presents radial and volar bowing of the distal phalanx (usually little finger) [19, 20]. The exact etiology is not known (suspected cartilaginous extension of the physis, L-shaped physis) [18, 19]. Diagnosis is made by clinical and radiologic evaluation [15, 21]. Treatment depends on the degree of deformity [19].

8.9 Clinodactyly

Clinodactyly is defined as angular deformity of the digit in the coronal plane (Fig. 8.10a–c) [1, 6–8, 22, 23]. It may be isolated or may be associated with the other congenital malformations (over 60 syndromes) [1, 6, 7, 23]. The angle of deviation defining clinodactyly varies from 8° to 15° (more than 20° according to some authors) [7, 23]. Clinodactyly occurs because of aberrant growth plates mostly in middle phalanx, and the most common clinical form is radial deviation of middle phalanx of the little finger [1, 7]. It is more aesthetic than functional problem, but in case of functional impairment and large angulation, surgical treatment should be performed [6, 22]. There are several treatment options such as opening or closing or

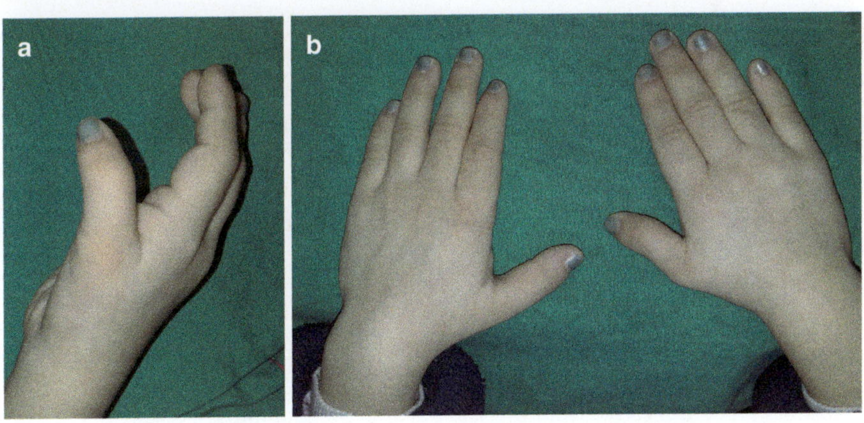

Fig. 8.10 Thumb clinodactyly: (**a**, **b**) clinical appearance; (**c**) radiography of both thumbs revealed right thumb congenital anomaly

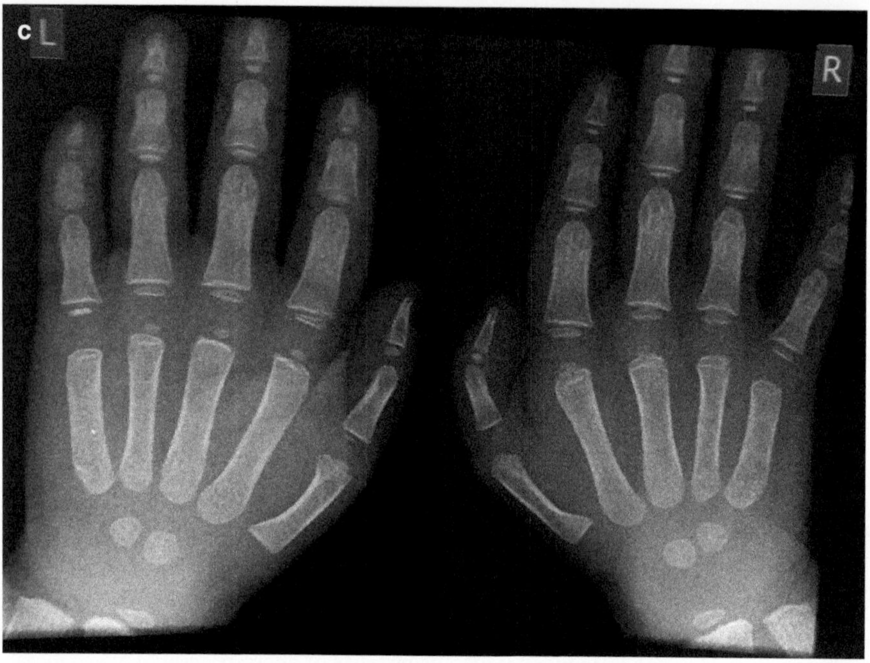

Fig. 8.10 (continued)

reverse wedge osteotomies, soft tissue rereleasing or tightening, and physiolysis with varying success [1, 7, 22, 23]. Postoperative immobilization depends on the used technique, and complications such as malunion are rare in children [7].

8.10 Camptodactyly

Camptodactyly is a contracture of proximal IPJ in the anteroposterior direction [1, 6–8]. It occurs as a consequence of the imbalance of flexors and extensors or due to circulatory disturbance, skin shortness, subcutaneous bands, and short flexors [1, 3, 7, 8]. Camptodactyly is mostly sporadic (30% of cases have familial background), fifth finger is affected in 70% of cases, and it can be part of many syndromes [1, 3, 7]. Patients with camptodactyly can be divided into three groups: newborn (male or female) patient, adolescent (mostly female), and patients associated with a variety of syndromes, and there is also Foucher classification into early and stiff, early and correctable, late and stiff, and late and correctible [6, 7]. Treatment is conservative (splinting), and if after 3–12 months of conservative treatment an extension lag of 60° exists, surgical treatment is indicated [1, 2, 7]. The surgical treatment includes procedures on the skin, arthrolysis, tenotomies and tendon transfers, osteotomies, and arthrodesis [1, 7].

8.11 Macrodactyly

Macrodactyly ("digital nerve-oriented benign neurofibroma") is rare congenital enlargement of one or several digits of the hands and feet with unknown etiology [2, 3, 6, 7, 14, 24, 25]. The incidence is around 0.2 per 10,000 births [17, 24]. There is slight male predomination, it is mostly unilateral, more than one digit can be involved, and it may be associated with various syndromes (Fig. 8.11) [1, 4, 21, 26, 27]. The finger grows as the child grows, and some authors make a distinction between static macrodactyly (with proportional growth) and progressive macrodactyly (with rapid growth) of the finger [1, 6, 17, 21]. Macrodactyly never involves one single anatomic unit (finger) of the hand, and the overgrowth components are the soft tissues (hypertrophies of other structures are secondary effects) [17]. Diagnostic procedures includes radiography, computerized tomography (CT), magnetic resonance imaging (MRI), and in some cases angiography and lymphography [27]. Surgical correction is individualized and very complicated [1, 5, 17, 21, 24, 26, 27]. It is best performed when the growth is finished, and it usually consists of multiple salvage procedure (such as radical excision of the soft tissue around the digital nerves, longitudinal splitting, or complete excision of digital nerve) or in extreme cases amputation of the digit [17, 21, 24, 25].

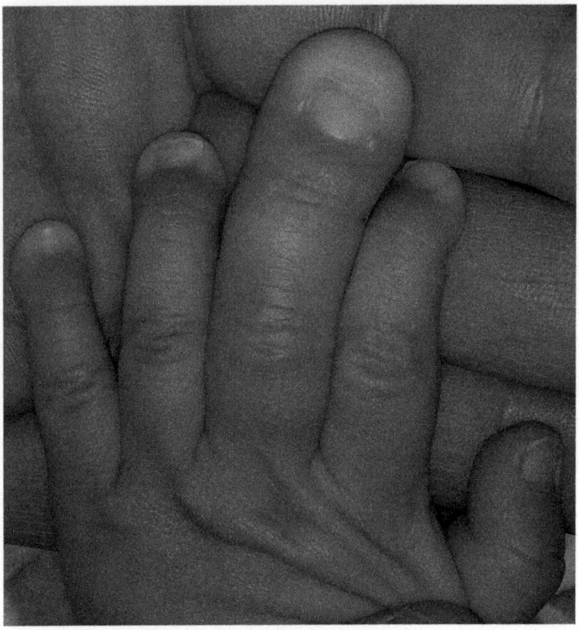

Fig. 8.11 Macrodactyly of the third finger

8.12 Thumb Hypoplasia

Hypoplasia of the thumb is a part of radial dysplasia and it involves all anatomical structures (Fig. 8.12) [4–6]. It occurs as isolated deformity or with other malformations and syndromes [1, 2, 6, 11]. The incidence of radial longitudinal deficiency is approximately 1:30,000 live births, with same incidence among sexes [2]. Modified Blauth classification of thumb hypoplasia includes five types in range of slight decrease in thumb size to complete absence of thumb [1, 2, 11]. Patients with type I and mild type II do not require surgical treatment, patient with IIIA type requires soft tissue surgery, and patients with Blauth type IIIB, IV, and V require pollicization (index finger act as a thumb) [2, 4, 5]. Optimal time for pollicization is the first and second year of life [2, 11].

8.13 Congenital Constriction Band Syndrome

The incidence of congenital constriction band syndrome (CCBS) is 1 per 15,000 [1, 21, 28, 29]. There is a widely accepted opinion that the cause of constriction band is intrauterine strips of amniotic membrane circling around the extremities [2, 3, 8, 11, 17, 28–30]. The syndactyly coexisting with constriction rings is hallmarked by a proximal sinus over the unseparated pair of fingers, producing so-called fenestrated syndactyly [2]. Patterson classified constriction band syndrome into simple (normal) constriction, constriction with soft tissue distal deformity, constriction with fusion of distal parts (acrosyndactyly), and amputation in utero, and there is also modified classification system of upper extremity constriction bands proposed by Hennigan [8, 29, 31]. If the constriction is mild, there is no need for surgery [1, 17]. If the edema is present distally, it should be released as soon as

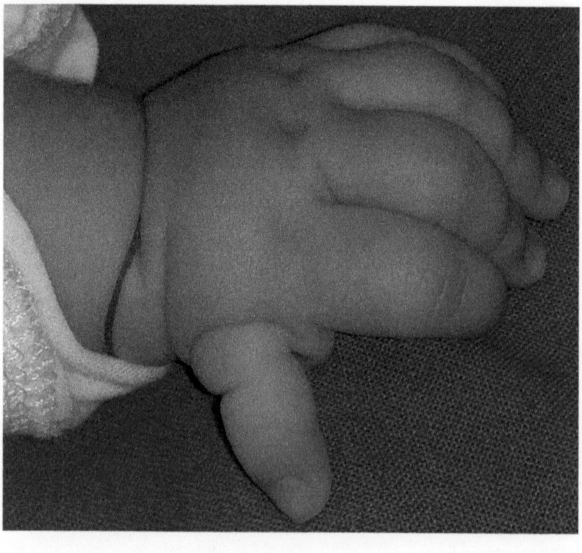

Fig. 8.12 Hypoplastic thumb of the left hand

possible (Fig. 8.13a–e) [17, 30, 31]. There are several surgical procedures proposed, including the release of the constrictions, the separation of the fenestrated syndactyly, and the treatment of the amputated digits [2, 3, 17, 29–31]. Surgery is usually performed as a single procedure or it can be performed in two stage 7 days apart [11, 28, 30, 31].

8.14 Congenial Trigger Thumb

Pediatric trigger thumb is one of the most common pediatric hand problems in practice [17, 32–34]. It represents a stenosing tenovaginitis of the flexor pollicis longus (FPL) tendon within its fibro-osseous tunnel, with the obstruction to tendon glide

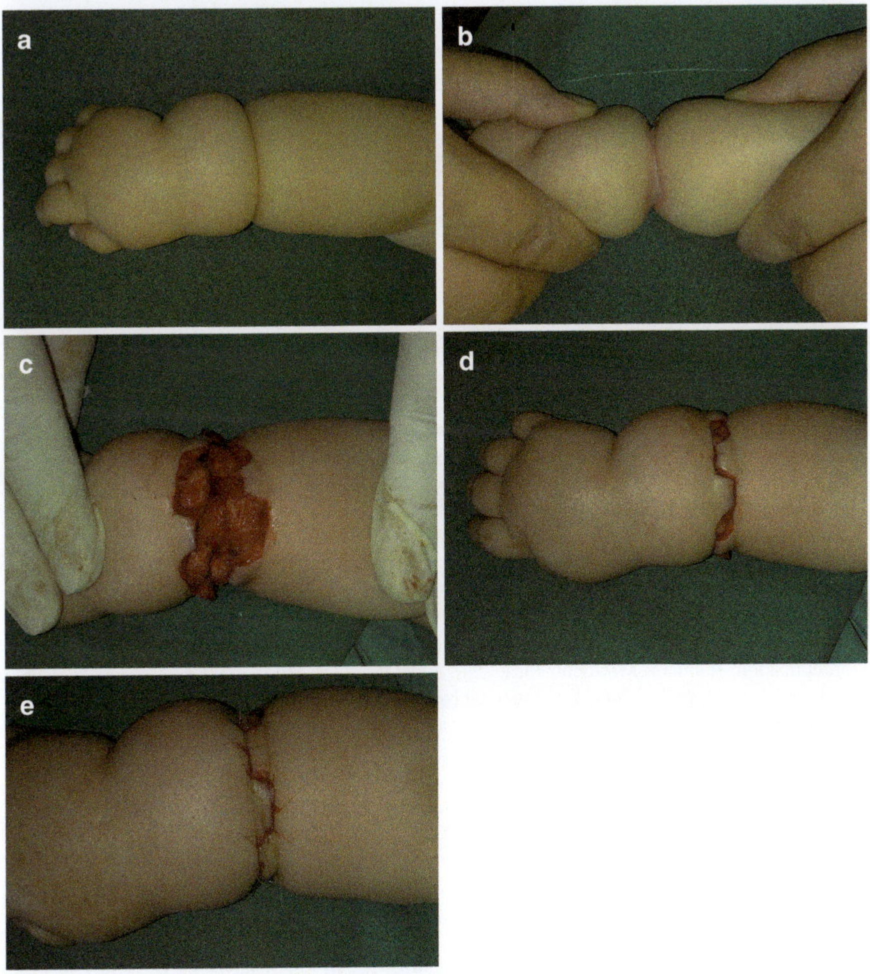

Fig. 8.13 Severe congenital constriction band reconstruction: (**a, b**) preoperative view with distal edema; (**c**) reconstruction with local flaps; (**d, e**) postoperative result

occurring at the A1 pulley (Notta node) [1, 17, 32–34]. Nonpainful triggering may be safely observed, with possible spontaneous resolution, and surgery is advised for persistent painful episodes of triggering (for more than 3 months) [17, 32–34].

References

1. Choi M, Sharma S, Louie O. Congenital hand abnormalities. In: Thorne H, Beasley RW, Aston SJ, Bartlett SP, Gurtner GC, Spear SL, editors. Grabb and Smith's plastic surgery. Philadelphia: Lippincott Williams & Wilkins; 2007. p. 856–63.
2. Little KJ, Cornwall R. Congenital anomalies of the hand-principles of management. Orthop Clin North Am. 2016;47(1):153–68.
3. Tonkin M, Oberg KZ. Congenital hand I: embryology, classification, and principles. In: Neligan PC, Gurtner GC, editors. Plastic surgery. St Louis: Elsevier, Saunders; 2013. p. 526–47.
4. Manske MC, Kennedy CD, Huang JI. Classification in brief: the Wassel classification for radial polydactyly. Clin Orthop Relat Res. 2016 Sep 9. [Epub ahead of print].
5. Guo B, Lee SK, Paksima N. Polydactyly: a review. Bull Hosp Jt Dis. 2013;71(1):17–23.
6. Kozin SH. Upper-extremity congenital anomalies. J Bone Joint Surg Am. 2003;85:1564–76.
7. Hovius SER. Congenital hand IV: disorders of differentiation and duplication. In: Neligan PC, editor. Plastic surgery. St Louis: Elsevier, Saunders; 2013. p. 603–33.
8. Manske PR, Oberg KC. Classification and developmental biology of congenital anomalies of the hand and upper extremity. J Bone Joint Surg Am. 2009;91-A(Suppl 4):3–18.
9. Faust KC, Kimbrough T, Oakes JE, Edmunds JO, Faust DC. Polydactyly of the hand. Am J Orthop (Belle Mead NJ). 2015;44(5):E127–34.
10. Malik S. Polydactyly: phenotypes, genetics and classification. Clin Genet. 2014;85(3):203–12.
11. Buck-Gramcko D. Congenital malformations of the hand and forearm. Chir Main. 2002;21(2):70–101.
12. Tada K, Kurisaki E, Yonenobu K, Tsuyuguchi Y, Kawai H. Central polydactyly-a review of 12 cases and their surgical treatment. J Hand Surg [Am]. 1982;7(5):460–5.
13. Christensen JC, Leff FB, Lepow GM, Schwartz RI, Colon PA, Arminio ST, Nixon P, Segel D, Leff S. Congenital polydactyly and polymetatarsalia: classification, genetics, and surgical correction. 1981. J Foot Ankle Surg. 2011;50(3):336–9.
14. Cooney WP, Wolf J, Holtkamp K, Dobyns JH. Congenital duplication of the thumb. Handchir Mikrochir Plast Chir. 2004;36(2–3):126–36.
15. Tonkin MA. Thumb duplication: concepts and techniques. Clin Orthop Surg. 2012;4(1):1–17.
16. Samson P, Salazard B, Magalon G. The "Bilhaut-Cloquet" technique for treatment of thumb duplication. Handchir Mikrochir Plast Chir. 2004;36(2–3):141–5.
17. Hung LK, Leung PC, Miura T. Congenital hand V: disorders of overgrowth, undergrowth, and generalized skeletal deformities. In: Neligan PC, Gurtner GC, editors. Plastic surgery. St Louis: Elsevier, Saunders; 2013. p. 634–50.
18. Temtamy SA, Aglan MS. Brachydactyly. Orphanet J Rare Dis. 2008;13:3–15.
19. Fairbank SM, Rozen WM, Coombs CJ. The pathogenesis of Kirner's deformity: a clinical, radiological and histological study. J Hand Surg Eur Vol. 2015;40(6):633–7.
20. Dykes RG. Kirner's deformity of the little finger. J Bone Joint Surg Br. 1978;60(1):58–60.
21. Krengel S, Fustes-Morales A, Carrasco D, Vázquez M, Durán-McKinster C, Ruiz-Maldonado R. Macrodactyly: report of eight cases and review of the literature. Pediatr Dermatol. 2000;17(4):270–6.
22. Medina JA, Lorea P, Elliot D, Foucher G. Correction of clinodactyly by early physiolysis: 6-year results. J Hand Surg [Am]. 2016;41(6):e123–7.

23. Piper SL, Goldfarb CA, Wall LB. Outcomes of opening wedge osteotomy to correct angular deformity in little finger clinodactyly. J Hand Surg [Am]. 2015;40(5):908–13. e1
24. Cerrato F, Eberlin KR, Waters P, Upton J. Presentation and treatment of macrodactyly in children. J Hand Surg [Am]. 2013;38A:2112–23.
25. Gluck JS, Ezaki M. Surgical treatment of macrodactyly. J Hand Surg [Am]. 2015;40(7):1461–8.
26. Uemura T, Kazuki K, Okada M, Egi T, Takaoka K. A case of toe macrodactyly treated by application of a vascularised nail graft. Br J Plast Surg. 2005;58(7):1020–4.
27. Kotwal PP, Farooque M. Macrodactyly. J Bone Joint Surg Br. 1998;80(4):651–3.
28. Habenicht R, Hulsemann W, Lohmeyer JA, Mann M. Constriction band syndrome ten-year experience with one-step correction of constriction rings by complete circular resection and linear circumferential skin closure. J Plast Reconstr Aesthet Surg. 2013;66:1117–22.
29. Homer LE, Mishra A, McArthur P. Amniotic constriction bands: a case series and proposed new classification system. Hand Surg. 2015;20(1):121–6.
30. Mutaf M, Sunay M. A new technique for correction of congenital constriction rings. Ann Plast Surg. 2006;57(6):646–52.
31. Hung NN. Congenital constriction ring in children: sine plasty combined with removal of fibrous groove and fasciotomy. J Child Orthop. 2012;6:189–97.
32. Soltanian H. Tenosynovitis In: Thorne H, Beasley RW, Aston SJ, Bartlett SP, Gurtner GC, Spear SL, editors. Philadelphia: Lippincott Williams & Wilkins; 2007. p. 826–29.
33. Akhtar S, Bradley MJ, Quinton DN, Burke FD. Management and referral for trigger finger/thumb. BMJ. 2005;331(7507):30.
34. Schaverien MV, Godwin Y. Paediatric trigger finger: literature review and management algorithm. J Plast Reconstr Aesthet Surg. 2011;64(5):623–31.

Syndactyly 9

9.1 Introduction

Syndactyly is defined as an abnormal interconnection between adjacent digits as a failure of differentiation of the mesenchymal structures [1, 2]. In normal anatomy, the distal end of the web lies on the palmar side roughly at the midlevel of the proximal phalanx [3]. Syndactyly can appear isolated, associated with other deformities in the upper or lower extremity, with polydactyly and/or clefting, or as part of a syndrome (Poland's, Apert's syndrome) [3–9]. Numerous techniques have been described for correction of syndactyly [7, 9].

9.2 Embryology

Around the day 26 (4 weeks after fertilization) the upper limb bud appears as an oblong ventrolateral bulge on the body wall between somites 9 and 12 [4, 5, 7, 10]. The emerging limb bud is composed of somatic lateral plate mesoderm covered by ectoderm [1, 4]. Subsequent limb bud growth and differentiation are controlled by distinctive regions—signaling centers: AER, apical ectodermal ridge (proximodistal growth); Wnt, Wingless type (dorsoventral growth); and ZPA, zone of polarizing activity (anteroposterior-radioulnar growth) [1, 3, 4, 7]. Digits are recognizable at 41–43 days and fully separate at 53 days [3, 10]. The process of apoptosis is needed for the separation of the fingers (it's mediated by bone morphogenetic protein 4—BMP-4) [3, 5]. These anomalies probably occur because of differentiation disturbances in the developing hand plate [3, 7].

A.M. Vlahovic, E.Q. Haxhija, *Pediatric and Adolescent Plastic Surgery for the Clinician*, DOI 10.1007/978-3-319-56004-5_9

9.3 Epidemiology

Syndactyly is one of the most common congenital hand malformations with an incidence of 1–2 per 2000 live births (most common in Caucasians) [2–4, 7–9]. About 50% of patients with syndactylia have bilateral involvement, males are more affected than females, and it is familial in 15–40% of cases [3, 4, 6, 7]. In isolated syndactyly, the third and fourth web are the most commonly involved [3, 6, 8].

9.4 Classification

Syndactyly can be classified as *simple* involving soft tissue only (incomplete that does not include fingertips and complete that does include fingertips), *complex* (with distal bone union), and *complicated* (with more than only distal bone fusion) (Figs. 9.1 and 9.2) [1, 5, 6, 8]. The formal syndactyly classification of

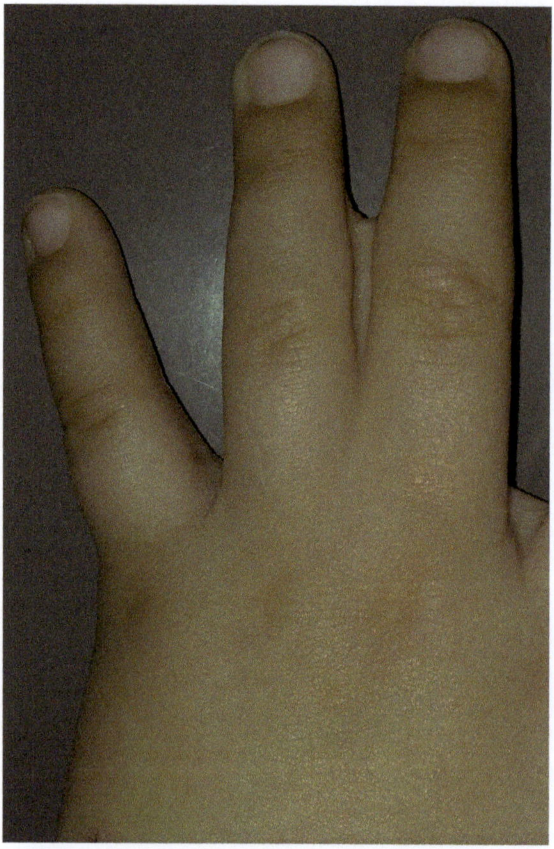

Fig. 9.1 Incomplete simple syndactyly of the third interdigital space

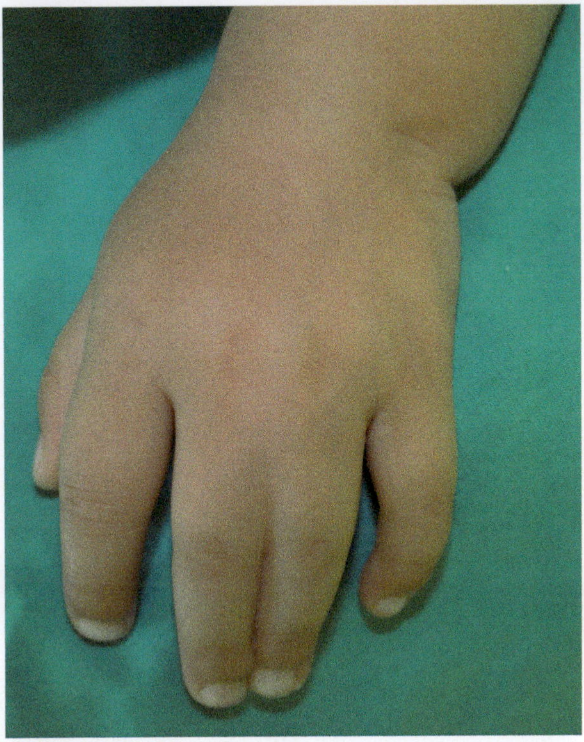

Fig. 9.2 Complete simple syndactyly of the third interdigital space

Temtamy and McKusick with five distinct subtypes has been expanded up to nine types and numerous subtypes [7].

Incomplete syndactyly is presented as the fusion of the fingers proximal to the distal phalanx [1, 3]. In the complete form of syndactyly, the nails can be separated with full pulps of the affected fingers, or there are conjoined nails, and when fingers are of unequal length, the longest finger will tend to bend more during growth [1, 3, 5–8].

Complex syndactyly (with distal bone fusion) can involve only two fingers when it is recognized by a tapered distal end with inward rotation of the fingers and abnormally ridged or confluent nails or more fingers can be involved when they are flat to very cupped with anomalous nails, abnormal bones, and joints (Fig. 9.3a, b) [3, 6]. *Complicated syndactyly* is a broad category characterized by abnormal osseous abnormalities including fusions, rudimentary bones, missing bones, abnormal joints, and sometimes crossbones [1, 5, 6]. Thumb-index syndactyly treatment is more complicated than finger syndactyly, and it is treated differently from other fingers [7].

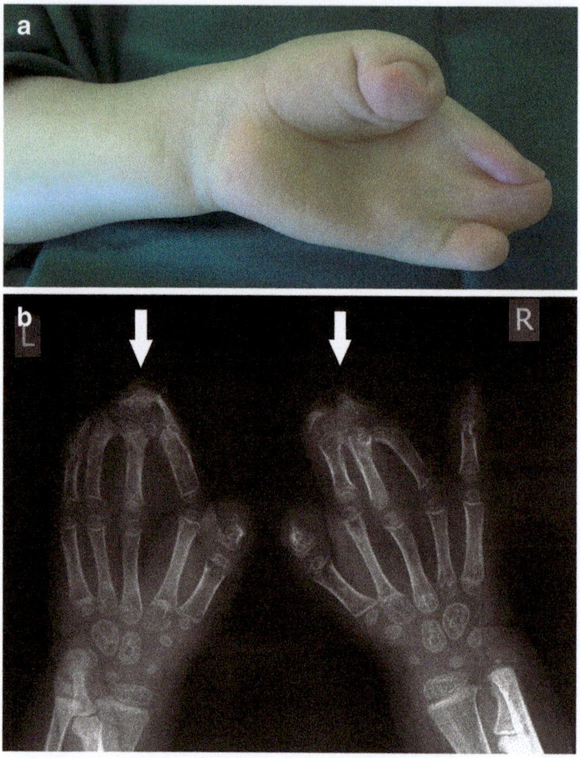

Fig. 9.3 Complex syndactyly of the hand in Apert's syndrome: (**a**) clinical appearance; (**b**) radiography of both hands revealing fusion of distal bones

9.5 Patient Presentation

Syndactyly can be present in a large variety of forms, and that is why good preoperative planning and thorough discussion with family are important [1–8]. The fingers can be normal or anomalous, and the number of affected fingers can differ, as well as the nature of involvement [1–7, 11–17]. In complicated syndactylies, careful assessment of each individual finger is necessary before the surgery [1, 3, 16]. Radiography of the affected hand should be performed to exclude skeletal deformities. Timing of surgery depends on the fingers involved and whether the syndactyly is cutaneous or not [1–8].

Early indications for surgery are thumb-index syndactyly, syndactylies between fingers of unequal length, and complex or complicated acrosyndactyly in order to prevent bone and joint deformities and asymmetric growth (Figs. 9.4a–c and 9.5a, b) [3, 6, 7].

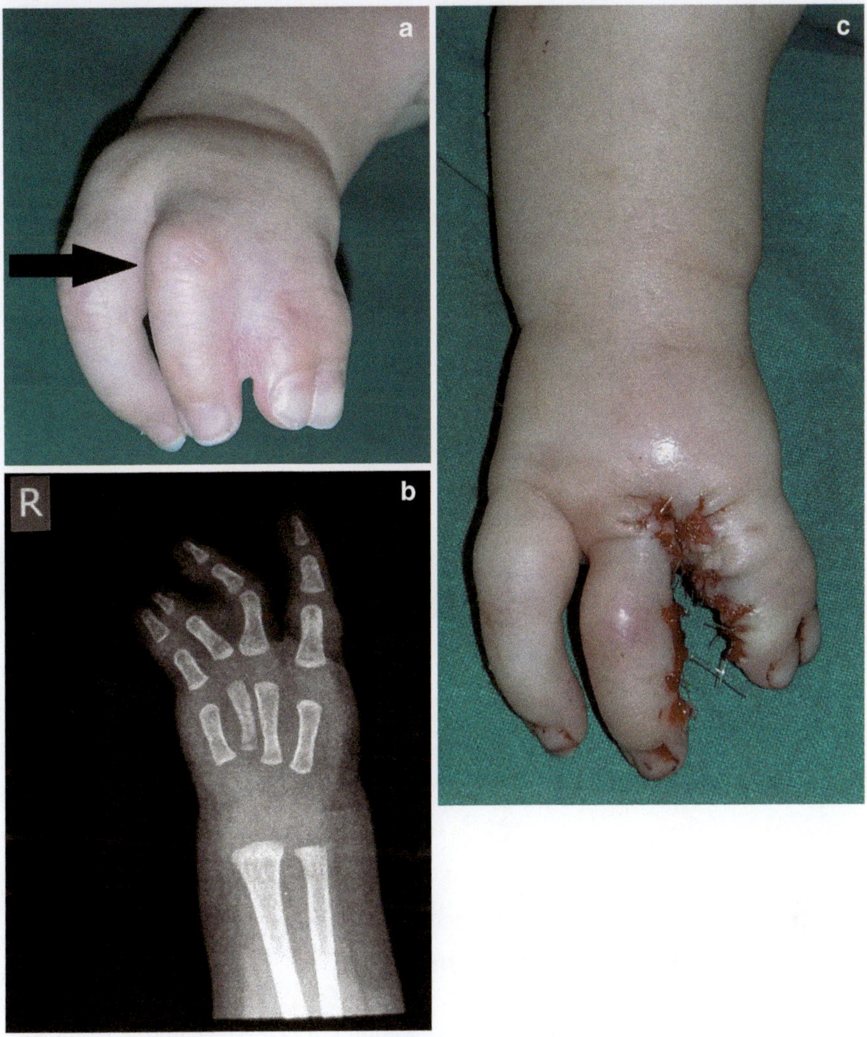

Fig. 9.4 Early indications for syndactyly correction: (**a**) flexion deformity of the middle finger caused by the fourth finger; (**b**) radiographic finding; (**c**) surgical treatment

Simple syndactyly release can be performed in children older than 6 months, but most surgeons will operate on these children between 1 and 2 years to prevent problems with anesthesia [3, 6, 7].

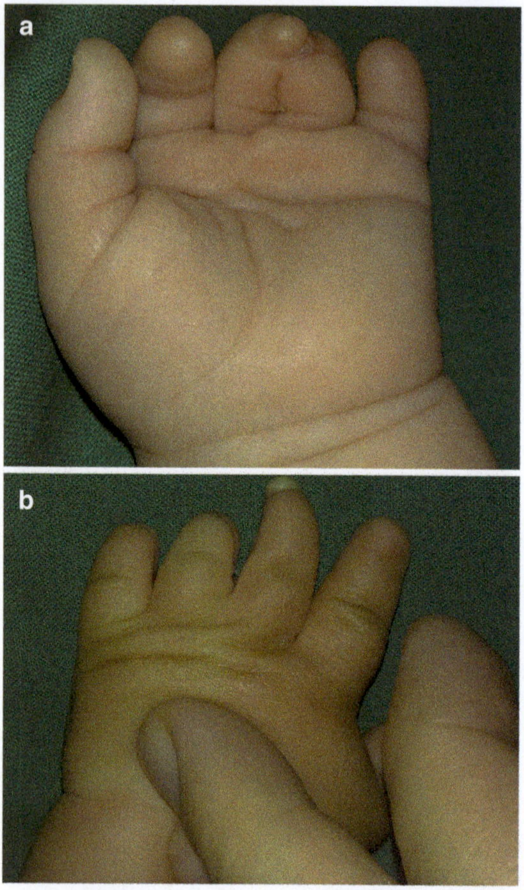

Fig. 9.5 Fenestrated syndactyly: (**a**) syndactyly of the distal part of the fingers with preoperative view; (**b**) postoperative result

9.6 Treatment/Surgical Technique

The release of syndactyly by classical technique implicates separation of the conjoined skin and subcutaneous tissue preserving integrity of the neurovascular bundles [4, 9, 12]. Techniques for separation of fingers include commissure reconstruction, digital incisions, and ways to outcome the lack of skin (Fig. 9.6a–h) [4, 6, 8]. The nail fusion can be corrected by opposing Z-flaps as described by Buck-Gramcko [4]. For safety reasons, two adjacent complete syndactylous fingers are not separated at the same time as vascular anatomy can be different [3, 4, 6]. In bilateral involvement, both hands should be operated at the same time [6].

9.6.1 Digital Incisions

Separation is carried out via dorsal and standard volar zigzag incisions, creating interdigitating flaps distal to the flap for web reconstruction and providing coverage

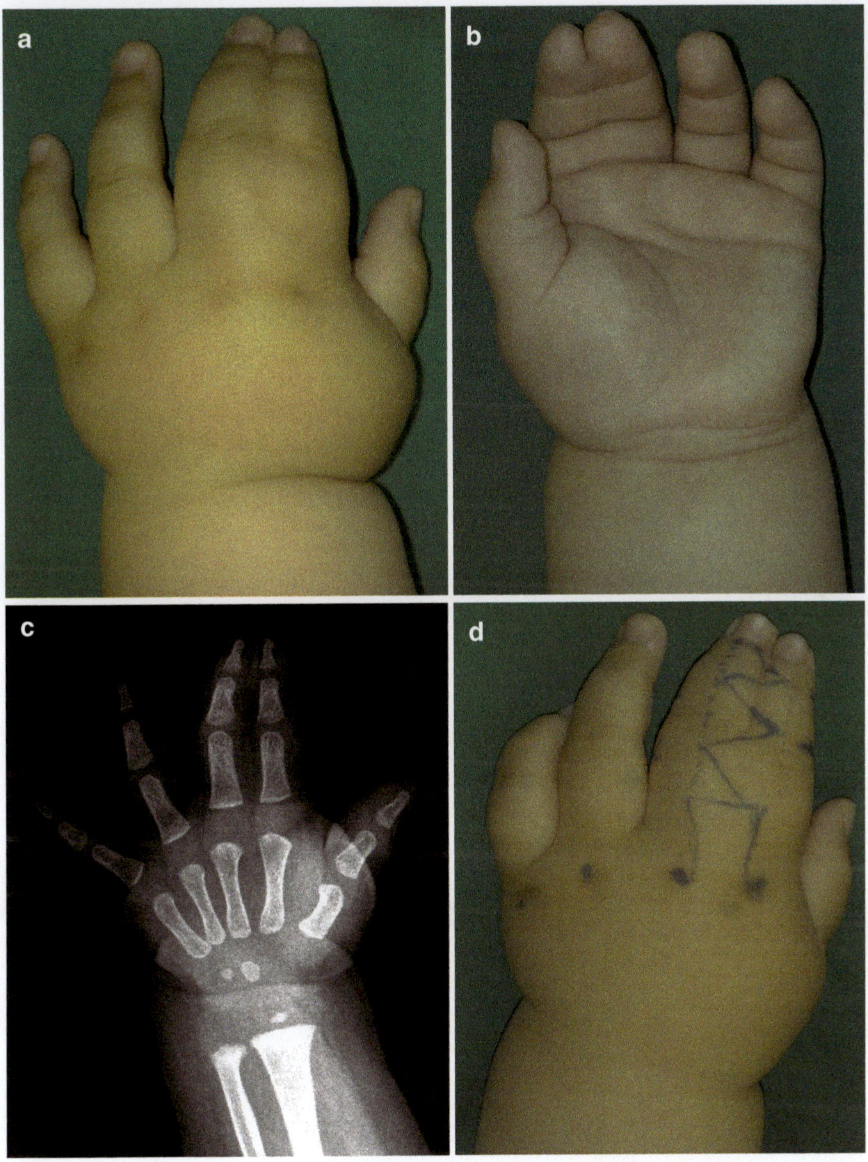

Fig. 9.6 Surgical treatment of syndactyly: (**a**) preoperative dorsal view; (**b**) preoperative palmar view; (**c**) preoperative radiography; (**d–f**) incision markings and incisions; (**g**, **h**) result

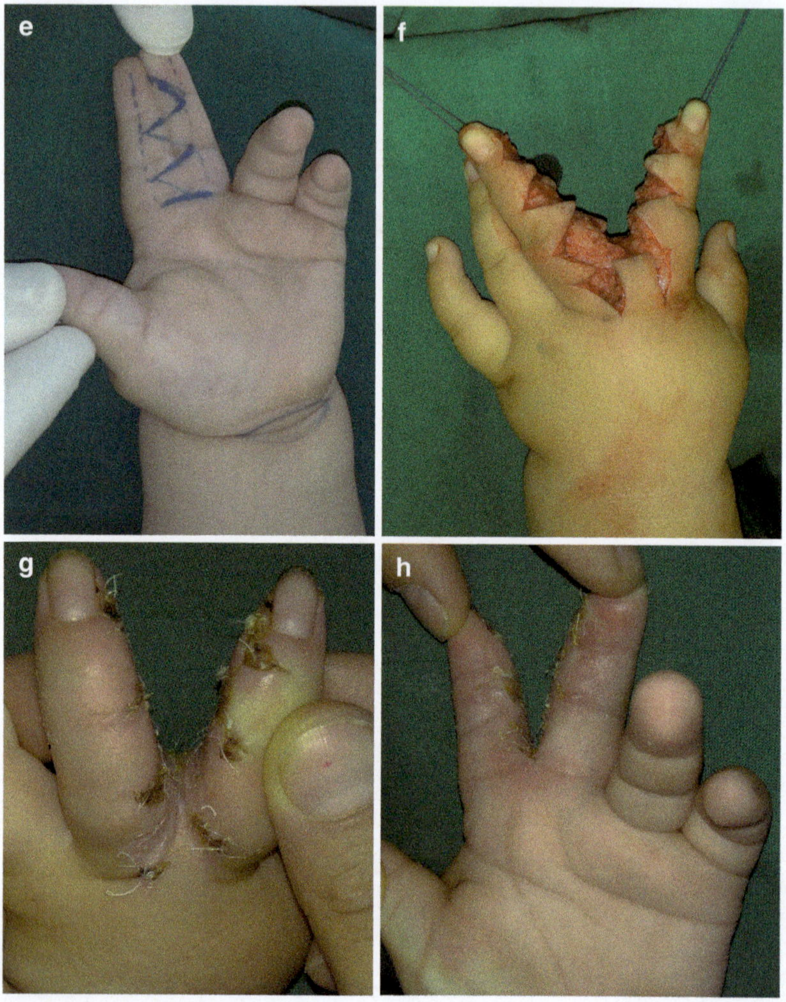

Fig. 9.6 (continued)

at the proximal IPJ [4, 14]. The triangular flaps can either be fully or partially interdigitated depending on the extent of the skin shortage [12, 15]. Some authors used modified zigzag incisions as longer, narrower, angled flaps or rectangular flaps joined with straight-line incisions [8, 14–16]. Digital defatting is also very important in surgical procedure to decrease the digital volume [8, 14]. It should be performed carefully, under loupe magnification, and there will be no consequences in flap vascularization or digital contour [14].

9.6.2 Creation of a Web

The key area of reconstruction in a syndactyly separation is the creation of the web using a local skin flap [1, 3–8, 16]. The web in syndactyly can basically be created by a dorsal flap, a palmar flap, or a combination of both [3, 4, 8, 14, 16]. In an effort to prevent skin grafts, dorsal metacarpal flaps have been used to create the web, followed by primary closure of the fingers (extended dorsal trilobed flap, V-Y dorsal MC flap, island commissural flaps) [8, 9, 11, 17]. For the first web, different kinds of Z-flaps, transposition flaps from the dorsum of the hand and index or thumb, and pedicled flaps and free flaps for the larger defects have been advocated [2].

9.6.3 Lateral Soft Tissue Defects

Digits in regular simple syndactyly offer less skin than needed for separated digits because the skin is not stretched between the fingers [8]. The residual defects on medial side of the fingers are usually covered by full-thickness skin grafts (FTSG) (less often by split-thickness skin grafts—STSG) [2–4, 14]. There is tendency for drawback of skin grafting because of several disadvantages (more time for surgery and healing, hyperpigmentation and hair growth, donor site scars) [2, 14]. There are several techniques for creating a new commissural flap [8, 9]. The tissue expansion has also been used, but it is mostly abandoned because of two-stage treatment and high rate of complications [8, 9, 14, 16].

9.6.4 Separation of the Fingertips

If the nails are separately developed in complete syndactyly, the pulp can be separated and the skin advanced to the rim (Buck-Gramcko technique) [4, 7]. Simple separation is often still possible if the nails are partly fused, and if the nails are conjoined, then nail wall reconstruction with flaps is necessary [4, 6, 7, 10, 16].

9.7 Postoperative Care

The dressings usually consist of paraffin gauze, applied on the wounds and grafts, followed by moist dressings, wet cotton wool, and an elastic bandage or above-elbow soft cast [3, 6, 7, 14, 16]. The first dressing and wound inspection differs among the authors (after 5–7 days or after 3 weeks), but it is best performed during the first 2 weeks after surgery [3, 7, 11, 14, 15]. Active motion, scar space and web massage, silicone scar pad, and occupational therapy are part of postoperative care [7].

9.8 Complications

Early complications mostly occur due to vascular compromise [7]. Infection with skin flaps and skin graft necrosis should be treated promptly [3, 7]. Web creep has been reported to be the most common late complication [3, 14]. Complications that occur by using skin grafts (skin contracture, hyperpigmentation, hypertrophic scaring) can be avoided by using dorsal metacarpal flaps or extended dorsal interdigital flaps and primary closure (Fig. 9.7a–c) [2, 3, 14]. Bony and nail deformities can also occur [7].

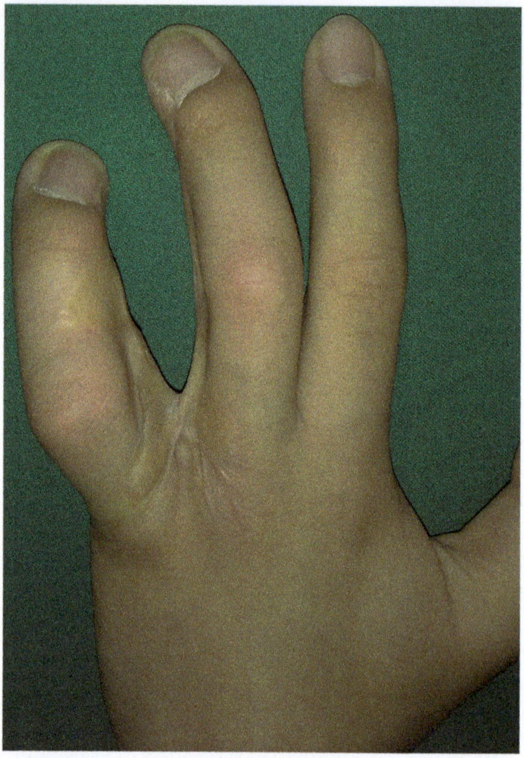

Fig. 9.7 Late complications after surgical treatment of syndactyly

Complications such as flexion contractures, rotation and lateral deviation, joint instabilities, and insufficient functioning of the individual separated fingers also occur, and that is why these patients should be followed till the end of growth [1, 3, 8, 11].

9.9 Secondary Procedures

Secondary procedures involve scar contracture release and re-deepening of webs [2, 7, 14]. In complicated syndactylies, ligament reconstructions, osteotomies, chondrodesis, and arthrodeses can be necessary [1–3, 6].

9.10 Poland's Syndrome

Alfred Poland had described a chest and hand deformity in 1841, and Patrick Clarkson named it Poland's syndrome in 1962 [18, 19]. The incidence of Poland's syndrome varies from 1:7000 to 1:100,000 [3, 13]. Poland's syndrome is mostly sporadic, with male predominance (3:1) and right side more involved [13, 20]. In familial form, both sides and sexes are equally affected [3, 13, 20].

In Poland's syndrome, patients present with a broad range of ipsilateral trunk, upper limb, and hand anomalies [1, 3, 13, 18, 20]. It is characterized in most cases by partial or complete underdevelopment or absence of sternocostal head of pectoralis major muscle and hypoplastic arm and hypoplastic hand with a simple syndactyly or symbrachydactyly [1, 13, 18–20]. The etiology of Poland's syndrome is unknown, and it occurs most probably because of interruption of the embryonic blood supply to the upper limb [3, 13, 20]. Hand anomalies in Poland's syndrome are classified into seven types ranging from normal hand to phocomelia-like deficiency with a significant number of patients having normal or near-normal hand [3, 11, 13].

For syndactyly and symbrachydactyly in Poland's syndrome surgical treatment, postoperative care, outcome, and complications are similar to syndactyly and symbrachydactyly (Fig. 9.8a–d) [1, 3, 11]. In syndactylous hypoplastic fingers, the separated individual fingers can be less functional than before the operation [3].

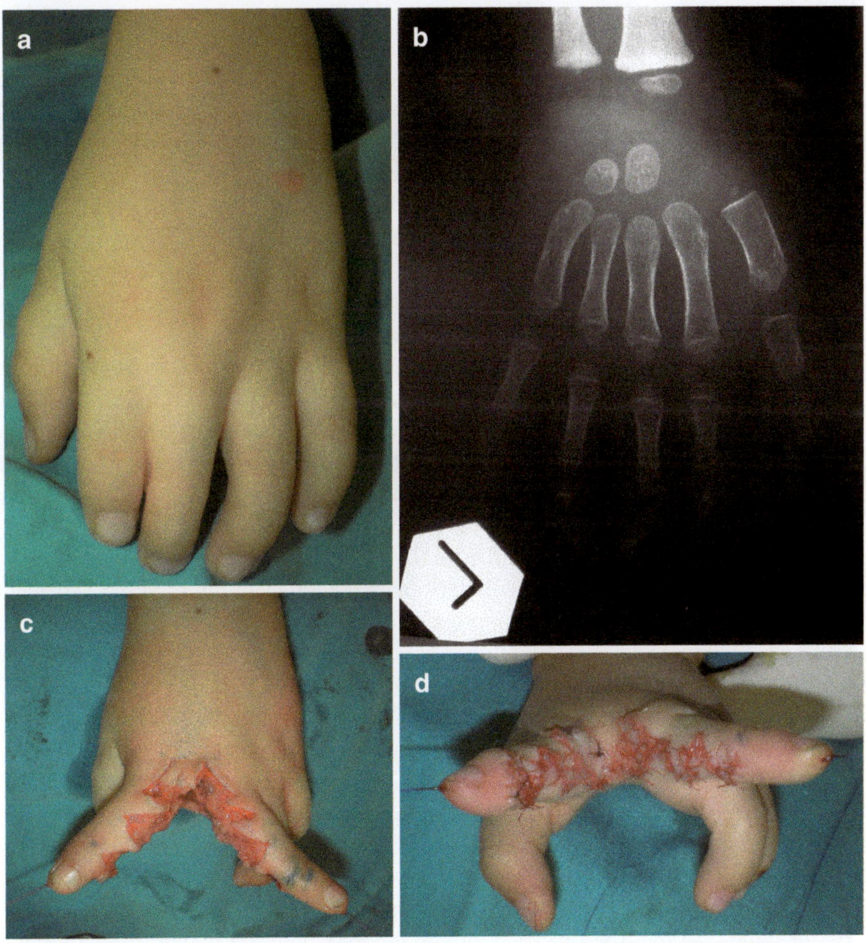

Fig. 9.8 Brachysyndactyly in Poland's syndrome: (**a**) preoperative view; (**b**) radiography revealing anomalous fingers; (**c**) zig-zag incisions and web construction; (**d**) postoperative result

9.11 Apert's Syndrome

Apert's syndrome is an autosomal dominant (AD) condition with the incidence of 1:65,000, caused by a mutation in the gene encoding fibroblast growth factor receptor 2 (FGFR2), characterized by craniosynostosis combined with acrosyndactyly and other deformation of all five digits [1, 3, 5, 6, 21, 22].

Hand anomalies in Apert's syndrome are classified by Upton (purely descriptive) and by van Heest et al. (guides surgical treatment) [1, 3, 5, 6, 22, 23]. In type I by Upton ("spade" hand), there is a radially deviated small thumb with a shallow first web; the index, long, and ring fingers display complete or complex syndactyly; and the little finger is attached by a simple complete or incomplete syndactyly [3, 5, 22, 23]. In type II ("mitten" or "spoon" hand), there is a radially deviated thumb with simple syndactyly of the first web, and second to fourth fingers are distally fused, creating a curve in the palm with divergent metacarpals, with the little finger like in Upton I type [3, 5, 23]. In type III hand ("rosebud" hand), there is complex syndactyly; the thumb and index, long, and ring fingers are distally fused with synostosis; the little finger is united to the ring finger by simple complete syndactyly; and the nail is broad and conjoined and overlies the bony fusion between the first to four digits (Fig. 9.9a–c) [2–4, 23]. Symphalangism at the proximal interphalangeal joints of the index, long, and ring finger is a persistent finding [22].

Patients with Apert's syndrome are usually treated in major craniofacial centers [1, 21]. Separation and correction of the thumb and other fingers in as few operations as possible are surgical goals [3]. There is a classical approach to the treatment of pansyndactyly in Apert's syndrome, with hand surgery performed at most cases at 9 months of age and 6 months after the treatment of craniostenosis [1, 6, 22].

Corrective hand surgery can be performed in three steps, and the procedure is performed bilaterally [22]. First procedure may include correction of clinodactyly (there are opinions that thumb clinodactyly does not influence on thumb function) and opening of the fourth space, [3, 22, 23]. Fingers with symphalangism can be separated by zigzag or straight incisions, and residual defects are covered with skin grafts [3, 22]. In the second and third procedures, the second web separation is performed, and if needed removal of the fourth digit and MC bone is performed [18]. Nail walls can be reconstructed with flaps from the adjacent finger pulp [22].

Fearon suggested a two-stage approach for pansyndactyly in Apert's syndrome realizing all fingers in two operations on all four extremities (first operation at 9–12 months and second 3 months later) with straight-line release of fingers (FTSG used for covering skin gap in proximal third or half of the finger), equal length dorsal and volar flaps for web space creation, and performance of midphalangeal osteotomies for older children (9–12 years) [21].

Harvey et al. performed preoperative imaging by bilateral CT angiography, enabling visualization of arterial anatomy, and this information is used by the surgeon to plan and execute single-stage syndactyly release of the entire hand, with dorsal rectangular flaps, straight-line incisions, and full-thickness skin grafts [23]. Tissue expansion for Apert's syndactyly in theory would seem ideally suited, but it

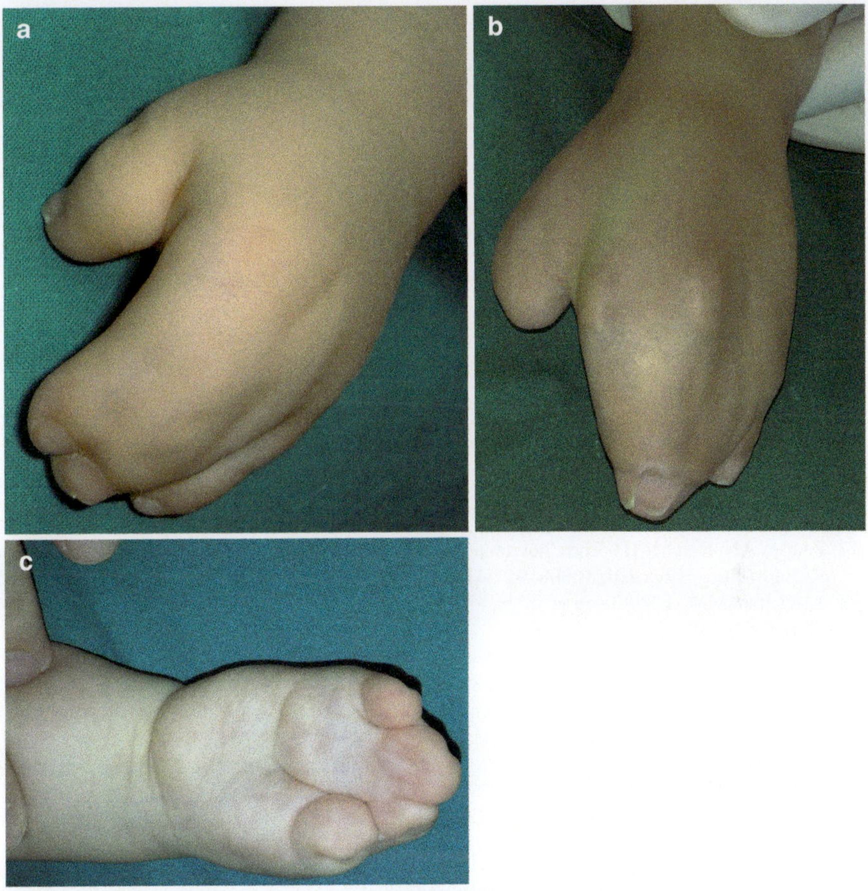

Fig. 9.9 Different types of syndactyly in Apert's syndrome: (**a**) type I ("spade hand"); (**b**) type II ("spoon hand"); (**c**) type III ("rosebud hand")

is not predictable, and there are unacceptable rates of complications [14, 24]. Absorbable skin sutures are placed for flaps and grafts [22].

Skin grafts are prone to maceration and infection (up to 22% partial skin graft loss), and secondary web contractures are common, with remarkable functional improvement in the hand despite poor joint motion [3, 22]. Secondary operations include web deepening and wedge osteotomies to correct the deviation [3].

References

1. Kozin SH. Upper-extremity congenital anomalies. J Bone Joint Surg Am. 2003;85:1564–76.
2. Deunk J, Nicolai JP, Hamburg SM. Long-term results of syndactyly correction: full-thickness versus split-thickness skin grafts. J Hand Surg Br. 2003;28(2):125–30.

3. Hovius SER. Congenital hand IV: disorders of differentiation and duplication. In: Neligan PC, Gurtner GC, editors. Plastic surgery. St Louis: Elsevier, Saunders; 2013. p. 603–33e4.
4. Choi M, Sharma S, Louie O. Congenital hand abnormalities. In: Thorne CH, Beasley RW, Aston SJ, Bartlett SP, Gurtner GC, Spear SL, editors. Grabb and Smith's plastic surgery. Philadelphia: Lippincott Williams & Wilkins; 2007. p. 856–63.
5. Manske PR, Oberg KC. Classification and developmental biology of congenital anomalies of the hand and upper extremity. J Bone Joint Surg Am. 2009;91-A(Suppl 4):3–18.
6. Buck-Gramcko D. Congenital malformations of the hand and forearm. Chir Main. 2002;21(2):70–101.
7. Little KJ, Cornwall R. Congenital anomalies of the hand-principles of management. Orthop Clin North Am. 2016;47(1):153–68.
8. Loréa P, Coessens BC. Evolution of surgical techniques for skin releases in the treatment of simple congenital syndactyly: a review. Eur J Plast Surg. 2001;24:275–81.
9. De Smet L, Van Ransbeeck H, Deneef G. Syndactyly release: results of the Flatt technique. Acta Orthop Belg. 1998;64(3):301–5.
10. Tonkin M, Oberg KZ. Congenital hand I: embryology, classification, and principles. In: Neligan PC, Gurtner GC, editors. Plastic surgery. St Louis: Elsevier, Saunders; 2013. p. 526–47e4.
11. Dy CJ, Swarup I, Daluiski A. Embriology, diagnosis, and evaluation of congenital hand anomalies. Curr Rev Muscoskelet Med. 2014;7:60–7.
12. Pandya AN, Belcher HJ. The Chevron technique for skin markings in syndactyly release. Plast Reconstr Surg. 1998;101(3):808–9.
13. Al-Qattan MM. Classification of hand anomalies in Poland's syndrome. Br J Plast Surg. 2001;54(2):132–6.
14. Greuse M, Coessens BC. Congenital syndactyly: defatting facilitates closure without skin graft. J Hand Surg [Am]. 2001;26(4):589–94.
15. Withey SJ, Kangesu T, Carver N, Sommerlad BC. The open finger technique for the release of syndactyly. J Hand Surg Br. 2001;26(1):4–7.
16. Jose RM, Timoney N, Vidyadharan R, Lester R. Syndactyly correction: an aesthetic reconstruction. J Hand Surg Eur Vol. 2010;35(6):446–50.
17. Niranjan NS, Azad SM, Fleming AN, Liew SH. Long-term results of primary syndactyly correction by the trilobed flap technique. Br J Plast Surg. 2005;58(1):14–21.
18. Clarkson JH, Harley OJ, Kirkpatrick JJ. Alfred Poland's syndrome: a tidy little controversy. J Plast Reconstr Aesthet Surg. 2006;59(9):1006–8.
19. Kulkarni D, Dixon JM. Congenital abnormalities of the breast. Womens Health. 2012;8(1):75–86.
20. Latham K, Fernandez S, Iteld L, Panthaki Z, Armstrong MB, Thaller S. Pediatric breast deformity. J Craniofac Surg. 2006;17(3):4564–7.
21. Fearon JA. Treatment of the hands and feet in Apert syndrome: an evolution in management. Plast Reconstr Surg. 2003;112(1):1–12; discussion 13–9.
22. Guero S, Vassia L, Renier D, Glorion C. Surgical management of the hand in Apert syndrome. Handchir Mikrochir Plast Chir. 2004;36(2–3):179–85.
23. Harvey I, Brown S, Ayres O, Proudman T. The Apert hand-angiographic planning of a single-stage, 5-digit release for all classes of deformity. J Hand Surg [Am]. 2012;37(1):152–8.
24. Ashmead D, Smith PJ. Tissue expansion for Apert's syndactyly. J Hand Surg Br. 1995;20(3):327–30.

Pigment Lesions 10

10.1 Introduction

The skin is comprised of two basic layers: the epidermis that contains four major cell types, keratinocytes, melanocytes, Langerhans cells, and Merkel cells, and dermis that contains nerves, blood vessels, lymphatics, muscle fibers, pilosebaceous, and apocrine and eccrine units [1]. Melanocytic nevi are moles with localized proliferations of pigment cells (melanocytes) in the skin [1, 2]. The exact mechanism how nevi develop in the skin is not known [2]. In children, pigmented lesions can pose significant diagnostic and therapeutic challenges [2–4]. By the end of 10 years, nevus count reaches more than 30 in white (5–10 in African, Asian, and Native American population) [3]. Melanocytic nevi presented at birth are named congenital melanocytic nevi (CMN), and all other nevi developed after birth are named acquired melanocytic nevi (AMN) (Fig. 10.1) [2–7].

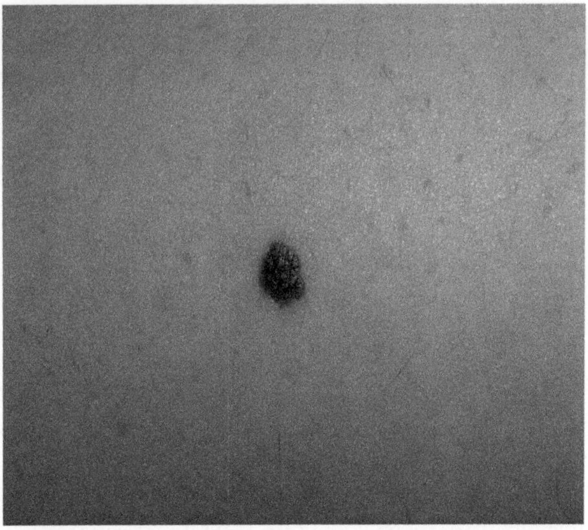

Fig. 10.1 Acquired melanocytic naevus

A.M. Vlahovic, E.Q. Haxhija, *Pediatric and Adolescent Plastic Surgery for the Clinician*, DOI 10.1007/978-3-319-56004-5_10

Melanoma is extremely rare in childhood, but there is tendency of rising incidence [2–4]. Ultraviolet (UV) light represents the primary environmental factor, increasing the number of total body nevi which positively correlates with melanoma risk [3, 4].

10.2 Congenital Melanocytic Nevi

Congenital melanocytic nevi (CMN) are classically defined as being present at birth, and they represent a disruption of the normal migration, proliferation, and differentiation of melanoblasts [2–6]. In the developing fetus, congenital melanocytic nevi CMN are thought to arise between the 5th and 24th week of gestation [2, 5].

The classification of CMN has been standardized and updated in 2012, based on size, location, number of satellite nevi, and additional morphologic characteristics [3, 7, 8]. The following characteristics of nevi are included: a) Size of CMN projected adult size: *Small* < 1.5 cm; *Medium*—M1: 1.5–10 cm, M2 > 10–20 cm; *Large*—(L1: >20–30 cm, L2: >30–40 cm); *Giant*—G1 > 40–60 cm, G2 > 60 cm; *Multiple medium* CMN—3 or more medium CMN without single, predominant CMN; b) Location of CMN: head, trunk, and extremities with subgroups; c) Number of satellite nevi: S0, no satellites S1 < 20 satellites, S2, 20–50 satellites, S3 > 50 satellites; and d) Additional morphologic characteristics: color, rugosity, nodules, and hairiness (Fig. 10.2a–d) [4, 8]. Approximately 2–3% of the neonates have CMN [3]. The incidence of large CMN is estimated at 1 in 20,000–50,000 live births [2, 3, 6, 9, 10]. The very large ("bathing trunk") CMN occur in approximately 1 in 500,000 live births [1, 11, 12].

CMN (small to medium sized) are usually present as round to oval pigmented lesions, with color that ranges from tan to black, with clear borders, and hypertrichosis [2, 3, 5]. Large CMN usually have irregular borders, multicolored pigment pattern, and rugose texture [1–5]; CMN undergo morphologic changes over time and become less or more pigmented, rugose, and verrucous and develop hypertrichosis [1, 3–6]. The evolution of CMN is especially intensive during first months of life [3, 6]. On dermatoscopy, CMN demonstrate reticular, globular, or reticuloglobular pattern [5]. Histologic findings of CMN include involvement by nevus cells of deep dermal appendages, neurovascular structures, deep dermis and subcutaneous fat, infiltration of nevus cells between the collagen bundles, and nevus cell-poor epidermal zone [5, 6]. The differential diagnosis for CMN includes AMN, epidermal nevus, nevus sebaceous, café au lait spot, and Mongolian spot [1, 5].

The exact risk for development of melanoma in CMN is not clear [5, 6]. The lifetime risk for melanoma arising in small CMN is between 0 and 5% (similar to AMN), and the risk for melanoma in large CMN is estimated to be between 5 and 10% [1, 3–6, 11, 13]. If there is CMN of 40–60 cm diameter in adult size, with a truncal location, numerous satellites nevi, and involvement of the leptomeninges, melanoma risk is high [2, 6]. The other features that indicate biopsy or excision include ulceration, uneven pigmentation, a change in shape, and nodularity [1]. Magnetic resonance imaging (MRI) screening of the central nervous system (CNS) early in life is recommended for the patients with high risk for malignant transformation [3, 5, 12].

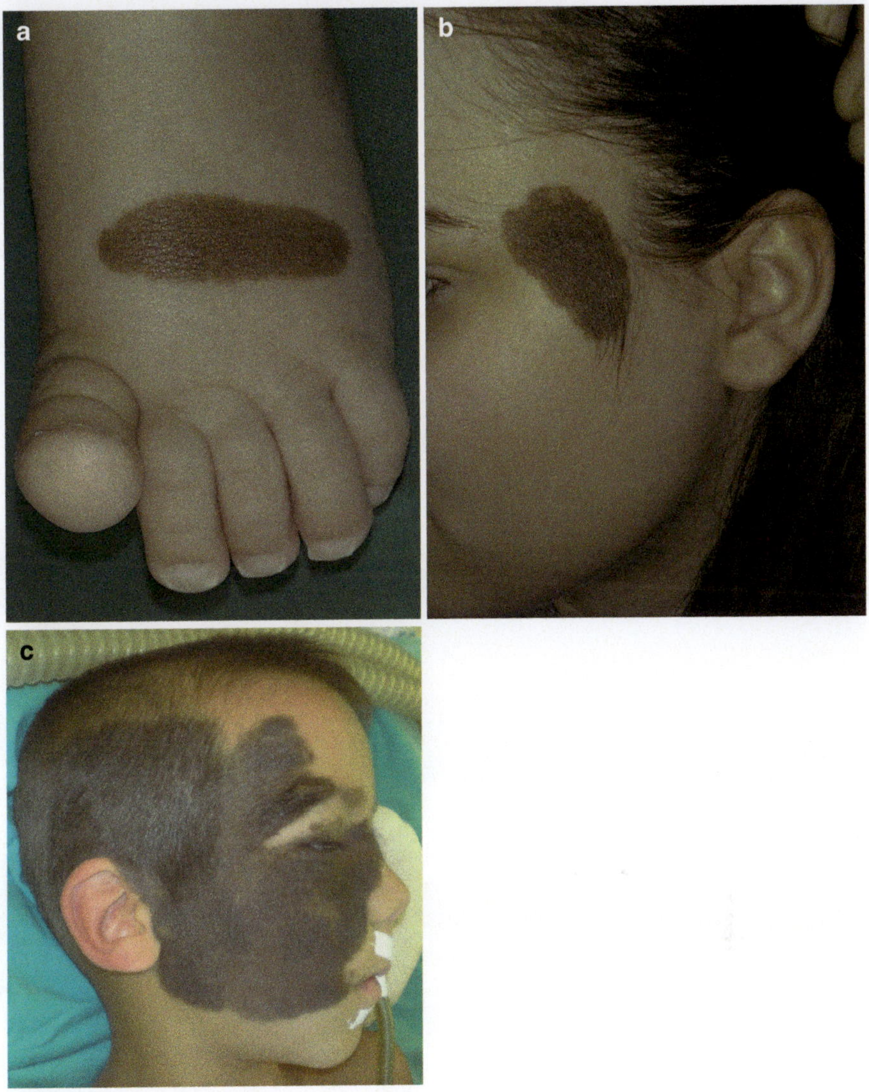

Fig. 10.2 Congenital melanocytic neavi: (**a**) small; (**b**) medium; (**c**) large; (**d**) giant congenital melanocytic nevus

Fig. 10.2 (continued)

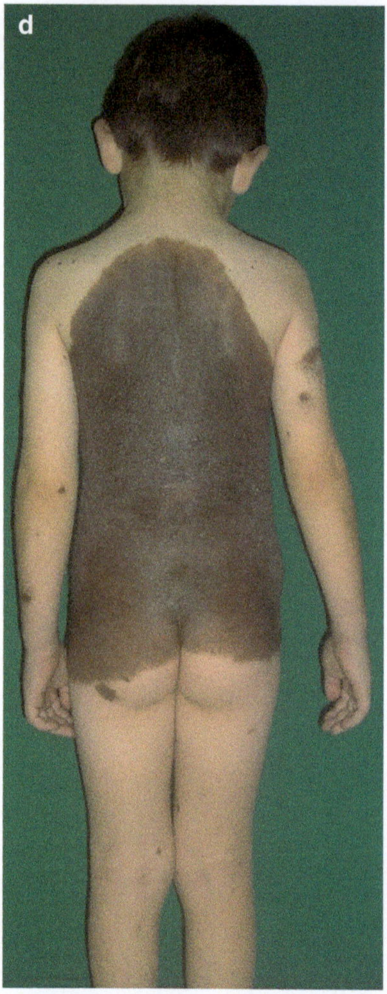

Neurocutaneous melanosis (NCM) is characterized by an excess deposition of melanocytes along the leptomeninges [1–7]. Congenital nevus-like nevus (CNLN) or "tardive" becomes evident during infancy or early childhood with features indistinguishable from those of true CMN [3, 13]. These nevi measuring 1.5 cm or larger are found in 1–4% of older children and adults [3, 6].

10.2.1 Treatment of CMN

There are many different strategies for treatment of patients with CMN with an ultimate goal that the clear, deep margin of resection has to be achieved [1–3, 5, 6, 8–16]. Approximately half of the malignancies that have occurred in large CMN

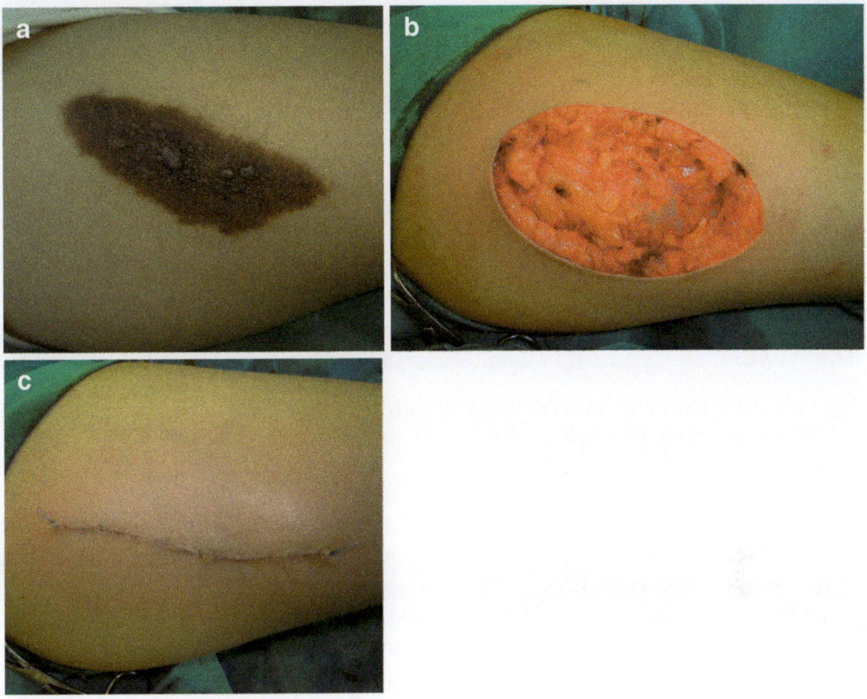

Fig. 10.3 Excision of congenital melanocytic nevus of the right femoral region: (**a**) preoperative view; (**b**) complete excision; (**c**) the result

developed in the first 3–5 years of life, and therefore, decisions regarding prophylactic removal should be made early in life [3, 6, 11].

Treatment decisions should be tailored to individual patients, taking into account lesion size, location, appearance, and leptomeningeal involvement [2, 3]. One-stage excision with primary closure is the mainstay of surgical management of small CMN (single easily excisable and facial CMN are offered surgery for cosmetic reasons) (Fig. 10.3a–c) [3, 6, 11]. Routine prophylactic excision of small and medium CMN is not recommended [2, 3, 6].

Many strategies have been advocated for the removal and reconstruction of large and giant CMN such as serial excision, tissue expansion, and excision with skin grafting and skin substitutes, sole or in combination [1–6, 8–16]. The guiding principles are elimination (reduction) of the risk for malignant transformation, preservation of function, and improving cosmetics [1, 3, 6, 13].

The juvenile skin does not have the laxity of an adult, making local flaps difficult to use in children [5]. Staged excision down to fascia, with a flap reconstruction (advancement, transposition, or rotational), after tissue expansion of uninvolved skin, represents the primary surgical approach for removal of large CMN (Fig. 10.4a, b) [3, 5, 6]. The donor site must match with color, texture, and contour of recipient site, and it has to be free of infection or scars [5]. Tissue

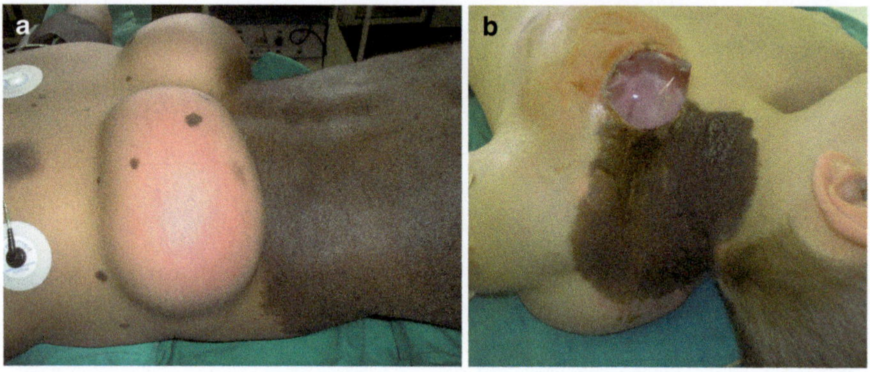

Fig. 10.4 Treatment of congenital melanocytic neavus with tissue expanders: (**a**) two expanders in lumbar region; (**b**) expander protrusion through wound dehiscence

expansion works better in infant and young child; however, some locations are not suitable for this technique (it is associated with more morbidity and a higher failure rate in the extremities) [15].

CMN can be managed effectively by serial excision (carefully in sensitive areas like periorbital or perioral because of possible distortion of these structures) with only one scar as a final result, avoiding morbidity from skin grafting and complications following tissue expansion [5, 16].

Excision and split-thickness skin graft (STSG) have usually poor aesthetic and functional outcome (back of the trunk is the only exception) (Fig. 10.5a–d) [3, 5, 16]. In the periorbital region and ear, full-thickness skin graft provide good match in both color and thickness for the recipient area [14]. Expanded full-thickness skin graft (FTSG) is an excellent choice for coverage of the dorsum of the hand and foot [5]. Other options for covering the wound after excision of giant CMN are autologous cultured skin substitutes (CSS) and artificial skin [11, 12].

Techniques such as curettage, dermabrasion, and laser therapy are used when excision is not feasible, but in that case there is a problem with recurrence because only the epidermis and upper pole of dermis are removed and nevomelanocytes remain in the dermis [3, 6]. Laser treatment is mostly used for treatment of facial CMN that are not amenable for surgical excision [6].

The optimal choice of treatment of CMN varies by body region [5, 10, 14]. Tissue expansion as a single or serial procedure is treatment of choice for scalp region [10, 11]. At the face, subunit principle has to be followed [5, 10]. For periorbital region, full-thickness graft and expanded full-thickness graft are used, leaving the residual brow nevus [5, 14].

Tissue expansion is very effective for anterior trunk, but it should not be used in the region of breast in females until the growth is finished, and for giant CMN

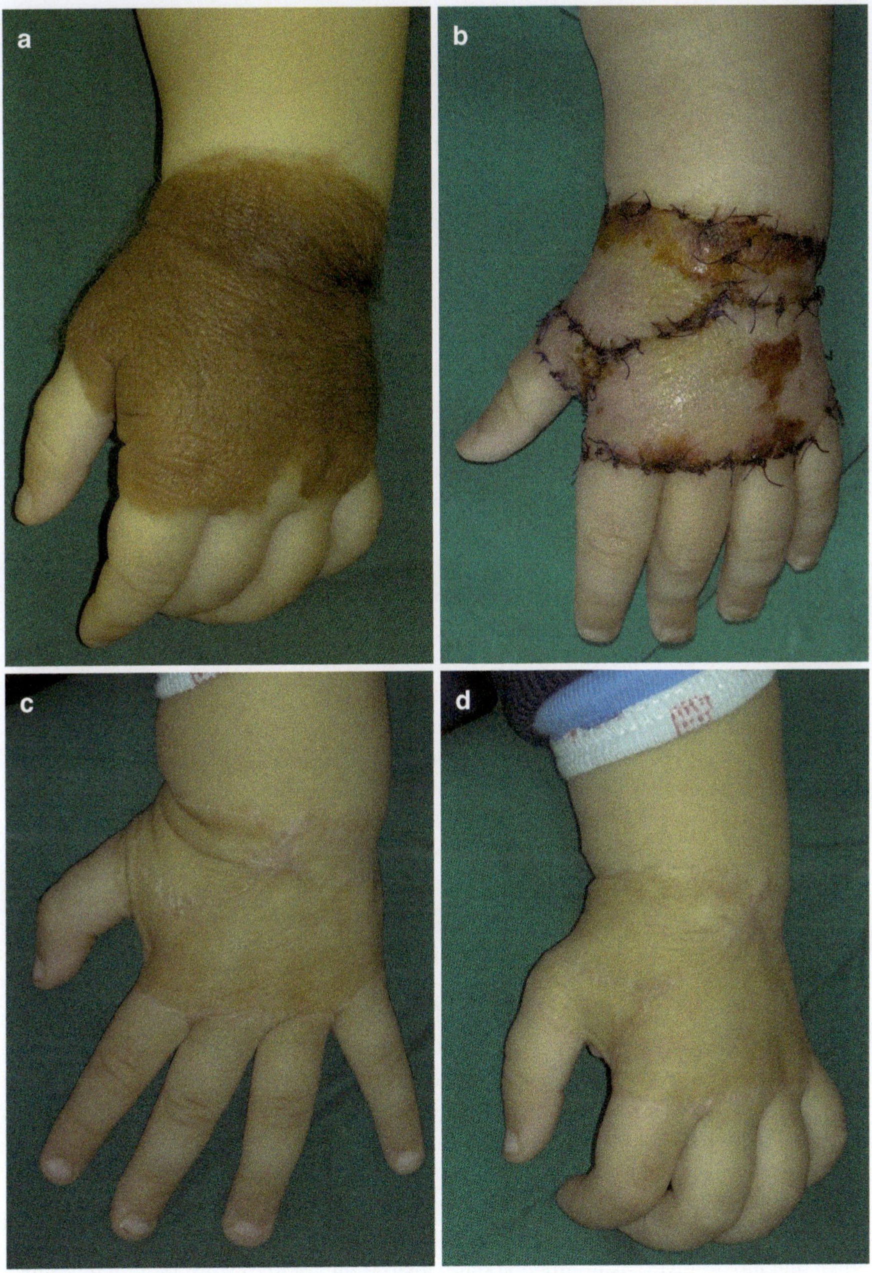

Fig. 10.5 Treatment of congenital melanocytic neavus with complete excision and placement of full-thickness skin grafts: (**a**) preoperative view; (**b**) skin grafts placement; (**c**, **d**) 6 months postoperatively

of the back, flanks, and abdomen, excision and split-thickness non-meshed graft give satisfactory result [5, 11].

For large and giant nevi on extremities, expanded local transposition flaps are used with best results [15]. Partial excision and skin grafting are proposed by some authors for the larger lesions distal to the knee or elbow, but after satisfactory early results pigmented cells "bleed" through the graft [5, 8, 15]. Artificial skin can also be used for covering of large full-thickness skin defects after excision of CMN [12].

Spontaneous lightening of CMN has been reported, and according to this sustaining of surgical treatment especially in the head region is advocated [3, 9].

10.3 Acquired Melanocytic Nevi

Acquired melanocytic nevi (AMN) are benign lesions and the most common type of melanocytic nevus [2]. Melanocytic nevi in children and adolescents have morphologic features and behavior that differ from nevi in adults [2–4]. Two pathways for evolution of melanocytic nevi are described: constitutional that gives rise to nevi with globular pattern (children, especially on the head and neck, and trunk), with predominantly dermal growth, and the acquired pathway that results in nevi with reticular pattern with predominantly junctional growth (especially in extremities) and most often develops during adulthood [3].

Ultraviolet light is the primary environmental influence on the number and location of nevi that develop during childhood [2–4]. Children with lightly pigmented skin have higher nevus counts, and several genes have been associated with nevus number and pattern [3, 4]. Most AMN appear gradually as children age (by 11–12 years of age); however, multiple nevi may appear suddenly or become more prominent in response to a variety of factors [2–4]. Atypical nevi usually begin to appear around puberty [3, 4].

A lifetime risk that any acquired mole transforms into melanoma is approximately 1:10,000 [3, 4]. There is increased risk for melanoma if there are more than 50 lesions, in case of presence of clinically atypical nevi, family history of melanoma, excessive sun exposure, lightly pigmented skin, and/or red hair, and these patients should be followed periodically with total body skin examination [2–4].

The key component of the ABCDE system (asymmetry, border irregularity, color variability, diameter > 6 mm, and evolving) that describes evolution of pigmented lesions is usually connected with histologic atypia in adults, but rarely in children [3]. Dermoscopic monitoring with close-up photographs is very helpful to distinguish melanocytic versus nonmelanocytic lesions and benign from malignant melanocytic lesions (to avoid unnecessary surgery) [2, 4]. Scalp, genital, and acral nevi

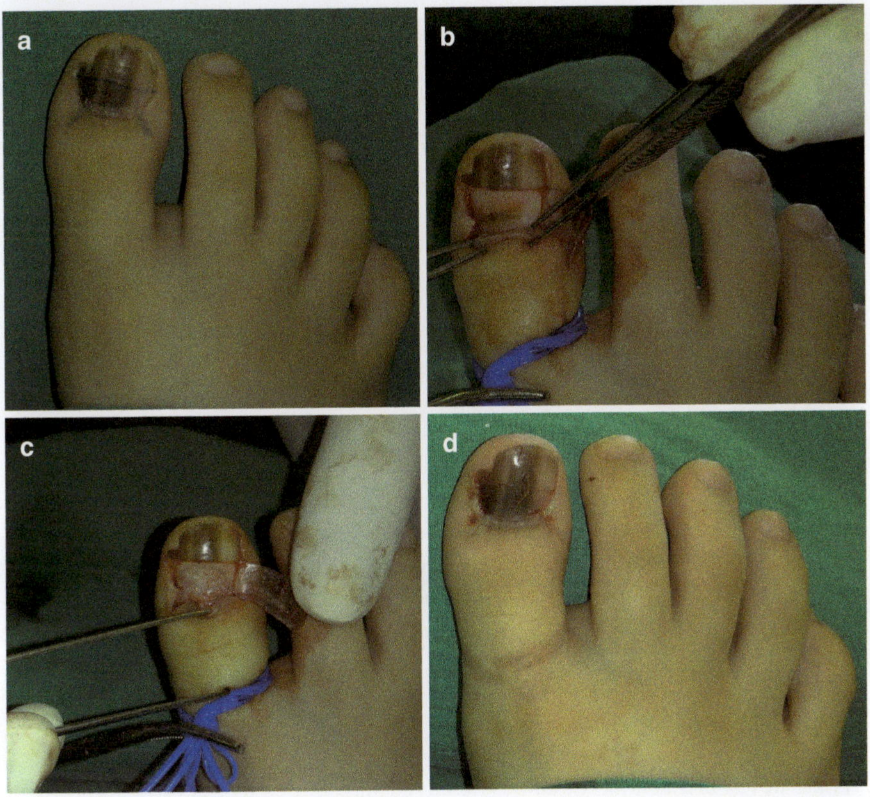

Fig. 10.6 Melanonychia of the right great toe: (**a**) preoperative view; (**b**) pigmented lesion revealed; (**c**) excision of the leasion; (**d**) postoperative view with nail left in place

(longitudinal melanonychia) do not exhibit worrisome behavior in children (Fig. 10.6a–d) [3]. Many children, especially during early adolescence, want nevi removed, and it should be performed only if there is psychosocial problem, atypical appearance, or irritation [2].

10.4 Speckled Lentiginous Nevus

Speckled lentiginous nevus (SpLN), nevus spilus, is considered to represent subtype of CMN [3, 6]. There are two distinct variants of SpLN: those with exclusively macular speckles and those with papular as well as macular speckles

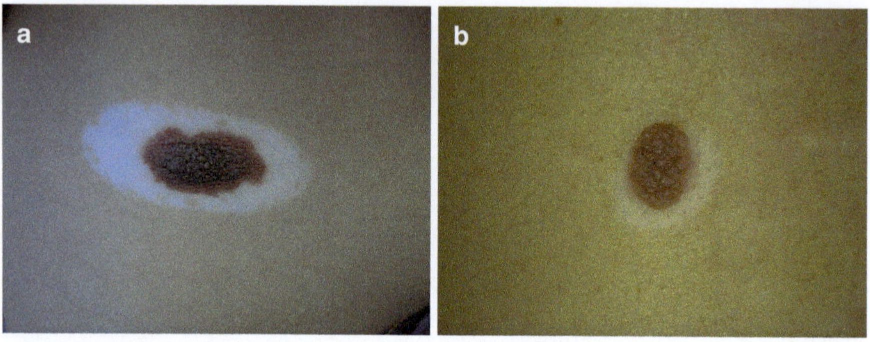

Fig. 10.7 Halo nevi: (**a, b**) different sizes of depigmentation zone

[6]. Large SpLN usually have sharp demarcation in the midline (reflecting embryonic development) [2, 3]. Different pigmented lesion can be superimposed with SpLN such as: café au lait, lentigines or banal-acquired nevi, Spitz, and blue nevi [2, 3, 6]. The risk of melanoma arising within a lesion is proportional to the size of SpLN [3].

10.5 Halo Nevus

A halo nevus is a benign melanocytic nevus surrounded by depigmentation with the incidence of about 5% among the children (Fig. 10.7a, b) [2, 17]. It appears usually as a single lesion, with the most common localization on the trunk [2]. Depigmentation is a result of immunologic destruction of melanocytes [2, 4, 17]. Halo nevi arise from a variety of histologic types of nevi (most of which are not dysplastic), and rarely it can be seen in patients with melanoma, multiple dysplastic nevi, and vitiligo [2, 17]. Most halo nevi regress over a period of months to years, leaving a depigmented macule [2, 4]. The excision is recommended only when clinical and/or pathologic features concerning malignancy are present [2, 4, 17].

10.6 "Café au lait" Macula

This is benign congenital macula with different color and size, most commonly seen after 2 years of life, and may occur as a part of neurofibromatosis or other syndromes (Fig. 10.8a, b) [18].

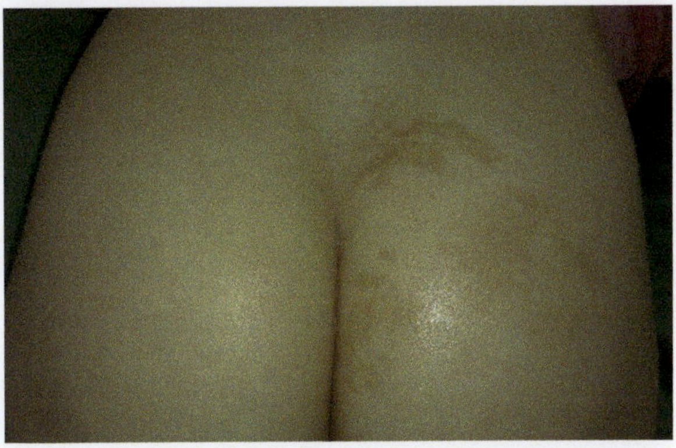

Fig. 10.8 Café au lait at gluteal region

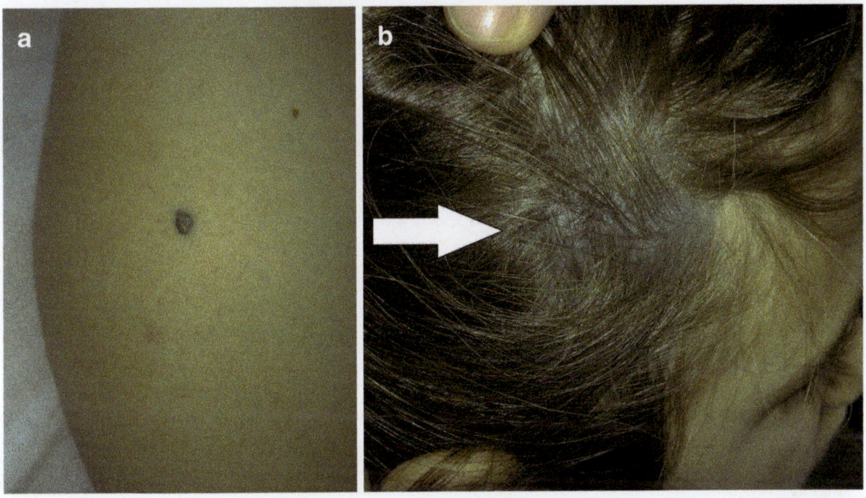

Fig. 10.9 Blue nevus: (**a**) right deltoid region localization; (**b**) large blue nevus at scalp region

10.7 Congenital Dermal Melanocytosis

The blue nevus, Mongolian spots, and nevi of Ota and Ito may represent melanocytes that have not migrated completely from the neural crest to the epidermis during the embryonic stage [2]. Blue nevus is melanocytic nevus derived from dendritic melanocytes in the dermis, and it arises during early childhood and adolescence as regular-shaped papules with melanoma risk especially for lesions located on the scalp (Fig. 10.9a, b) [2, 6, 19]. A Mongolian spot is benign congenital birthmark

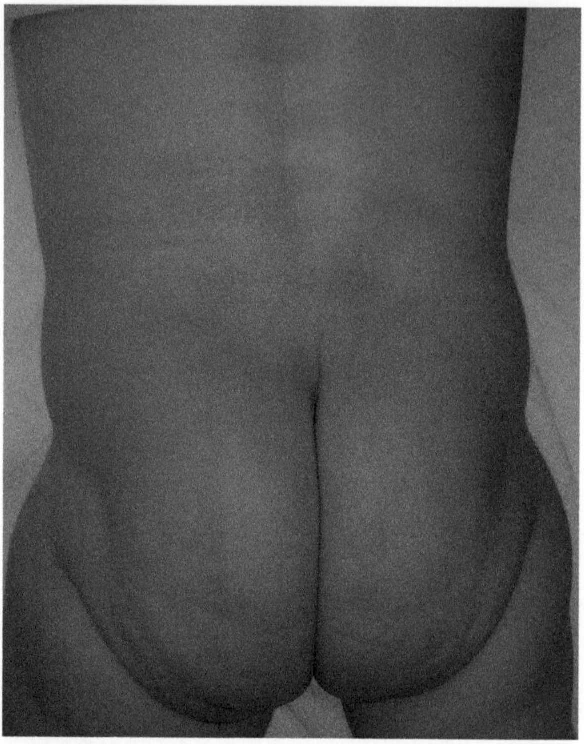

Fig. 10.10 Mongolian spot of the lumbar region

(dermal melanocytosis) with irregular shape, most commonly located in the lumbosacral and gluteal area (Fig. 10.10) [19]. Nevus of Ota is blue or gray patch benign lesion that occurs in the distribution of the branches of the trigeminal nerve, with onset at birth or around puberty [2, 19]. Nevus of Ito frequently occurs with nevus of Ota, and it is located on the shoulder area [2].

10.8 Spitz Nevus

Spitz nevus (spindle cell nevus) is benign, melanocytic nevus described by Sophie Spitz in 1948 [2, 20]. It occurs more common in children than adults, and the incidence is unknown [2–4]. The vast majority of Spitz nevi begin as small, well-circumscribed, pink papules that grow rapidly [2, 3]. It has higher cytologic atypia compared to other nevi [4]. Spitz nevi occur commonly in the head and neck region (followed by torso and extremities) [2].

Biopsy is indicated in any age for Spitz nevi with atypical features (size more than 8–10 mm, excessive growth, asymmetry, or ulceration) or if they arise in post-pubertal patients with the same techniques and management principles as to atypical melanocytic nevi [3, 4, 18]. If the excision is incomplete, and the histology finding confirms Spitz nevus, there is no need for re-excision in children [3].

An atypical spitzoid neoplasm (ASN) represents a type of melanocytic lesion with borderline histologic features indistinguishable from those of melanoma and an uncertain malignant potential [2, 3].

Spitz nevi, ASN, and spitzoid melanoma belong to spectrum that is biologically distinct from banal nevi, dysplastic nevi, and melanoma, with specific molecular markers, and several immunohistochemical stains proposed for use in assessing these lesions [2, 3, 19, 21].

10.9 Atypical Melanocytic Nevus

Atypical melanocytic nevi are acquired usually sporadic lesions smooth, 5 and 10 mm in size, may have irregular borders, vary in color (brown to black to pink), and tend to occur in sun-exposed areas [1, 2, 4, 21, 22]. In children, changing atypical nevi should be sampled and examined microscopically [2]. Children and adults (2% normal population) can have "atypical mole syndrome" that includes 100 or more melanocytic nevi, one or more melanocytic nevi with at least 8 mm diameter, and one or more melanocytic nevi with atypical features, and they are at increased risk for development of melanoma (Fig. 10.11) [2, 22].

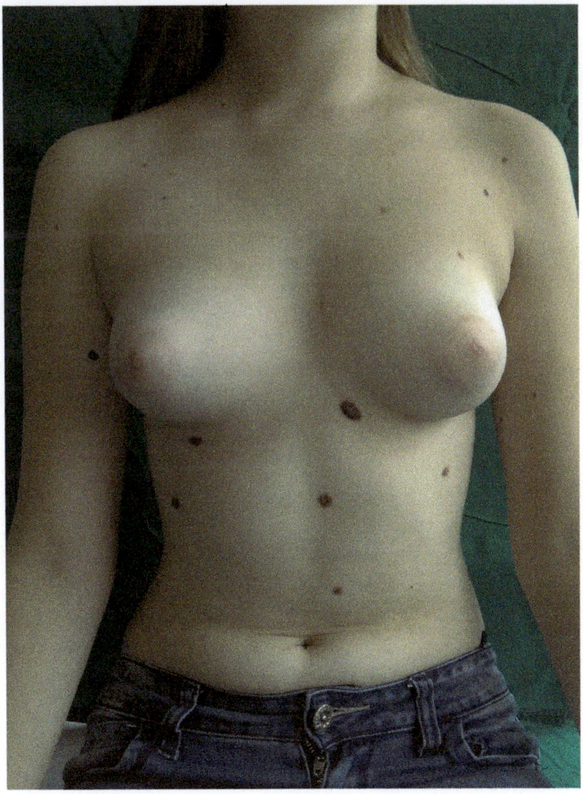

Fig. 10.11 Melanocytic syndrome

10.10 Melanoma

Melanoma in children is rare with approximately 0.5% of melanomas occurring in the individuals younger than 20 years of age and less than 0.05% in patients younger than 10 years of age [4, 19, 23–25]. There is a rising incidence of melanoma in adolescents and adults in a past few decades [3, 4, 21, 24]. The term pediatric melanoma encompasses diagnostically and biologically heterogeneous group of patients aged less than 18 years at diagnosis [19]. Melanoma is relatively common tumor in older adolescents, and it carries a similar prognosis and clinical course as adult melanoma [19, 24]. Generally, melanoma is morphologically classified as lentigo maligna, superficial spreading, nodular, and acral lentiginous type [22]. Lesions of "adult type" are more frequent in pubertal and postpubertal years, and there are also prognostic differences between histologically similar tumors in very young and older patients [2].

Pediatric melanoma can be divided into four age groups: congenital, infantile, birth to 1 year, childhood, 1 year to puberty, and adolescent [24]. Congenital and transplacental melanomas describe spreading of melanoma from the mother to placenta and the fetus [23, 24].

A family history of melanoma and the presence of multiple melanocytic nevi represent important risk factors for the development of melanoma in patients under 15 years of age [4, 19, 25]. Amelanosis, bleeding, color uniformity, diameter variability, and de novo development are the most common pediatric melanoma characteristics [2, 24]. Cutaneous childhood melanoma can be divided also into lesions occurring in the setting of CMN and lesions unassociated with CMN [21]. Melanoma arising in patients with giant CMN often develops in puberty, while conventional superficial spreading melanoma is almost exclusively a disease of white adolescents [13, 22].

There are two major groups of cutaneous melanocytic proliferation arising in the setting of a CMN in childhood: *atypical junctional proliferation in CMN and nodular dermal proliferation* [23]. Melanomas unassociated with CMN tend to be amelanotic or nodular, presenting as a rapidly growing "bump" that may mimic a pyogenic granuloma, keloid, or wart rather than a changing nevus (Fig. 10.12a–d) [3, 23]. Melanoma can be confused with other pigmented or vascular lesions [2, 24]. They are usually not present with the traditional ABCDE criteria [23]. Concern about new or changing melanocytic nevus in a child often prompts parents and pediatrician to request evaluation by a dermatologist or surgeon [3]. Superficial spreading melanoma becomes after 10 years an increasingly frequent diagnosis, and the lesion typically occurs in the intermittently sun-exposed skin of the trunk and proximal extremities [23]. The staging system for pediatric melanoma is the same as adult melanoma, and the approach is similar as for the adults [23, 24].

Surgical excision is therapy of choice, with adjunctive therapies that include chemotherapy, radiation therapy, and immunotherapy [2, 4, 24]. The use of sentinel lymph node (SLN) biopsy has increased despite no clinical or prognostic evidence to support it [2, 19, 26, 27]. Survival in pediatric patients is generally similar to adult patients [24].

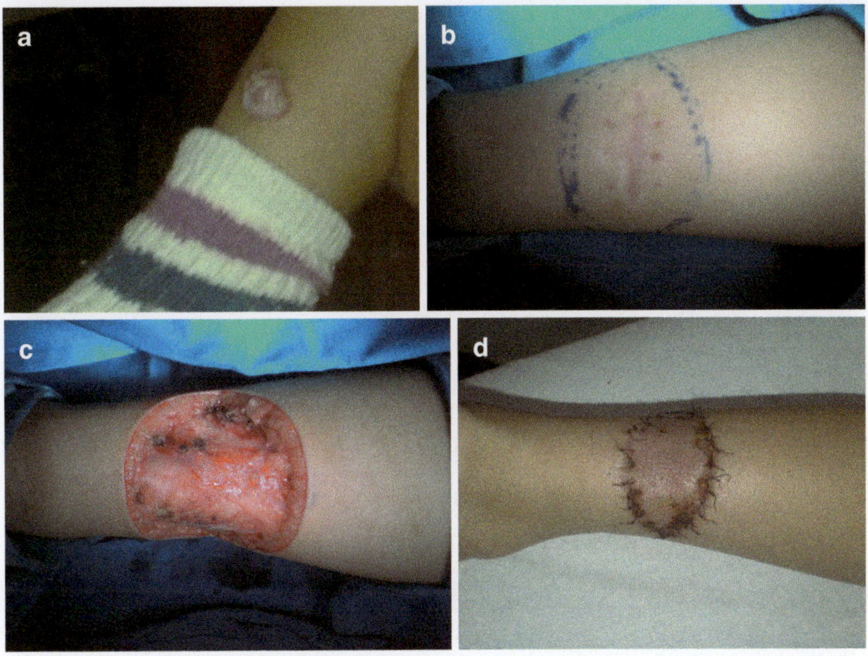

Fig. 10.12 Melanoma of the crural region: (**a**) preoperative picture made by parents before primary surgery; (**b**) histopathology revealed presence of melanoma—postoperative scar; (**c**) wide excision at reoperation; (**d**) skin graft placement

References

1. Culliford A, Hazen A. Dermatology for plastic surgeons. In: Thorne CH, Beasley RW, Aston SJ, Bartlett SP, Gurtner GC, Spear SL, editors. Grabb and Smith's plastic surgery. Philadelphia: Lippincott Williams & Wilkins; 2007. p. 105.
2. Russak JE, Dinulos James GH. Pigmented lesions in children. Semin Plast Surg. 2006;20(3):169–79.
3. Schaffer JV. Update on melanocytic nevi in children. Clin Dermatol. 2015;33(3):368–86.
4. Hawryluk EB, Liang MG. Pediatric melanoma, moles, and sun safety. Pediatr Clin N Am. 2014;61(2):279–91.
5. Bauer BS, Adler N. Congenital melanocytic nevi. In: Neligan PC, Gurtner GC, editors. Plastic surgery. St Louis: Elsevier, Saunders; 2013. p. 837–54.
6. Price HN, Schaffer JV. Congenital melanocytic nevi-when to worry and how to treat: facts and controversies. Clin Dermatol. 2010;28(3):293–302.
7. Krengel S, Scope A, Dusza SW, Vonthein R, Marghoob AA. New recommendations for the categorization of cutaneous features of congenital melanocytic nevi. J Am Acad Dermatol. 2013;68(3):441–51.
8. Gosain AK, Santoro TD, Larson DL, Gingrass RP. Giant congenital nevi: a 20-year experience and an algorithm for their management. Plast Reconstr Surg. 2001;108(3):622–36.
9. Kinsler V, Bulstrode N. The role of surgery in the management of congenital melanocytic naevi in children: a perspective from Great Ormond Street Hospital. J Plast Reconstr Aesthet Surg. 2009;62:595–601.

10. Zaal LH, van der Horst CM. Results of the early use of tissue expansion for giant congenital melanocytic naevi on the scalp and face. J Plast Reconstr Aesthet Surg. 2009;62(2):216–20.
11. Warner PM, Yakuboff KP, Kagan RJ, Boyce S, Warden GD. An 18-year experience in the management of congenital nevomelanocytic nevi. Ann Plast Surg. 2008;60(3):283–7.
12. Shiestl C, Stiefel D, Meuli M. Giant naevus, giant excision, eleg(i)ant closure? Reconstructive surgery with Integra Artificial Skin to treat giant congenital melanocytic naevi in children. J Plast Reconstr Aesthet Surg. 2010;63(4):610–5.
13. Vourc'h-Jourdain M, Martin L, Barbarot S. Large congenital melanocytic nevi: therapeutic management and melanoma risk: a systematic review. J Am Acad Dermatol. 2013;68(3):493–8. e1–14.
14. Margulis A, Adler N, Bauer BS. Congenital melanocytic nevi of the eyelids and periorbital region. Plast Reconstr Surg. 2009;124(4):1273–83.
15. Kryger ZB, Bauer BS. Surgical management of large and giant congenital pigmented nevi of the lower extremity. Plast Reconstr Surg. 2008;121(5):1674–84.
16. Hassanein AH, Rogers GF, Greene AK. Management of challenging congenital melanocytic nevi: outcomes study of serial excision. J Pediatr Surg. 2015;50(4):613–6.
17. Weyant GW, Chung CG, Helm KF. Halo nevus: review of the literature and clinicopathologic findings. Int J Dermatol. 2015;54(10):e433–5.
18. Shah KN. The diagnostic and clinical significance of café-au-lait macules. Pediatr Clin N Am. 2010;57(5):1131–53.
19. Harrison-Balestra C, Gugic D, Vincek V. Clinically distinct form of acquired dermal melanocytosis with review of published work. J Dermatol. 2007;34(3):178–82.
20. Luo S, Sepehr A, Tsao H. Spitz nevi and other Spitzoid lesions part II. Natural history and management. J Am Acad Dermatol. 2011;65(6):1087–92.
21. Haley JC, Hood AF, Chuang TY, Rasmussen J. The frequency of histologically dysplastic nevi in 199 pediatric patients. Pediatr Dermatol. 2000;17(4):266–9.
22. Ariyan S, Berger A. Melanoma. In: Neligan PC, Gurtner GC, editors. Plastic surgery. St Louis: Elsevier, Saunders; 2013. p. 743–85.
23. Wood BA. Paediatric melanoma. Pathology. 2016;48(2):155–65.
24. Jen M, Murphy M, Grant-Kels JM. Childhood melanoma. Clin Dermatol. 2009;27(6):529–36.
25. Livestro DP, Kaine EM, Michaelson JS, Mihm MC, Haluska FG, Muzikansky A, et al. Melanoma in the young: differences and similarities with adult melanoma: a case-matched controlled analysis. Cancer. 2007;110(3):614–24.
26. Kim J, Sun Z, Gulack BC, Adam MA, Mosca PJ, Rice HE, Tracy ET. Sentinel lymph node biopsy is a prognostic measure in pediatric melanoma. J Pediatr Surg. 2016;51(6):986–90.
27. Howman-Giles R, Shaw HM, Scolyer RA, Murali R, Wilmott J, McCarthy SW, Uren RF, Thompson JF. Sentinel lymph node biopsy in pediatric and adolescent cutaneous melanoma patients. Ann Surg Oncol. 2010;17(1):138–43.

Benign Skin and Soft Tissue Tumors 11

11.1 Introduction

Pediatric tumors are highly varied in origin and clinical presentation [1]. Benign skin and skin-associated soft tissue tumors can be classified simply into those that are epithelial, cutaneous appendage, neural crest, or mesenchymal origin and inflamatory lesions [2, 3]. From radiological point of view regarding imaging features, they can be divided into tumors of the epidermis and dermis, tumors of subcutaneous tissue, and tumors associated with fascia overlying the muscle, and there are also metastatic tumors, other tumors and tumorlike lesions, and inflamatory lesions [3]. Pediatric masses can have their origin due to errors along the pathways of embryological development [2]. Possibility that benign tumors can have malignant alteration has always to be considered [2, 4, 5].

Pediatric skin and soft tissue tumors are not uncommon [1, 2, 5–9]. History and thorough clinical examination, child age at presentation, location of the tumor, and rate of growth are essential diagnostic criteria [4, 6–8]. Clinical examination must asses the site, number of lesions, consistency (shape, size, elevation status, surface status, color, hardness, alignment), mobility, subjective symptoms of patient, and the time course of the appearance of the lesion [1, 4, 8]. The imaging of soft tissue tumors can be unspecific, and radiography, ultrasonography (US) including Doppler, computerized tomography (CT), and magnetic resonace imaging (MRI) usually provide much information about the characteristics of a mass [1, 3, 4, 8]. Benign and malignant tumors can be difficult to distinguish in children [4, 6]. If diagnostic procedures are not adequate to establish the diagnosis, after careful inspection and palpation, the biopsy should be performed [1, 4, 8]. Diagnosis and management of cutaneous defects that occur during embryogenesis are very difficult, and they require appropriate physical exam, laboratory testing, and often imaging studies [9].

A.M. Vlahovic, E.Q. Haxhija, *Pediatric and Adolescent Plastic Surgery for the Clinician*, DOI 10.1007/978-3-319-56004-5_11

11.2 Developmental Defects

11.2.1 Cranial Defects

Midline diverticulum of the dura normally projects anteriorly (fonticulus frontonasalis) and anteroinferiorly (prenasal space), and they closed during normal development leaving frontonasal suture and foramen cecum [2, 10]. If this dural diverticulum stays adherent to ectoderm, anomalies such as dermoid and epidermoid cyst, nasal dermal sinus, nasal gliomas, and cephalocele may occur [10]. Cephaloceles are persistent dural diverticula containing intracranial contents that herniated through the cranial defect [9, 10]. Meningocele contains meninges and cerebrospinal fluid, while protrusion of meninges and brain tissue through skull defect is called meningoencephalocele [9]. Heterotopical glial tissue is the presence of brain tissue in the scalp without an open cranial defect [9, 11]. Imaging studies for cranial defects include US, MRI, and CT, and if occult central nervous system (CNS) connection is identified, neurosurgeon consult should be obtained [2, 9].

11.2.2 Nasal Defects

Tumors in this region are uncommon, and they are not allowed to be excised or biopted before the diagnostic is performed [9]. Ultrasound can determine characteristic of the lesion (solid or cystic), and MRI is the diagnostic tool of choice to determine connection of skin or subcutaneous lesion with CNS [9, 10, 12–14]. Treatment of lesions in this region requires multidisciplinary approach [9–15].

11.2.2.1 Nasal Dermoid Cyst and Sinus

Nasal dermoid cyst and sinus (NDCS) is a rare developmental anomaly with an incidence of 1:20,000 to 1:40,000 births that can be present as cyst, sinus, or fistula and may have intracranial extension in 4–45% [10–14]. Pathogenesis involves the incomplete obliteration of neuroectoderm in the developing frontonasal region [2, 12]. It is mostly present as nasal dorsum mass (79%) and may be associated with sinus opening [2, 12–14]. Intermitent discharge of the sebaceous material and recurrent infection are common, with hair protruding through a punctum as a pathognomonic sign [12]. Progressive enlargement of a nasal dermoid can cause soft tissue and skeletal deformity, local infection, meningitis, and brain abscess [12]. Different imaging modalities, such as CT and MRI are used to determine extent of the lesion and intranasal or intracranial extension [13, 14]. There is a classification of nasal dermoids into superficial, intraosseous, intracranial extradural, and intracranial intradural [14]. On histologic exam, nasal dermoid is characterized as well-defined cyst lined by squamous epithelium of ectodermal origin with adnexal structures of mesodermal origin [12, 13].

Complete excision is the treatment of choice (Figs. 11.1a–f and 11.2a–d) [12, 13]. If there is no sinus opening in the skin, open rhinoplasty approach is recommended, and if there is sinus tract opening, it must be excised (with small excision)

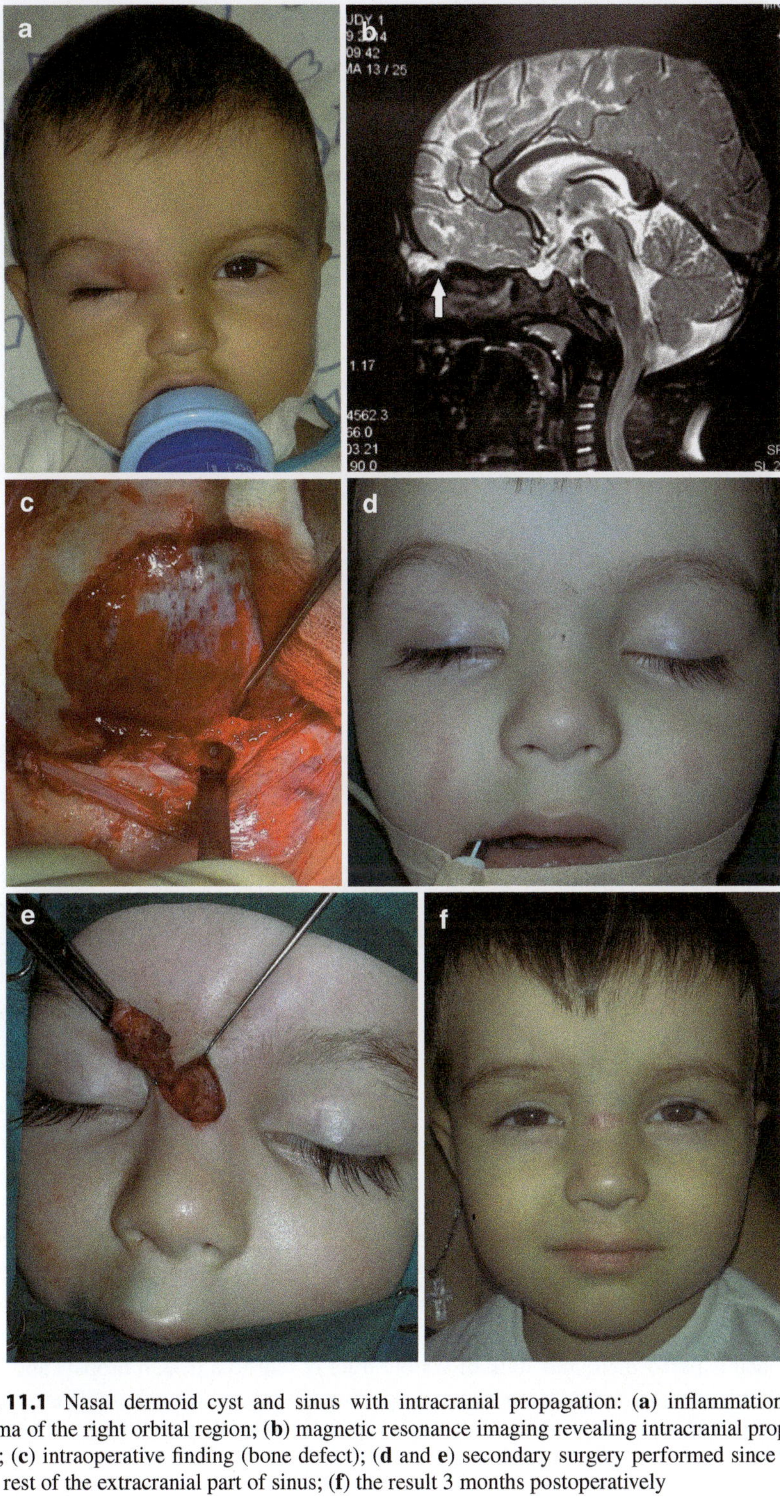

Fig. 11.1 Nasal dermoid cyst and sinus with intracranial propagation: (**a**) inflammation and edema of the right orbital region; (**b**) magnetic resonance imaging revealing intracranial propagation; (**c**) intraoperative finding (bone defect); (**d** and **e**) secondary surgery performed since there was rest of the extracranial part of sinus; (**f**) the result 3 months postoperatively

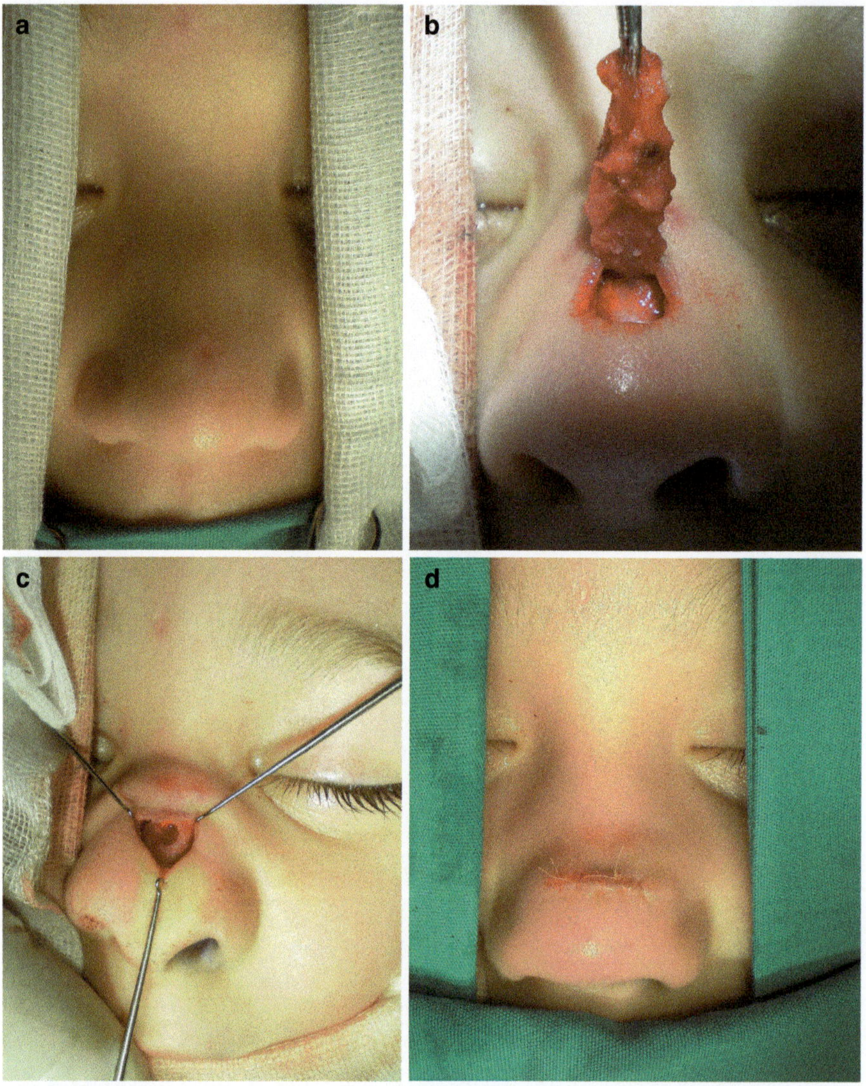

Fig. 11.2 Nasal dermoid sinus excision: (**a**) sinus opening at nasal dorsum; (**b**) intraoperative view; (**c**) complete excision of the sinus; (**d**) postoperative view

along with sinus tract which is excised through open rhinoplasty approach or endoscopic approach [2, 13]. In case of sinus extension deep to the nasal bones, nasal osteotomy is recommended in vertical manner so the tract can be followed proximally [2, 12, 13]. When intracranial extension is present, first, the extracranial approach is performed, and stalk of visible tract is sent to a frozen biopsy, and if it is positive, the intracranial approach is performed via bicoronal incision ("keystone" approach) or via endoscopic endonasal skull base surgery (EESS) [12, 13].

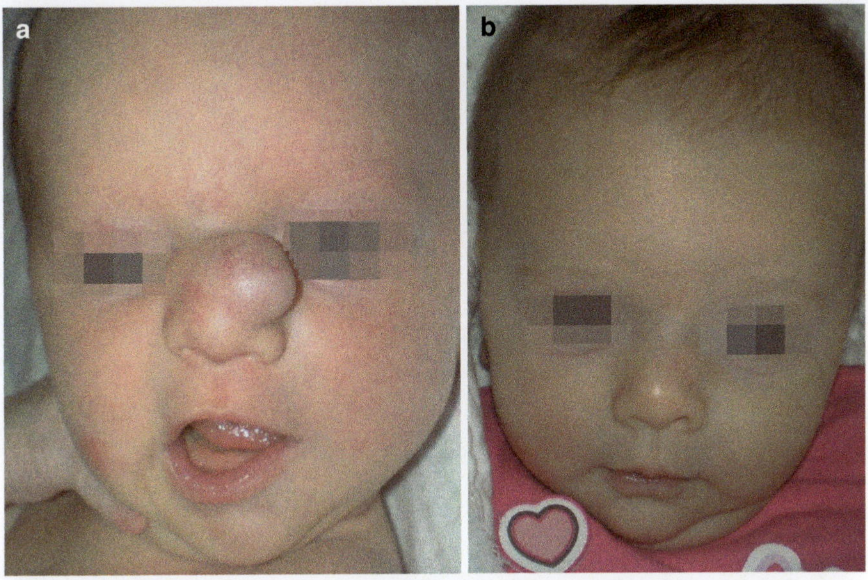

Fig. 11.3 Nasal ectopic glial tissue excision: (**a**) lesion of the left nasal region; (**b**) postoperative result

11.2.2.2 Nasal Glioma (Nasal Heterotopic Glial Tissue)

Nasal glioma is a rare congenital malformation that presents mature brain tissue isolated from the cranial cavity or spinal canal [9, 11, 15]. It is derived from either entrapped neuroectodermal tissue or a nasal encephalocele which later becomes disconnected [11, 15]. Imaging studies such as CT, MRI, and nasal endoscopy are used to differentiate nasal glioma from encephalocele (biopsy or aspiration is contraindicated) [11]. The treatment of choice is surgical excision (for intranasal glioma, transnasal endoscopic approach is recommended) (Fig. 11.3a, b) [11, 15].

11.2.2.3 Dermal Sinus Tracts

Dermal sinus tract ("ectodermal inclusion cysts") is result of incomplete sequestration of the neuroectoderm and somatic ectoderm, and it can occur from the occiput to sacrum [2, 16, 17]. They are most commonly presented with hypertrichosis, skin tags, and abnormal pigmentation [1]. MRI is the main diagnostic tool, and treatment is surgical (Fig. 11.4a–c) [1, 2, 16, 17].

11.2.3 Sinus Preauricularis and Accessory Tragus

These are common anomalies presented as an epithelial-lined sinus "pit," skin tag, or a skin tag containing cartilage ("accessory tragus") [18]. Accompanied anomalies of urinary tract are present in 8.6% of the patients with these anomalies, and US

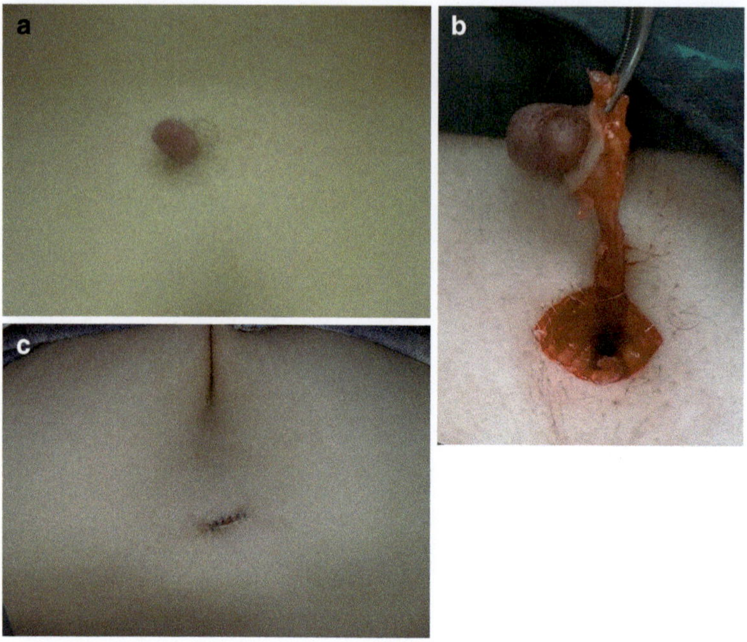

Fig. 11.4 Dermal sinus tract excision: (**a**) clinical appearance; (**b**) excision of the sinus tract; (**c**) postoperative view

of urinary tract should be performed [9]. The treatment is surgical because of aesthetic reasons in case of accessory tragus and to prevent infections and further complication for sinus (Fig. 11.5a–d) [9, 18].

11.2.4 Neck Anomalies

Pediatric neck masses present diagnostic and therapeutic challenge, requiring extensive knowledge of the anatomy, the embryology, and the pathology [10, 19–30]. In children, most lesions are benign, either congenital or inflammatory [20].

11.2.4.1 Thyroglossal Duct Cyst

The thyroid gland develops during third gestational week (GW) in form of ventral diverticulum from the endoderm of the first and second branchial pouches [2, 26]. As the median thyroid anlage descends caudally, a tract forms the thyroglossal duct [23, 24, 26]. Thyroglossal duct typically involutes between 7 and 10 GW, and thyroglossal duct cyst (TGDC) remnant is formed if the tract persists or fails to obliterate, along any portion of the thyroid descent (base of the tongue and pyramidal lobe of the thyroid [2, 23, 24, 26].

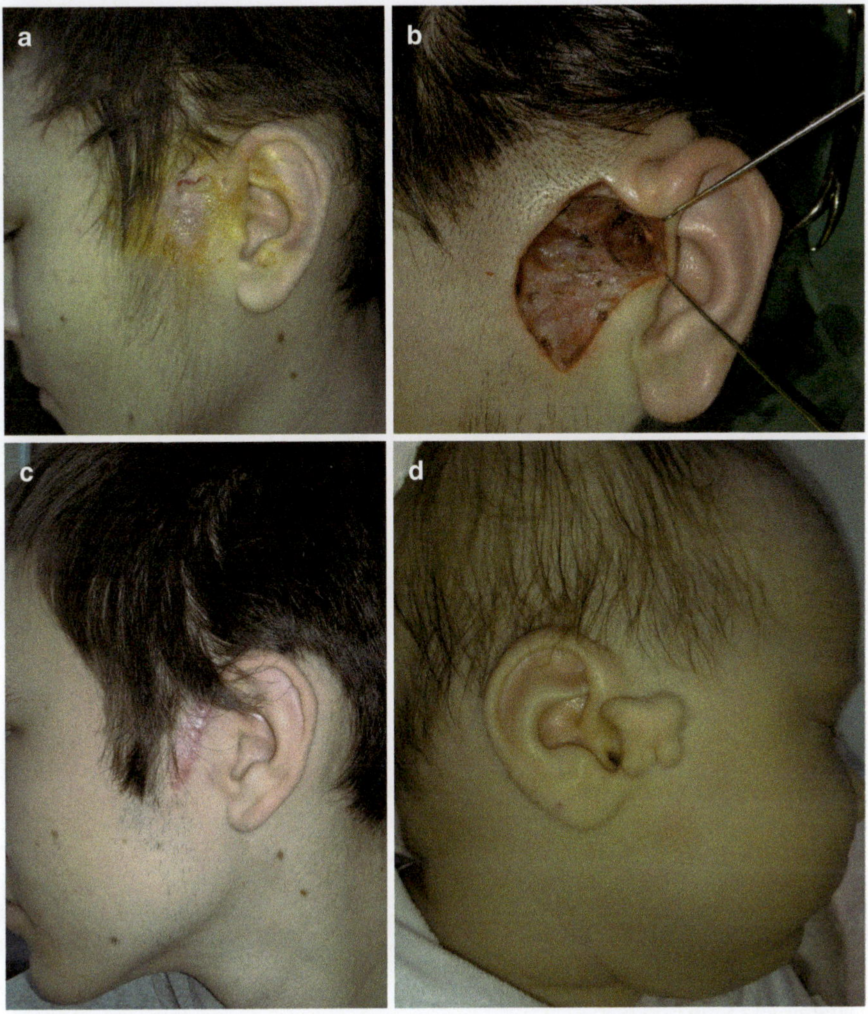

Fig. 11.5 Excision of preauricular sinus: (**a**) inflammation of preauricular region; (**b**) complete excision; (**c**) postoperative result; (**d**) accessory tragus

TGDC anomalies are the most common congenital anomaly of the neck and the second most common neck mass found in children (50% is manifested until 10 years of life) [19, 23, 24, 26]. TGDC remnants occur in approximately 7% of population and both sexes are equally affected [24, 26]. TGDC is most commonly located ahead of thyrohyoid membrane and in suprahyoid region, but it can also be located anywhere from the base of the tongue to thyroid gland [2, 26]. The cyst is always primary anatomical presentation and the sinus is secondary [2].

Clinically, in most cases, there is asymptomatic, cystic neck mass, and near one third of patient is presented with infection, and one forth is presented with draining sinus (incorrectly used term fistula) [2, 23, 24, 26]. Lateralization of TGDC can

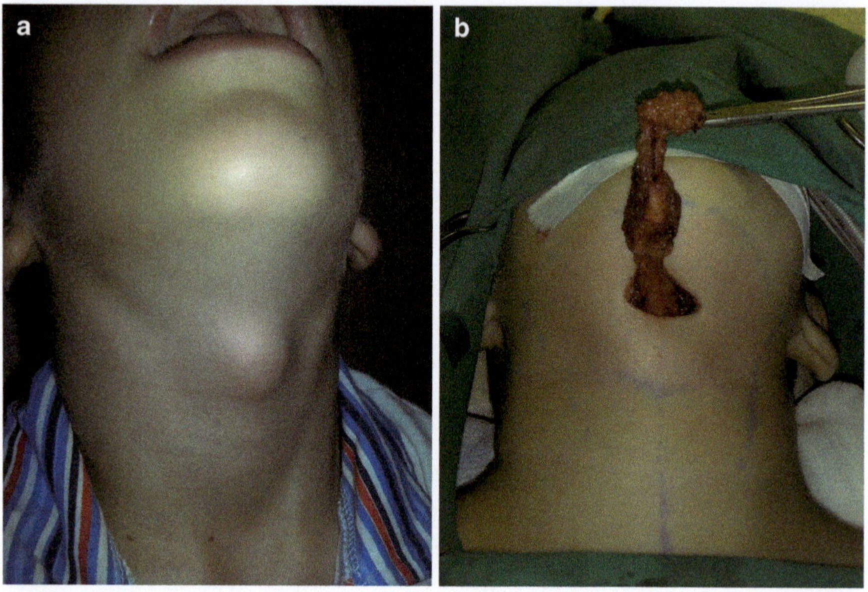

Fig. 11.6 Thyroglosal duct cyst excision: (**a**) preoperative view; (**b**) complete excision by Sistrunk procedure

occur in 10–16% of cases [23, 24]. Histologically, TGDCs are lined by respiratory and/or squamous epithelium [20, 24]. It is important to rule out the ectopic thyroid gland (sometimes the TGDC can occur within the thyroid gland) [24]. Malignant alteration is present in 1% of cases (papillary thyroid carcinoma, squamous cell carcinoma) [19, 23, 24].

Imaging includes US, CT, or MRI, and sometimes thyroid scintigraphy and screening of thyroid-stimulated hormone TSH are indicated [23, 26, 30]. Differential diagnosis includes dermoid cyst, epidermoid cyst, lymph node, lipoma, and thyroid adenoma [23, 24, 26, 30].

Treatment is surgical excision by the Sistrunk procedure [2, 23, 24, 26]. After identification of cyst, the channel is followed up to the hyoid bone, excision of the hyoid bone is performed, and the tract is ligated near its proximal origin (Fig. 11.6a, b) [2, 23, 30]. Complications of the procedure include bleeding, hematoma, and infection [23, 24]. Recurrence is reported in range of 2.6–5% (and up to 47%), and "extended" Sistrunk procedure should be performed in that case [2, 19, 22, 24, 26, 30]. There are also reports of successful treatment of TGDC with 99% sterile ethanol [21].

11.2.4.2 Branchial Arch Anomalies

Branchial arch anomalies (BAA) present 20–30% of the excised cervical masses in children, and they are the most common lateral neck masses [19, 26]. Branchial anomalies (BAs) can present as cyst (80%), sinus, or fistula, and they result from the maldevelopment of the branchial apparatus which consists of grooves-ectoderm, arches-mesoderm, and pouches-endoderm during the embryonic period [2, 26, 27,

30]. BAs are typically present in infancy and childhood, but it can be diagnosed for the first time at any age with males and females equally affected [19, 27, 28, 30].

Diagnosis is made in more than half of cases by anamnestic data and physical examination, and sometimes additional radiographic studies are needed [9, 27]. On histology, first arch BAs are lined with squamous epithelium, and the second and third arch anomalies are composed of squamous and respiratory epithelium [19, 27, 29, 30]. US, CT, MRI, fistulography, and direct laryngoscopy are the diagnostic tools used for BAAs, and definitive treatment is surgical [19, 27–30].

Second BAAs present 70–95% of all BAs [2, 9, 19, 26, 28, 30]. The second BA forms the hyoid bone and the adjacent structures, and the second pouch-endodermal layer forms the epithelium of palate tonsil and the supratonsillar fossae [19, 26]. The majority of SBAAs are cyst (divided into four types by Bailey) [30]. Treatment of the second BAA cysts is surgical (Fig. 11.7a–c) [27, 28]. Second BAA can form

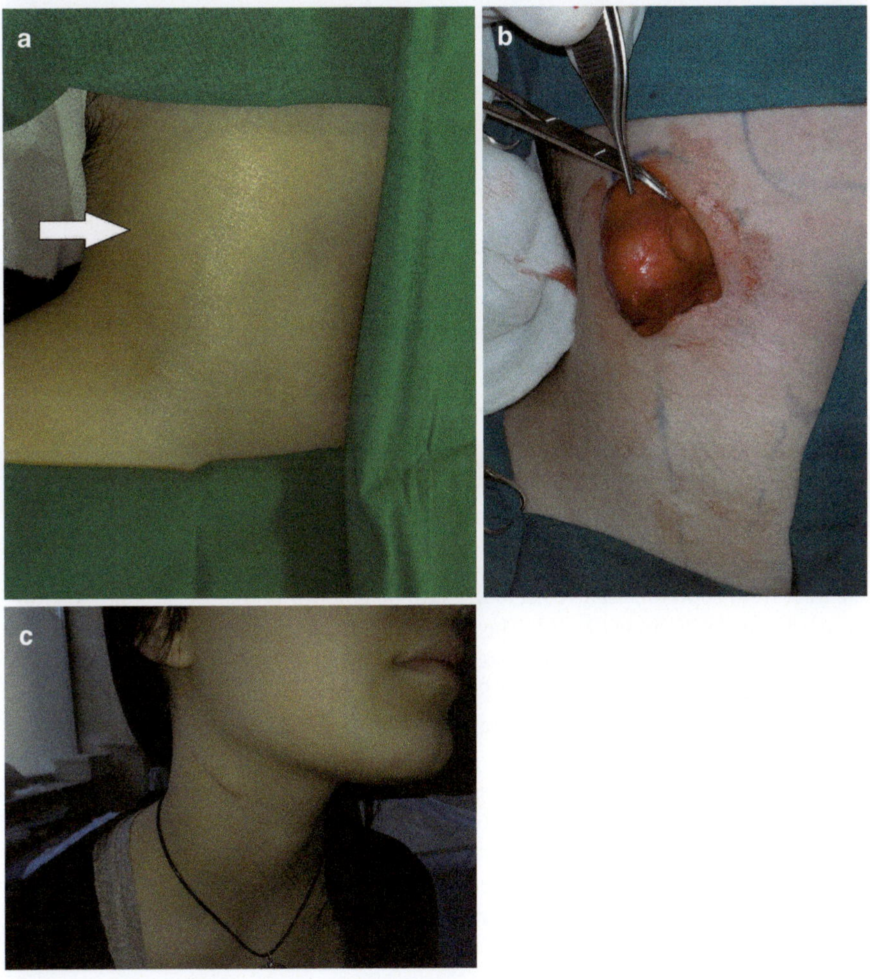

Fig. 11.7 Second branchial arch cyst excision: (**a**) preoperative view of the right lateral neck region; (**b**) excision of the cyst; (**c**) acceptable scar 2 months postoperatively

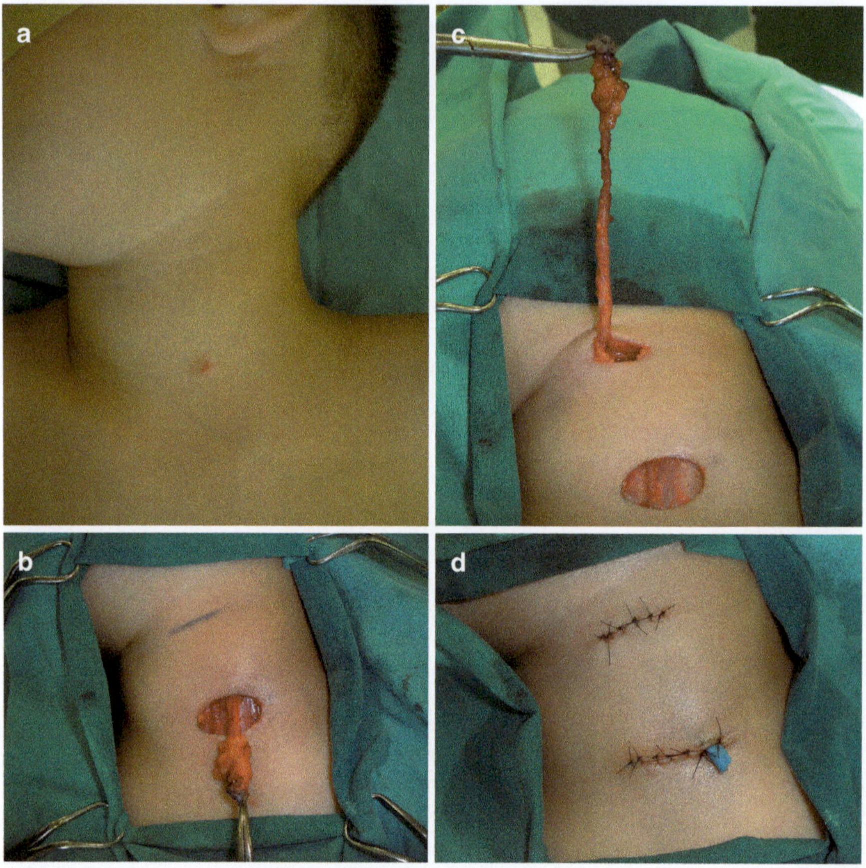

Fig. 11.8 Second branchial arch fistula excision: (**a**) preoperative view (fistula opening at left side of the neck region); (**b**) complete excision of the fistula through stepladder excision; (**c**) postoperative view

the tract from supratonsillar fossa to the skin on anterior border of the sternocleidomastoid muscle (SCM) [19, 26]. The fistulae of second BA are typically presented at infancy or childhood, and cysts are presented in older age, mostly as nontender, soft mass, deep to anterior border of SCM, manifested after respiratory infection [2, 9, 26]. Excision of fistula can be performed through single or through stepladder incision (Fig. 11.8a–c) [19, 26–28].

First BAAs present 1–8% of branchial cleft anomalies; they are located in proximal part of the neck in parotid region or submandibulary, always superior to the hyoid bone, mostly presented as cysts [2, 18, 19, 26]. Belanky and Medin divide first BAAs into type I, with the tract passing laterally or superiorly to the facial nerve without opening into the external auditory canal and type II with the tract passing superiorly or superomedially to the facial nerve (inconsistent relationship) with opening into external auditory canal, and there is also classification of first BAAs proposed by Work and Arnot [19, 26, 28, 30]. Preauricular cyst and sinus can be misdiagnosed for first BAAs [18]. Treatment of these anomalies is surgical and challenging because of their proximity to the facial nerve (facial nerve palsy is described in 10–40% of cases) [1, 19, 26–28].

Third and fourth BAAs are rarest among brancial arch anomalies with cranial origin at pyriform sinus and with close proximity with the thyroid gland at inferior part [2, 19, 26, 29, 30]. Third and fourth branchial arch anomalies are presented at any age, usually as lateral neck mass or suppurative thyroiditis, and in most cases on the left side [19, 28–30]. They are differentiating by their relationship with the superior laryngeal nerve and common carotid artery, by their opening at the pyriform sinus, and by the presence of thymic and thyroid tissue [28, 29]. Diagnostic tools include US, barium swallow, CT, and MRI [2, 27, 28, 30]. Complete excision is golden standard with chemocauterization of pyriform fossa sinuses and with hemithyroidectomy in some cases [26, 28–30]. There are also reports of successful treatment by sclerosation of BA cysts with OK-432 [29].

11.2.4.3 Cervical Chondrocutaneous Branchial Remnants (CCBRs)

Cervical chondrocutaneous branchial remnants (CCBRs) are rare congenital, benign neck anomalies arising from branchial arch, probably from remnants of the first or second arch [31–33]. They are dysgenetic tumors (choristomas) originating from dislocated tissue and always have central cartilages, elastic or hyaline (Fig. 11.9a, b) [31, 32]. CCBRs are rare in contrast to the similar preauricular tags; they do not communicate with other structures of the neck, and approximately one third have associated anomalies [9, 31–33]. The treatment of choice is complete surgical excision [9, 18, 32].

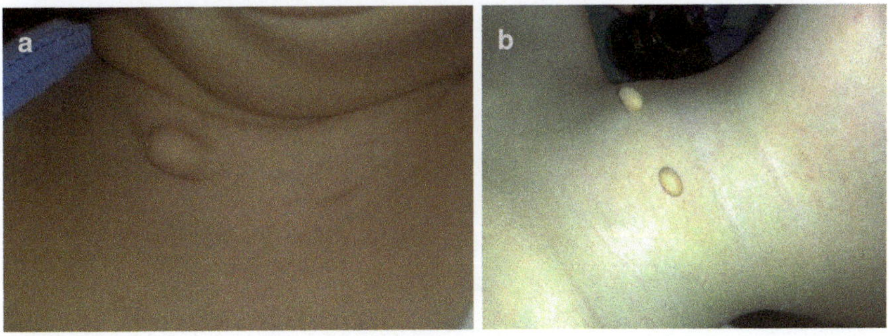

Fig. 11.9 Chondrocutaneous branchial remnant: (**a**) unilateral; (**b**) bilateral

11.3 Benign Skin Tumors

11.3.1 Benign Lesions of Epidermal Origin

Epidermal nevi are common hamartomatous lesions, presented as verrucous papulae usually in a linear configuration, mostly on extremities with most lesions consisted of skin-colored to brown papillomatous papules or plaques distributed along Blaschko's lines [2, 34]. The histopathology of epidermal nevus resembles hyperplasia of keratinocytes and skin appendages [34]. Treatment options are topical treatment with corticosteroids, cryotherapy, laser treatment, or surgical excision [2, 34].

11.3.2 Benign Lesions of Dermal Origin

11.3.2.1 Hair Follicles

Epithelioma calcificans is initially described by Malhebrae and Chanentais in 1880, and it is known as pilomatricoma from 1977 [1, 35]. It is derived from the hair follicle matrix cells, and in 40% it occurs under 10 years of life [1, 5, 34, 35]. It is slow-growing, irregularly contoured, mobile, but rock hard mass found in the deep dermis or subcutaneous layer of the skin [2, 3, 34, 35]. A bluish or reddish hue is a key to diagnosis [35]. It is mostly located in head and neck region, followed by the upper extremities and trunk, and there is female predominance [34, 35]. US is the only diagnostic tool needed in most cases [1, 34]. It is often misdiagnosed for epidermoid or dermoid cyst, calcified lymph node, and sebaceous cyst [34, 35]. Surgical excision is treatment of choice with low recurrence rate (1–6%) (Fig. 11.10a, b) [1, 34, 35].

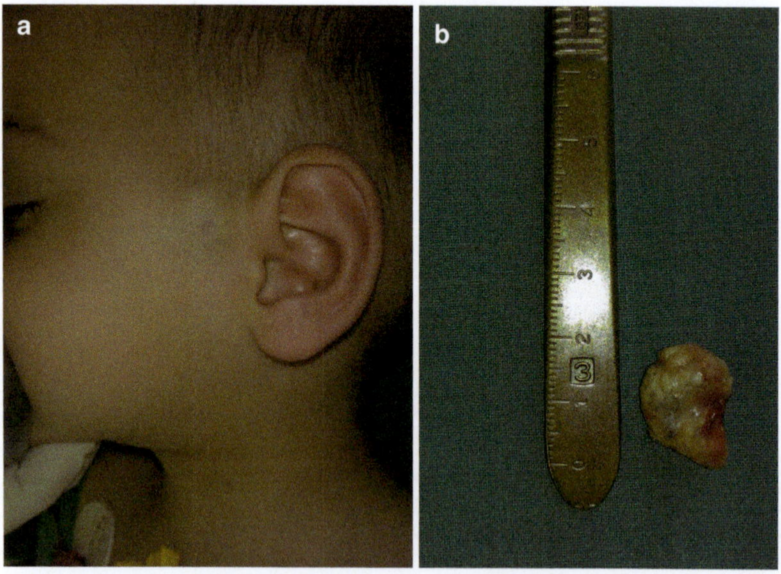

Fig. 11.10 Pilomatricoma excision: (**a**) preoperative view of the left preauricular region; (**b**) complete excision of pilomatricoma

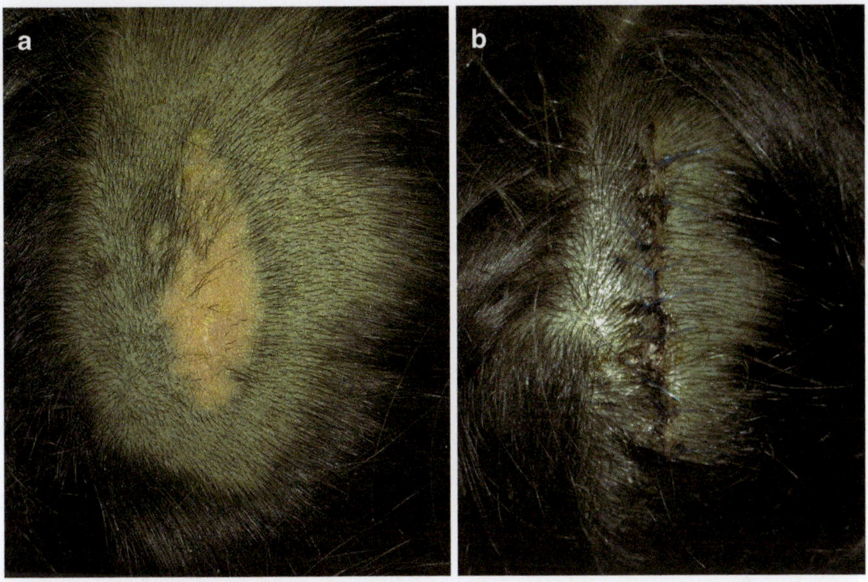

Fig. 11.11 Nevus sebaceous of the scalp: (**a**) preoperative view; (**b**) complete excision

11.3.2.2 Sebaceal Gland Tumors

Nevus sebaceous of Jadassohn is well-defined hairless tan or yellow-orange plaque present on the scalp, head, or neck that occurs sporadically, with similar incidence in males and females [35, 36]. During adolescence the lesion becomes more prominent due to hyperplasia of sebaceous and apocrine glands [36]. Secondary tumors arise within the nevus sebaceous (fortunately malignances are very rare) [2, 34, 36]. The diagnosis of nevus sebaceous is made based on clinical appearance and by histopathological exam (after excision), and differential diagnosis includes epidermal nevus, juvenile xanthogranuloma, and congenital aplasia cutis [35, 36]. Treatment of nevus sebaceous is surgical, especially if there are any irregular areas in lesion (Fig. 11.11a, b) [2, 35, 36].

11.3.2.3 Cysts

Epidermal inclusion cyst is solitary, noncompressible, slow-growing, papular, or nodular lesion, often seen in pediatric population [3, 34]. They are lined by well-differentiated stratified squamous epithelium and enlarged by cellular proliferation and desquamation of keratinized debris into the center of the cyst [2, 10]. A central punctum is a clue to the diagnosis [34]. Rupture of the cyst wall may cause inflammation [2, 3, 34]. Complete excision is treatment of choice [2, 10, 34].

Dermoid cysts arise as nontender, yellowish, subcutaneous nodule that develops along the embryonic lines of closure [2, 37]. According to the classification of New and Erich, dermoid cysts are classified into three pathologic types: acquired implantation (resemble epidermal cysts), congenital teratoma (embryonic germinal epithelium of all three types), and congenital inclusions (dermoid cysts of the head and neck) which are further divided into four anatomical groups, periorbital, dorsum of

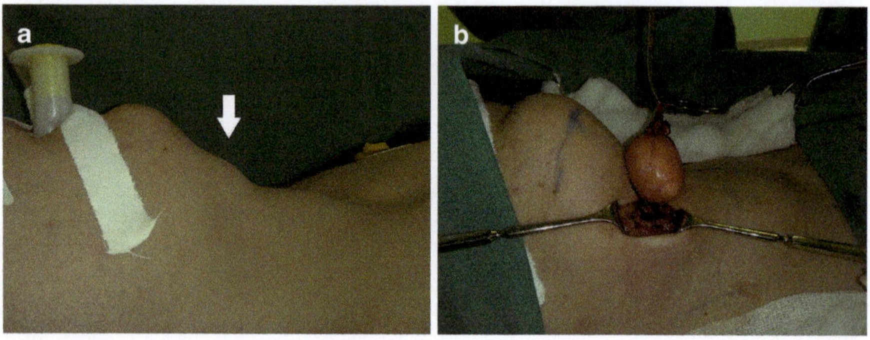

Fig. 11.12 Dermoid cyst of the anterior neck region: (**a**) preoperative view; (**b**) complete excision

the nose, submental region, and suprasternal, thyroidal, and occipital region [2, 10, 37]. Dermoid cysts occur in around 60% of cases on the lateral third of the eyebrow [2, 10, 34, 37]. Because of local growth, there can be pressure erosion of the bone [34]. Dermoid cysts are derived from ectoderm and mesoderm; they are lined by keratinizing squamous epithelium but include dermal structures such as hair follicles, sweat glands, apocrine glands, and sebaceous glands [10, 37]. The lipid material in cysts is derived from sebaceous secretions [2, 10]. Diagnosis is usually made by US, and CT and MRI are used to rule out both intracranial and intraorbital extension [34, 37]. Treatment of choice is early surgical excision, it is site dependent, and it can be open or endoscopic (Fig. 11.12a, b) [10, 34, 37].

11.3.3 Benign Soft Tissue Tumors

Benign soft tissue tumors are classified according to the tissue involved, and there is an updated classification of soft tissue tumors of the World Health Organization (WHO) presented in 2013 [38].

11.3.3.1 Benign Tumors of Fibrous Origin

Pediatric fibroblastic and myofibroblastic tumors are relatively common group of soft tissue proliferation [8, 39, 40]. There are several types of fibromatoses in pediatric population presenting as benign, intermediate-locally aggressive, and intermediate-rarely metastasizing [8, 39, 40]. Infantile myofibroma (solitary, multicentric, or generalized) is the most common fibrous tumor of infancy and lipofibroma, and desmoid fibromatoses are not so common [7–9, 34, 39]. Solitary lesions are erythematous to purple, mobile, rubbery, or firm subcutaneous tumors [9]. Surgical excision is the treatment option if there is complication such as obstruction of vital structures [7–9, 34, 39]. Dermatofibroma (benign fibrous histiocytoma) is a common cutaneous nodule, characterized by proliferation of fibroblast, histiocytes, and vascular endothelial cells, and frequently develops on the lower extremities, and

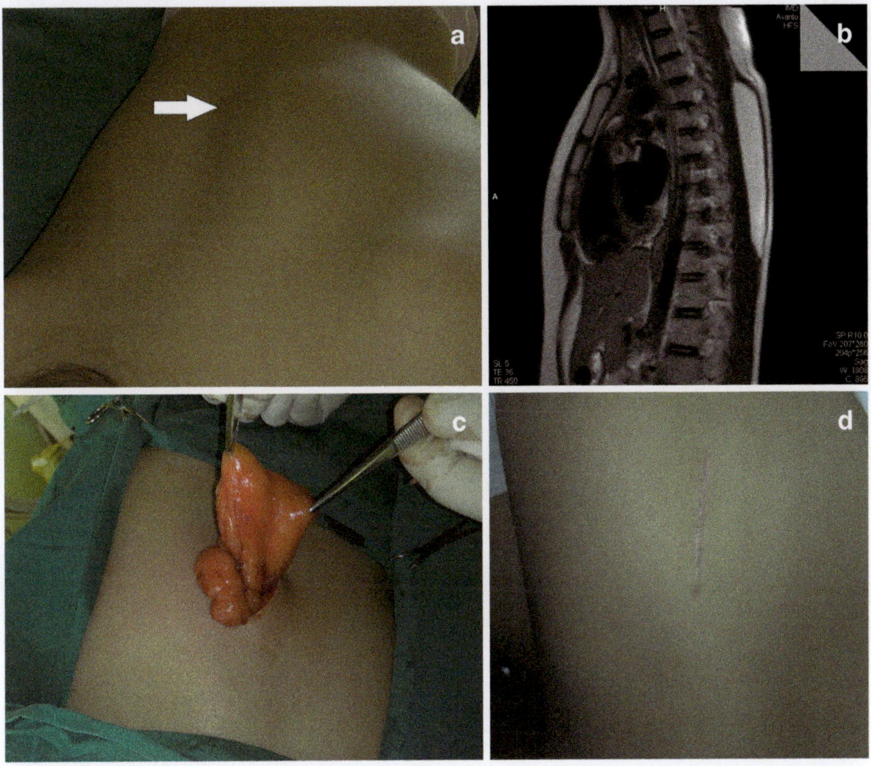

Fig. 11.13 Lipoma excision: (a) preoperative view; (b) magnetic resonance imaging of the dorsum; (c) intraoperative view; (d) postoperative result

excision is rarely indicated [2, 41]. Juvenile xanthogranuloma mostly occurs in pediatric population as infantile and adolescent/adult type [41].

11.3.3.2 Benign Tumors of Fat Origin

Lipoma is relatively uncommon benign tumor in pediatric population, consisting of mature adipose cells [3, 8, 34]. They most commonly arise at puberty as well as circumscribed, solitary, or multiple lesions, localized within the subcutaneous or deeper tissues, preferentially on the neck, shoulders, back, and abdomen [2, 8, 34]. Treatment is surgical excision with the pseudocapsule (Fig. 11.13a–d) [2, 8].

11.3.3.3 Benign Tumors of Muscle Origin

Leiomyoma (cutaneous or subcutaneous) is a tumor that is derived from the smooth muscles in the skin, including the arrector muscle of the hair and vascular smooth muscle, and rhabdomyoma is benign tumor of the striated muscle that occurs in children as fetal rhabdomyomas [1, 2, 8].

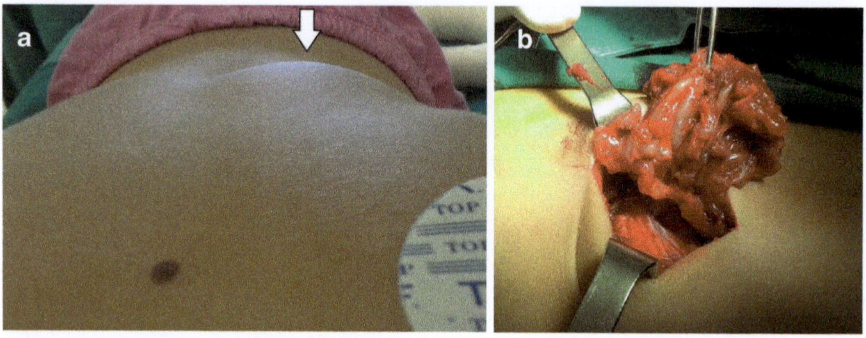

Fig. 11.14 Plexiform neurofibroma: (**a**) tumor of the left dorsal region; (**b**) complete excision

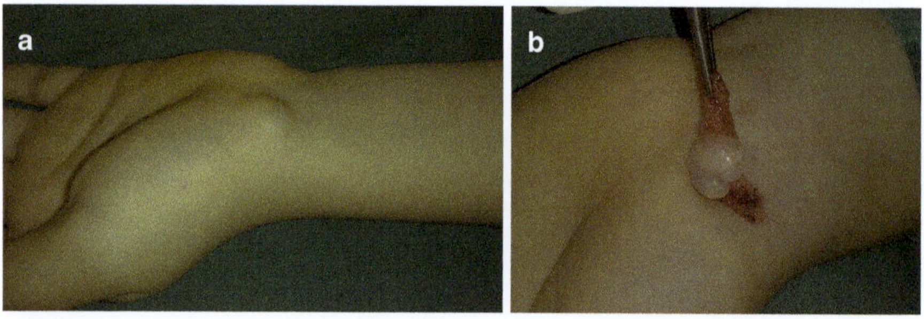

Fig. 11.15 Ganglion of the right radiocarpal region excision: (**a**) preoperative view; (**b**) intraoperative view

11.3.3.4 Benign Tumors of Nerve Sheath

They rise in anatomical nerve route and usually lead to nerve function disorder [2, 3, 8, 42]. The two most common peripheral nerve sheath tumors are neurofibroma (NF) and schwannoma [7, 42]. Neurofibromas arise from the connective tissue of peripheral nerve sheaths (composed of Schwann cells, fibroblasts, mast cells, and perineural cells), and they can appear as localized, diffuse, and plexiform neurofibromas (16–40% of patients with NF) (Fig. 11.14a, b) [1–3, 7, 8]. Plexiform neurofibromas are associated with neurofibromatosis I [7, 42]. Shwannomas and granular cell tumor are rarely seen in children [1, 7, 8].

11.3.3.5 Benign Tumor of Synovial Tissue

Ganglion is cystic swelling containing gel-like material, overlying a joint capsule, ligament, tendon sheaths, or a bone [43–46]. Pathogenesis is unclear but is most probably because of mucin production as a reaction to stress [46]. It is a common lesion in pediatric population with unknown incidence [43–46]. Unlike in adults a majority of ganglion cyst in children is found in volar aspect [44, 45]. US is the first imaging modality and an MRI can also be used [45]. Open surgical excision offers significantly lower chance of recurrence compared with aspiration in the treatment of wrist ganglions (Fig. 11.15a, b) [43, 44].

11.4 Infective Lesions

11.4.1 Hidradenitis Suppurativa

Hidradenitis suppurativa is a chronic, recurrent, inflammatory disease that affects apocrine gland-bearing sites [47, 48]. This is a disease of follicular unit involving aberrant cutaneous cellular immunity likely in response commensal bacteria; deep dermal, painful abscesses ultimately heal leaving fibrosis and induration of the skin [18, 47, 48]. HS can have a significant influence on a qualiy of life [47–49]. It is very rare among the children under 10 years of age, (less than 2% of all cases are

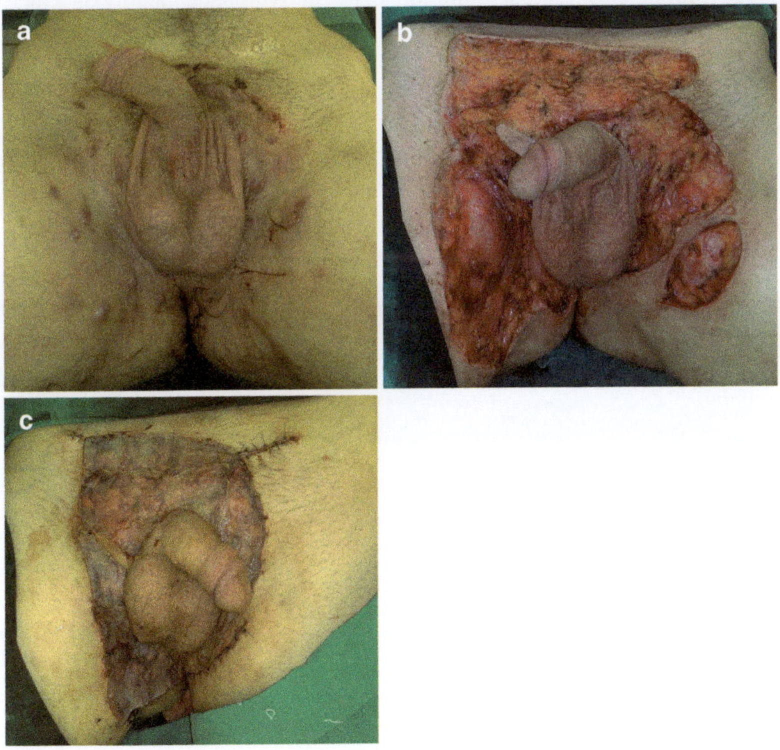

Fig. 11.16 Severe hidradenitis of the pubic and anogenital region: (**a**) preoperative view; (**b**) complete excision of the lesion; (**c**) defect reconstruction with split-thickness skin graft placement

pediatric) with 2:1 female to male ratio [47, 49]. Diagnosis of HS is made by clinical appearance with the groin and axilla as most affected regions [48, 49]. There is classification by Hurley into three stages according to extent of the disease in the tissue [49]. The treatment depends on the severity of the disease, and it includes conservative treatment (chlorhexidine wash, azelaic acid, clindamycin 1% lotion, or solution), antibiotics (clindamycin, doxycycline, rifampicin), anti-inflammatory agents, CO_2 laser, and surgery (Fig. 11.16a–c) [47–49].

11.4.2 Lymphadenopathy

Cervical lymphadenopathy is common among pediatric population [50–52]. Bacterial lymphadenitis is usually acute and unilateral; *Staphylococcus aureus* and *Streptococcus agalactiae* and pyogenes are the most common causative organisms, and submandibular nodes are affected in 50% of patients [1, 50, 51]. Diagnostic includes blood tests, imaging (US, CT, MRI), and fine needle aspiration biopsy (FNAB) or open biopsy (which is golden standard; largest node should be excised) [50, 51]. Near one third of acutely infected lymph nodes suppurate requiring incision and drainage [1]. Most common cervical lymphadenopathy is caused by

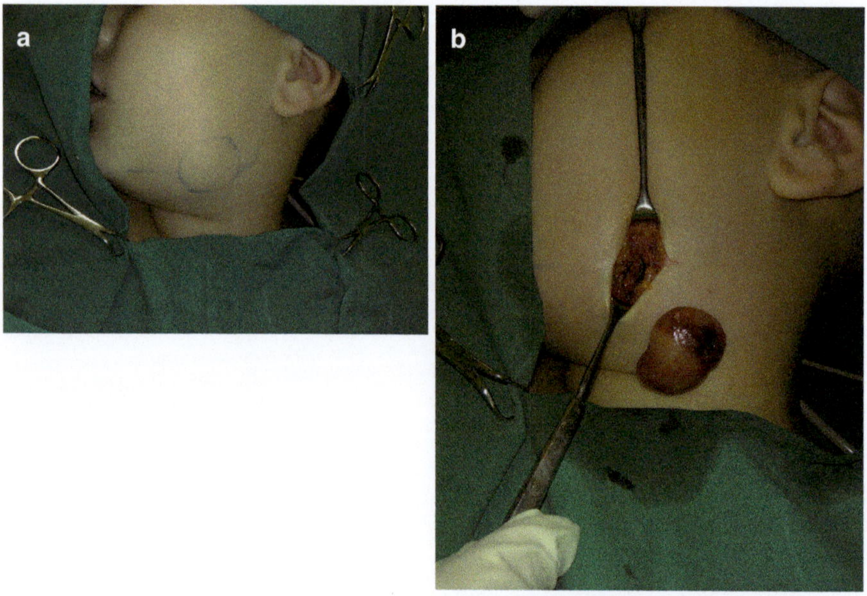

Fig. 11.17 Neck lymphadenopathy: (**a**) preoperative view; (**b**) excision of the submandibular lymph node

bacterial or viral infection, but also atypical mycobacterial infection, infectious mononucleosis, and cytomegalovirus have to be considered in differential diagnosis [50]. Differential diagnosis includes wide spectrum of benign and malignant causes (Fig. 11.17a, b) [1, 50, 51].

Cat scratch disease is the most common cause of chronic regional lymphadenopathy affecting the head and neck region in children caused by *Bartonella henselae* [1, 3, 50–53]. Lymphadenopathy is mostly localized on the upper extremity followed by the neck and jaw [53]. Antibiotic therapy and surgical excision are treatment options in symptomatic patients [1, 53].

References

1. Kapur S, Bentz ML. Pediatric tumors. In: Neligan PC, Gurtner GC, editors. Plastic surgery. St Louis: Elsevier; 2013. p. 877–92.
2. Ogawa R. Benign and malignant nonmelanocytic tumors of the skin and soft tissue. In: Neligan PC, Gurtner GC, editors. Plastic surgery. St Louis: Elsevier; 2013. p. 707–42.
3. Beaman FD, Kransdorf MJ, Andrews TR, Murphey MD, Arcara LK, Keeling JH. Superficial soft-tissue masses: analysis, diagnosis, and differential considerations. Radiographics. 2007;27(2):509–23.
4. Brisse HJ, Orbach D, Klijanienko J. Soft tissue tumours: imaging strategy. Pediatr Radiol. 2010;40(6):1019–28.
5. Knight PJ, Reiner CB. Superficial lumps in children: what, when, and why? Pediatrics. 1983;71(2):147–53.
6. Vacanti JP, Cusick RA. Tumors of soft tissues. In: O'Neill JA, Rowe MI, Grosfeld JL, Fankalsrud EW, Coran AG, editors. Pediatric surgery. St Louis: Mosby; 1998. p. 1911–24.
7. Laor T. MR imaging of soft tissue tumors and tumor-like lesions. Pediatr Radiol. 2004;34(1):24–37.
8. Thacker MM. Benign soft tissue tumors in children. Orthop Clin North Am. 2013;44(3):433–44.
9. Farvolden D, Sweeney SM, Wiss K. Lumps and bumps in neonates and infants. Dermatol Ther. 2005;18(2):104–16.
10. Tranvinh E, Yeom KW, Iv M. Imaging neck masses in the neonate and young Infant. Semin Ultrasound CT MR. 2015;36:120–37.
11. Penner CR, Thompson L. Nasal glial heterotopia: a clinicopathologic and immunophenotypic analysis of 10 cases with a review of the literature. Ann Diagn Pathol. 2003;7(6):354–9.
12. Rahbar R, Shah P, Mulliken JB, Robson CD, Perez-Atayde AR, Proctor MR, et al. The presentation and management of nasal dermoid: a 30-year experience. Arch Otolaryngol Head Neck Surg. 2003;129(4):464–71.
13. Herrington H, Adil E, Moritz E, Robson C, Perez-Atayde A, Proctor M, Rahbar R. Update on current evaluation and management of pediatric nasal dermoid. Laryngoscope. 2016;126(9):2151–60.
14. Hartley BE, Eze N, Trozzi M, Toma S, Hewitt R, Jephson C, Cochrane L, Wyatt M, Albert D. Nasal dermoids in children: a proposal for a new classification based on 103 cases at Great Ormond Street Hospital. Int J Pediatr Otorhinolaryngol. 2015;79(1):18–22.
15. Rahbar R, Resto VA, Robson CD, Perez-Atayde AR, Goumnerova LC, McGill TJ, Healy GB. Nasal glioma and encephalocele: diagnosis and management. Laryngoscope. 2003;11(12):2069–77.

16. Lam S, Barry J, Dauser RC. Dermal sinus tract: clinical presentation and imaging findings. Pediatr Neurol. 2014;51(5):747–8.
17. Tisdall MM, Hayward RD, Thompson DN. Congenital spinal dermal tract: how accurate is clinical and radiological evaluation? J Neurosurg Pediatr. 2015;15(6):651–6.
18. Nofsinger YC, Tom LW, LaRossa D, Wetmore RF, Handler SD. Periauricular cysts and sinuses. Laryngoscope. 1997;107(7):883–7.
19. Christison-Lagay E. Complications in head and neck surgery. Semin Pediatr Surg. 2016;25(6):338–46.
20. Hamoir M, Berbheim N, Poorten VV, Chantrain G, Laer CV, Hamans A, Deron P. Initial assessment of neck mass in children. B-ENT. 2005;1(Suppl 1):126–8.
21. Chung MS, Baek JH, Lee JH, Choi YJ, Yoon JH, Nam SY, et al. Treatment efficacy and safety of ethanol ablation for thyroglossal duct cysts: a comparison with surgery. Eur Radiol. 2016; [Epub ahead of print]
22. Pastore V, Bartoli F. “Extended” Sistrunk procedure in the treatment of recurrent thyroglossal duct cysts: a 10-year experience. Int J Pediatr Otorhinolaryngol. 2014;78(9):1534–6.
23. de Tristan J, Zenk J, Künzel J, Psychogios G, Iro H. Thyroglossal duct cysts: 20 years' experience (1992–2011). Eur Arch Otorhinolaryngol. 2015;272(9):2513–9.
24. Thompson LD, Herrera HB, Lau SK. A clinicopathologic series of 685 thyroglossal duct remnant cysts. Head Neck Pathol. 2016;10(4):465–74.
25. Patel NN, Hartley BEJ, Howard DJ. Management of thyroglossal tract disease after failed Sistrunks procedure. J Laryngol Otol. 2003;117:710–2.
26. LaRiviere CA, Waldhausen JH. Congenital cervical cysts, sinuses, and fistulae in pediatric surgery. Surg Clin North Am. 2012;92(3):583–97.
27. Schroeder Jr JW, Mohyuddin N, Maddalozzo J. Branchial anomalies in the pediatric population. Otolaryngol Head Neck Surg. 2007;137(2):289–95.
28. Waldhausen JH. Branchial cleft and arch anomalies in children. Semin Pediatr Surg. 2006;15(2):64–9.
29. Kim MG, Lee NH, Ban JH, Lee KC, Jin SM, Lee SH. Sclerotherapy of branchial cleft cysts using OK-432. Otolaryngol Head Neck Surg. 2009;141(3):329–34.
30. Koch BL. Cystic malformation of the neck in children. Pediatr Radiol. 2005;35:463–77.
31. Begovic N, Simic R, Vlahovic A, Kravljanac D, Djuricic S, Mijovic T. Cervical chondrocutaneous branchial remnants-report of 17 cases. Int J Pediatr Otorhinolaryngol. 2014;78(11):1961–4.
32. Nielsen LJ, Von Rosen K, Jakobsen LP. Cervical chondrocutaneous branchial remnants: a case report. Eplasty. 2016;16:ic17.
33. Klockars T, Kajosaari L. Cervical chondrocutaneous branchial remnants. Cleft Palate Craniofac J. 2017;54(2):223–6.
34. Fogelson SK, Dohil MA. Papular and nodular skin lesions in children. Sem Plast Surg. 2006;20(3):180–91.
35. Price HN, Zaenglein AL. Diagnosis and management of benign lumps and bumps in childhood. Curr Opin Pediatr. 2007;19(4):420–4.
36. Rosen H, Schmidt B, Lam HP, Meara JG, Labow BI. Management of nevus sebaceous and the risk of Basal cell carcinoma: an 18-year review. Pediatr Dermatol. 2009;26(6):676–81.
37. Pryor SG, Lewis JE, Weaver AL, Orvidas LJ. Pediatric dermoid cysts of the head and neck. Otolaryngol Head Neck Surg. 2005;132(6):938–42.
38. Fletcher CD. The evolving classification of soft tissue tumours - an update based on the new 2013 WHO classification. Histopathology. 2014;64(1):2–11.
39. Coffin CM. Fibroblastyc-myofibroblastic tumors. In: Mitchell CW, editor. Pediatric soft tissue tumors, a clinical, pathological, and therapeutic approach. Baltimore: Williams & Wilkins; 1997. p. 133–78.
40. Sargar KM, Sheybani EF, Shenoy A, Aranake-Chrisinger J, Khanna G. Pediatric fibroblastic and myofibroblastic tumors: a pictorial review. Radiographics. 2016;36(4):1195–214.

41. Coffin CM. Fibrohistyocytic tumors. In: Mitchell CW, editor. Pediatric soft tissue tumors, a clinical, pathological, and therapeutic approach. Baltimore: Williams & Wilkins; 1997. p. 179–213.
42. Coffin CM, Dehner LP. Neurogenic tumors of soft tissue. In: Mitchell CW, editor. Pediatric soft tissue tumors, a clinical, pathological, and therapeutic approach. Baltimore: Williams & Wilkins; 1997. p. 80–132.
43. Gude W, Morelli V. Ganglion cyst of the wrist: pathophysiology, clinical picture, and management. Curr Rev Muscoskelet Med. 2008;1:205–11.
44. Simon Cypel TK, Mrad A, Somers G, Zuker RM. Ganglion cyst in children: reviewing treatment and recurrence rates. Can J Plast Surg. 2011;19(2):53–5.
45. Bracken J, Bartlett M. Ganglion cysts in the paediatric wrist: magnetic resonance imaging findings. Pediatr Radiol. 2013;43(12):1622–8.
46. Coffin CM. Synovial based tumors and synovial sarcoma. In: Mitchell CW, editor. Pediatric soft tissue tumors, a clinical, pathological, and therapeutic approach. Baltimore: Williams & Wilkins; 1997. p. 295–310.
47. Liy-Wong C, Pope E, Lara-Corrales I. Hidradenitis suppurativa in the pediatric population. J Am Acad Dermatol. 2015;73(5 Suppl 1):S36–41.
48. Alikhan A, Lynch PJ, Eisen DB. Hidradenitis suppurativa: a comprehensive review. J Am Acad Dermatol. 2009;60(4):539–61.
49. Scheinfeld N. Hidradenitis Suppurativa in prepubescent and pubescent children. Clin Dermatol. 2015;33(3):316–9.
50. Rosenberg TL, Nolder AR. Pediatric cervical lymphadenopathy. Otolaryngol Clin North Am. 2014;47(11):721–31.
51. Brown RE, Harave S. Diagnostic imaging of benign and malignant neck masses in children-a pictorial review. Quant Imaging Med Surg. 2016;6(5):591–604.
52. Locke R, Comfort R, Kubba H. When does an enlarged cervical lymph node in a child need excision? A systematic review. Int J Pediatr Otorhinolaryngol. 2014;78:393–401.
53. Klotz SA, Ianas V, Elliott SP. Cat-scrath disease. Am Fam Physician. 2011;83(2):152–5.

Malignant Skin and Soft Tissue Tumors 12

12.1 Introduction

Malignant skin tumors in pediatric population are extremely rare (1–2% of all skin tumors excised); however the possibility of a malignant soft tissue lesion must be systematically considered [1–7]. Worrisome mass have following risk factors: rapid growth, ulceration, fixation or deep localization on fascia, rough texture, hard structure, size larger than 3 (5) cm, onset in neonate, and high vascularity [1, 5–7].

The most common skin malignancies that affect children are rhabdomyosarcoma (RMS), fibrosarcoma (FS), synovial sarcoma (SS), neuroblastoma (NB), malignant peripheral nerve sheath tumor, and cutaneous lymphomas [1, 2, 6, 7, 8]. Pediatric plastic surgeon can be involved in managing of cervical teratoma, which is mostly histologically benign lesion, but represents significant challenge for treatment [9–11].

Semi-malignant pediatric tumors include fibromatoses, dermatofibrosarcoma protuberans (DFSP), and vascular tumors (hemangioendothelioma and tufted angioma) [1, 12]. Recently there is significant progress made in treatment of malignant lesions in children, with increasing number of survivors [13].

12.2 Rhabdomyosarcoma

Rhabdomyosarcoma (RMS) is a rapidly growing malignant soft tissue tumor of mesenchymal origin (cells committed to becoming skeletal muscle) that rarely involves the skin [2–5, 8, 14–21]. Cutaneous appearance is secondary to extension from the soft tissue into the dermis [5]. It is the most common of the pediatric soft tissue sarcoma, and it accounts for 4–8% of all malignancies in children less than 15 years of age (the peak incidence of RMS is between 1–4 and 2–6 years) [2, 3, 5, 7, 8, 14, 17, 19, 21]. Congenital RMS is extremely rare, and only 0.4% of patients are under 1 month of life [17, 19]. The lesion is in near 40% of cases located in head and neck region, followed by genitourinary tract, and extremities

A.M. Vlahovic, E.Q. Haxhija, *Pediatric and Adolescent Plastic Surgery for the Clinician*, DOI 10.1007/978-3-319-56004-5_12

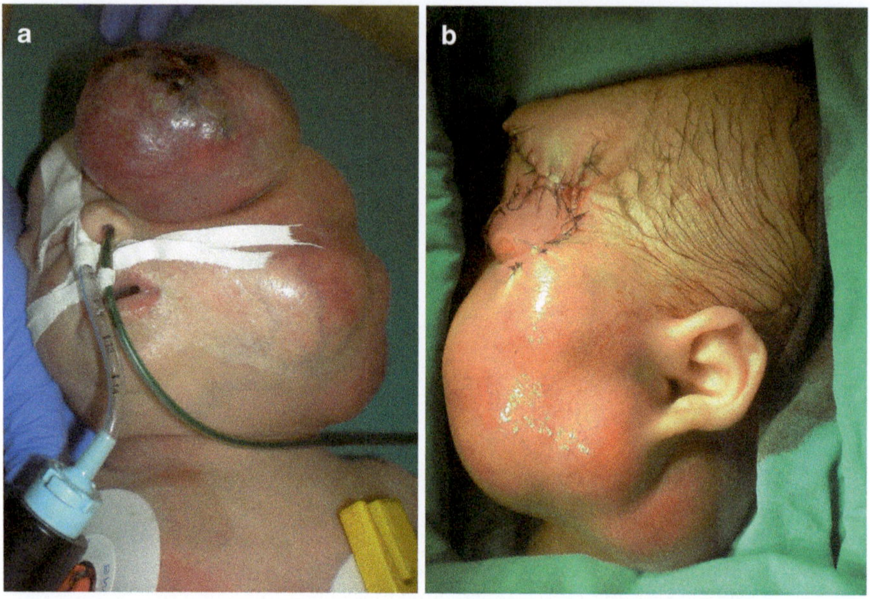

Fig. 12.1 Rhabdomyosarcoma of the head: (**a**) intraoperative view; (**b**) tumor biopsy

[2, 3, 17, 21]. The clinical appearance varies from small cutaneous nodule to an extensive fast-growing tumor (it is often overlooked or misdiagnosed for infection, lymphatic malformation, or hemangioma) [4, 5, 16–18]. There are four groups of RMS according to the Intergroup Rhabdomyosarcoma Study based on whether tumor is localized or metastatic and whether or not it is resectable [2].

Fine needle biopsy, core needle biopsy, and incisional or excisional biopsy are used as diagnostic tools for rhabdomyosarcoma, followed by light microscopic examination, immunohistochemistry, electron microscopy, and cytogenetic analysis [5, 17–19]. Magnetic resonance imaging (MRI) and computerized tomography (CT) are used for tumor and lymph node evaluation [3, 8, 20, 21]. There are three histologic types of RMS: embryonal, alveolar, and undifferentiated (pleomorphic) [2, 3, 8, 17]. Embryonal tumors are found in 80–85% of cases and they mostly occur at birth, and alveolar occurs at adolescent period (worse prognosis) (Fig. 12.1a, b) [2, 3, 15]. RMS can be present in syndromes such as Li-Fraumeni and Beckwith-Wiedemann syndrome [3, 18]. Metastasis of RMS is primarily by hematogenous route [17, 19].

Treatment of RMS includes chemotherapy, radiation therapy, and surgery [2, 3, 5, 8]. Radiotherapy and chemotherapy are treatment of choice for local control of the primary lesion, regression of tumor size, and for unresectable tumors [2, 3, 8, 17]. Primary excision should be attempted only if complete excision can be accomplished without significant consequences, and secondary excision may be considered after chemotherapy [2–4]. Poor prognosis occurs if the diagnosis of RMS is established during infancy or adolescence, if there is alveolar histology, and if there is metastatic disease at the time of presentation [3–5, 8].

12.3 Infantile Fibrosarcoma

Infantile fibrosarcoma (IF) is classified as nonrhabdomyosarcoma malignant mesenchymal tumor (the second most common childhood sarcoma involving the skin), with the incidence of 5 per million infants less than 1 year of age [5, 22, 23].

IF affects children primarily before the age of 2, representing 5–10% of all sarcomas in children younger than 1 year of age, and congenital fibrosarcoma has clinical signs before 3 months of age [22, 23]. In most cases the tumor represents as bulging, locally destructive, rapidly growth mass mostly on the lower extremities and trunk with a very low rate of metastases [5, 20, 22–24]. Skin involvement is usually secondary [5].

Differential diagnosis includes RMS, vascular tumors and malformations, and infections [5, 23]. Surgical removal has remained a primary component of the treatment with adjuvant chemotherapy (preoperatively or postoperatively) (Fig. 12.2a–h) [22, 23]. There is small difference in disease-free survival between the patients who had positive tumor margins and those who did not, meaning that “heroic” surgery should be avoided [22]. The overall 10-year surviving rate is 90% [23].

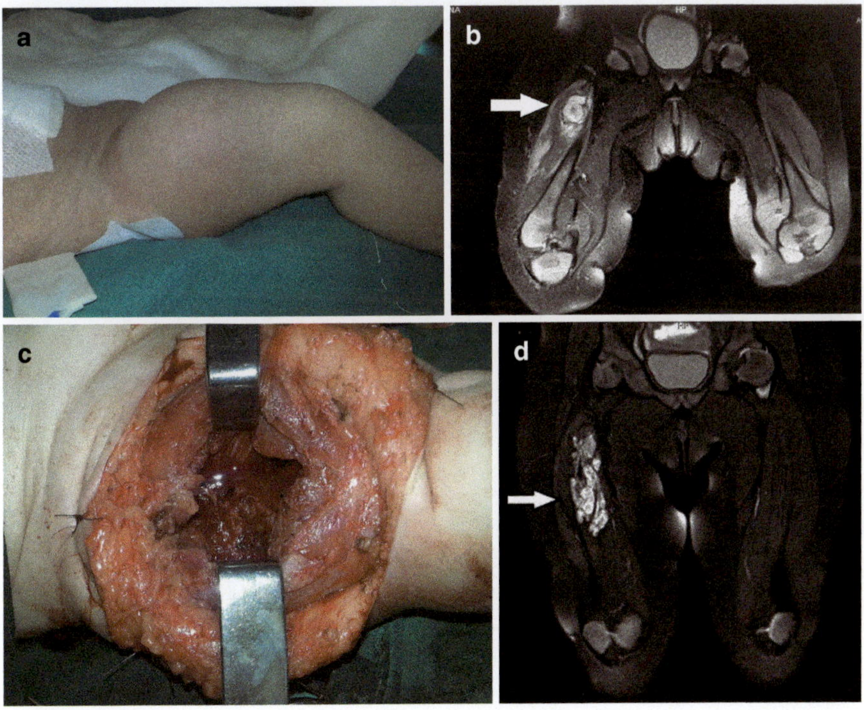

Fig. 12.2 Infantile fibrosarcoma of the right femoral region: (**a**) preoperative view; (**b**) magnetic resonance imaging finding; (**c**) tumor biopsy; (**d**) magnetic resonance imaging finding prior definitive surgery; (**e** and **f**) excision of the tumor; (**g**) 2-year postoperative finding; (**h**) magnetic resonance imaging finding revealing no presence of tumor

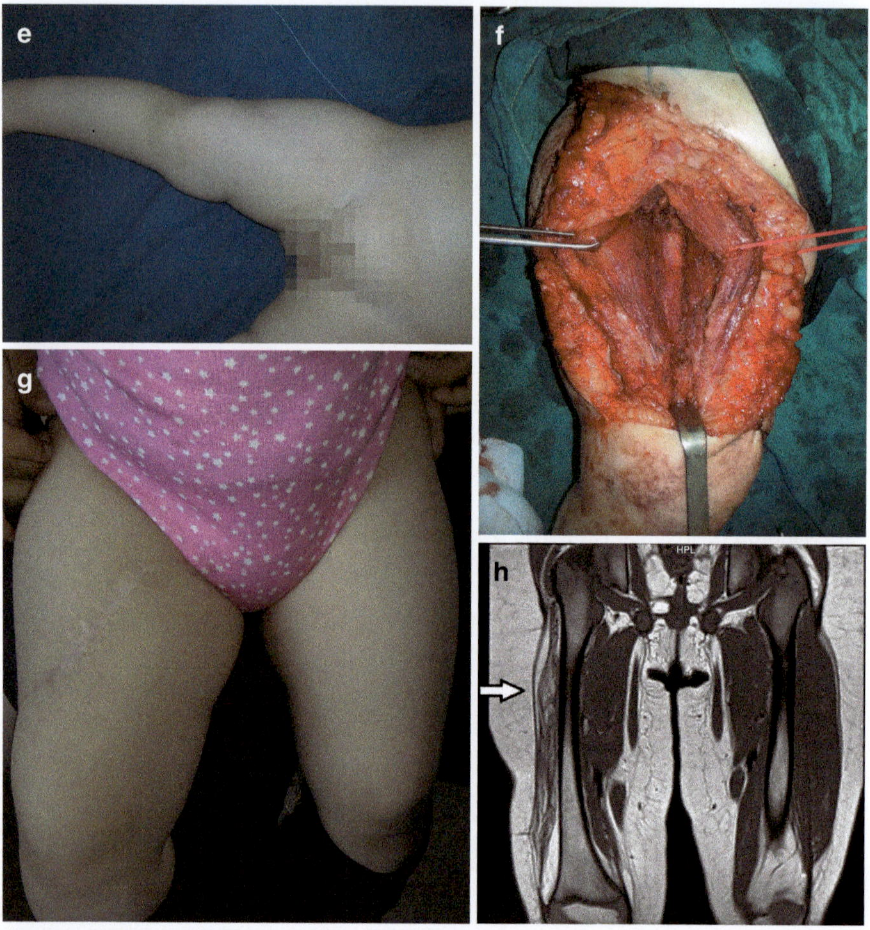

Fig. 12.2 (continued)

12.4 Cervical Teratoma

Teratomas are rare and unusual tumors derived from all three germ cell layers (ectoderm, endoderm, and mesoderm) [9–11, 20, 25]. Congenital teratoma is usually found in sacrococcygeal region, and head and neck region is affected in 5% of cases [9–11, 20]. The incidence is reported to be between 1 in 20,000 and 40,000 live births [9, 10, 20]. The tumors may be diagnosed in the antenatal, perinatal, and postnatal period [11, 25]. Antenatal diagnosis is crucial because it optimizes the preparedness of the clinical personnel in attendance at the delivery of these children to execute whatever intervention is required to secure the airway [9–11, 25]. There is maternal polyhydramnios in near one third of prenatally diagnosed cervical teratoma on routine ultrasonography (US) [10, 11, 25]. Although usually histologically benign, the mortality rate for untreated tumors is 80–100% [10, 11]. The major risk posed by large cervical teratomas is that of neonatal airway obstruction [9, 11, 25].

Multidisciplinary approach is very important for these children [9–11]. Both ex utero intrapartum treatment (EXIT) and operation on placental support (OOPS) procedures have been performed for cervical teratoma to secure the airway [9, 11, 25]. Preoperatively CT scanning or MRI should be performed in stabile patients [11].

Definitive treatment of these tumors is surgical excision, and it should be performed promptly because of respiratory and other complications (Fig. 12.3a–d)

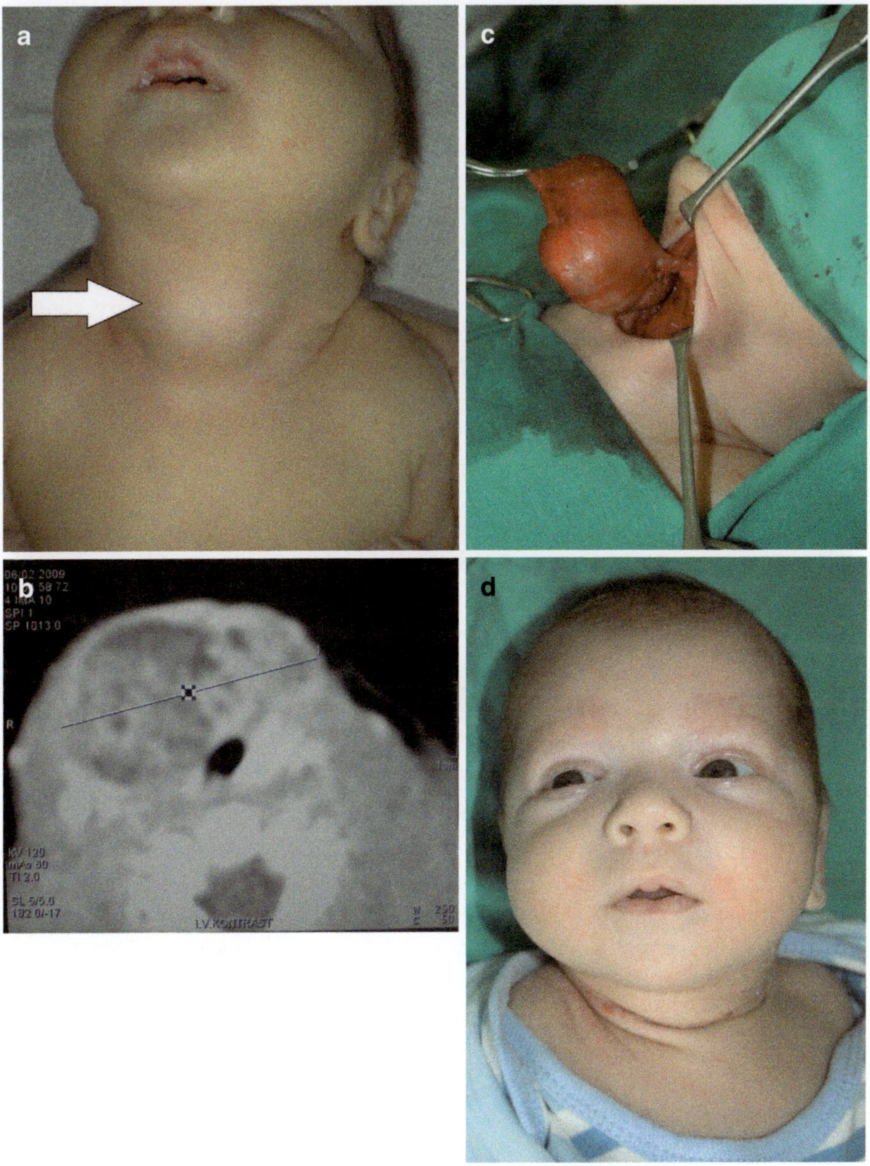

Fig. 12.3 Cervical teratoma: (**a**) preoperative view; (**b**) computerized tomography finding; (**c**) intraoperative view; (**d**) postoperative scar at lower anterior neck region

[9–11, 25]. They are pseudo-encapsulated and should be treated easily, and excision of the thyroid cartilage, pharyngeal wall, and thyroid parenchyma is sometimes required [9–11]. Operative mortality rate nowadays is low, with injury of regional nerves reported postoperatively [11].

12.5 Cutaneous Neuroblastoma

Neuroblastoma (NB) is one of the most common solid malignant tumors in children (50% of malignancies in infants), derived from the primitive neural crest cells of the sympathetic nervous system, with the incidence of 10 per million births [4, 5, 25–27]. NB mostly occurs in the abdomen (80%), and around 5% are primarily located in cervical region [12, 20, 21, 26]. Primary cervical neuroblastoma can be presented with Horner syndrome, cranial nerve palsy IX–XII, heterochromia iridis, and compression of vital cervical organs; diagnosis is made by US, CT, and MRI, and it has favorable prognosis [20]. Primary cutaneous neuroblastoma is extremely rare in children (most commonly there are cutaneous metastases from primary adrenal tumor) presenting as bluish, hard, and painless nodules or papule [1, 5, 12]. After compression there is central pale region "icy blanch" secondary to local catecholamine release [5, 27]. Clinically cervical NB presents as a palpable indolent mass in the lateral neck with compression on vital neck structures [27]. Diagnostic evaluation includes genetic analysis, immunophenotyping, serum and urine catecholamines and lactate dehydrogenase (LDH) levels, and metaiodobenzylguanidine (MIBG) scan (to rule out metastasis) [4, 5, 26, 27]. N-myc amplification with 10 or more copies per haploid genome is considered as highly unfavorable factor [27]. Radiological evaluation including US, MRI, and CT is necessary to evaluate the exact extension of the tumor [5, 21, 26, 27]. Treatment of neuroblastoma includes combination of surgery, chemotherapy, and radiation (Fig. 12.4a, b) [4, 5]. Surgery is the treatment of choice for localized neuroblastoma without N-myc amplification [4, 26, 27].

12.6 Dermatofibrosarcoma Protuberans (DFSP)

Dermatofibrosarcoma protuberans (DFSP) (also called giant cell fibroblastoma and low-grade sarcoma) is a rare soft tissue tumor with low- to intermediate-grade malignancy, characterized by high rates of local recurrence yet low risk of

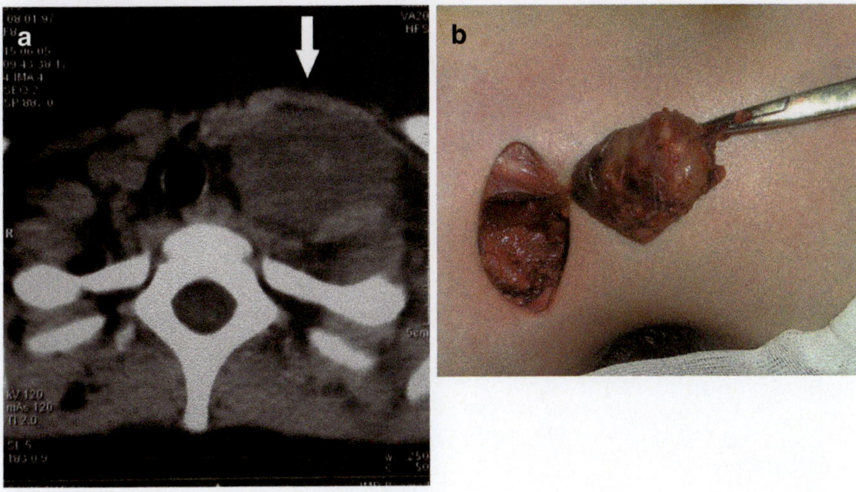

Fig. 12.4 Neuroblastoma metastases, cervical localization: (**a**) preoperative radiological finding; (**b**) tumor excision

metastasis [5, 12, 15, 28]. It is in most cases located on the trunk and the proximal portion of the limbs [4, 5, 12]. Pediatric DFSP is reported between 6 and 20% in literature [4, 12]. DFSP in children demonstrated atypical variations and in that way mimics keloids, vascular anomalies, or fibrosarcoma [4, 12, 15]. The initial presentation of the DFSP is of an asymptomatic, nodular plaque, ranging from 1 to 5 cm, which is fixed to the skin [5, 12]. The main characteristic of DFSP is its capacity to invade surrounding tissue to considerable distance from the central focus of the tumor [12].

The treatment of choice for nonmetastatic DFSP is complete surgical resection (classically or by Mohs micrographic surgery) with margin at least 2–5 cm (Fig. 12.5a–f) [4, 5, 12, 15]. After complete excision, the defect can be reconstructed by direct sutures, skin grafts, and local or distant flaps [5, 12]. Dermatofibrosarcoma protuberans is immunoreactive for CD34 (differentiating from dermatofibroma) and S-100 protein-negative (differentiating from neurofibromas) [4, 5]. The recurrence rate ranges from 0 to 30% and grows with narrower excision border [4, 12]. Radiotherapy should be used in cases of microscopic residual disease or as an adjuvant therapy [12].

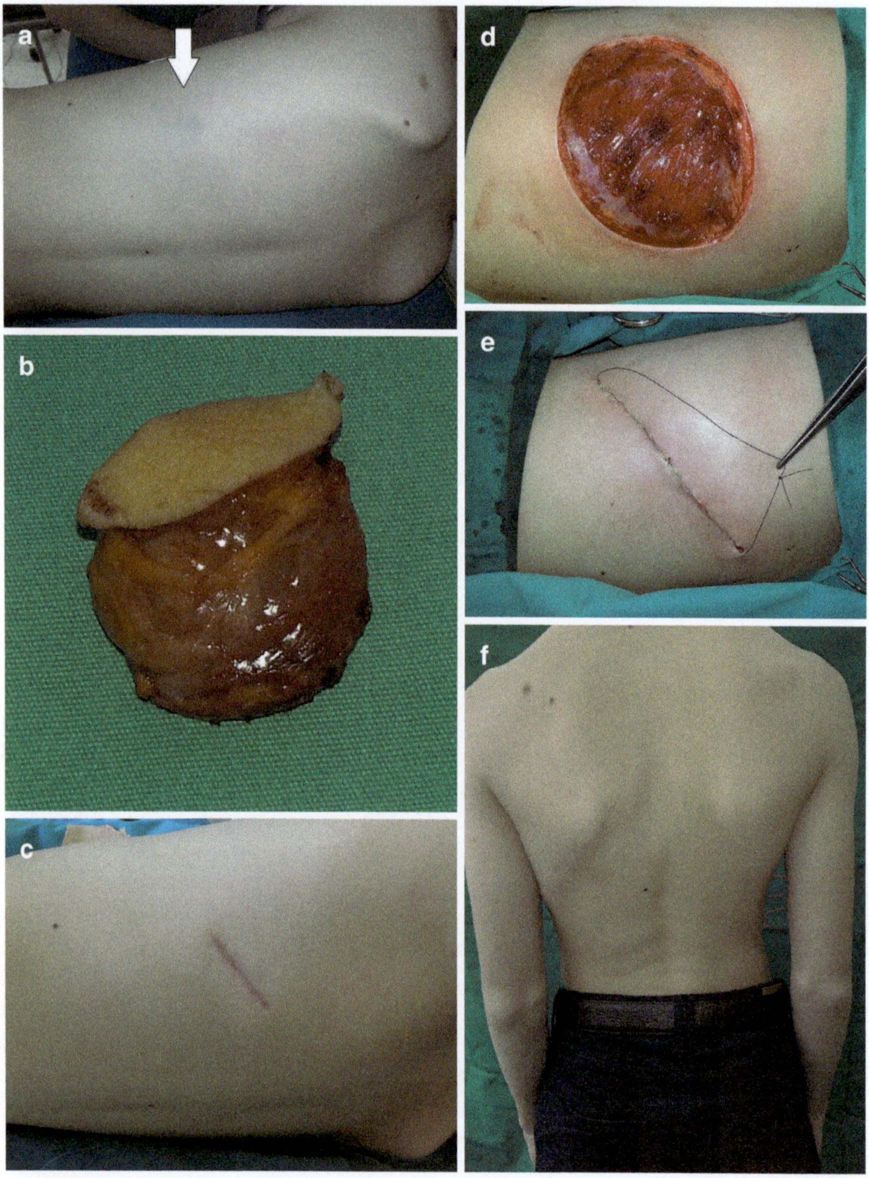

Fig. 12.5 Dermatofibrosarcoma protuberans: (**a**) tumor of left dorsal region; (**b**) tumor excision; (**c**) second excision (tumor presence on the resection margins after first procedure); (**d**) wide excision at second surgical procedure; (**e**) postoperative view; (**f**) 2-year follow up

12.7 Synovial Sarcoma

Synovial soft tissue sarcomas arise from the synovioblastic differentiation of pluripotent mesenchymal stem cells, and they represent 8–10% of all malignant somatic soft tissue neoplasms [3, 8, 29–32]. The incidence per year is 0.7 per million [28]. They are in most cases presented as solitary, well-circumscribed lesions in the upper or lower extremities [3, 8, 27]. They never arise within the joint (since the cells of origin are not synovial) [8, 28].

The most common symptom is a painless mass that has existed for several weeks to years, and there is calcification in up to 30% of cases [3]. The treatment of choice is surgical excision with tumor-free margins of 1–3 cm with adjuvant chemotherapy and radiotherapy depending on initial tumor size, respectability, and primary site (Fig. 12.6a–d) [3, 8, 30, 32]. The overall survival rate with surgery and radiation therapy is shown to be 76% at 5 years and 57% at 10 years [3, 30].

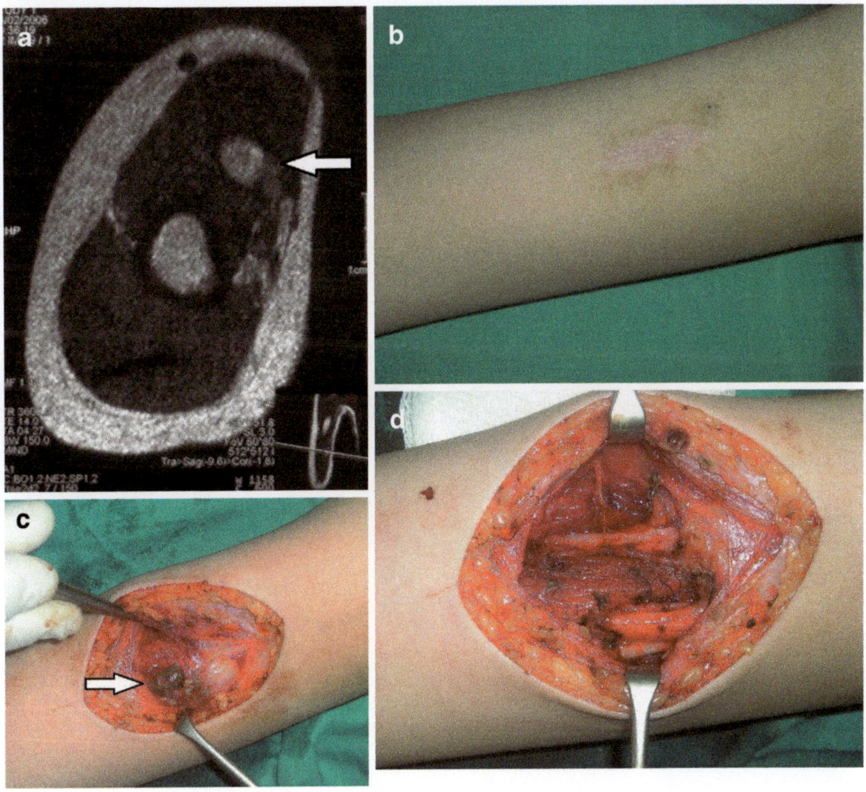

Fig. 12.6 Synovial sarcoma of the right brachial region excision: (**a**) magnetic resonance imaging finding; (**b**) preoperative view (the child was previously treated in other hospitals); (**c** and **d**) excision of tumor

12.8 Lymphoma

Lymphoma is commonly presented as cervical mass [21]. On clinical examination grounds, nodes larger than 2 cm, hard nodes, and supraclavicular nodes along with weight loss, fever, and organomegaly are highly suspected for malignancy [30]. Lymphomas are the most common pediatric cancer, divided into Hodgkin lymphoma (HL) and non-Hodgkin lymphoma (NHL) and further subdivided according to the cell line involved [2, 21, 23, 33–35]. The incidence of Hodgkin lymphoma (HL) is 50 per million; it has a peak of distribution in adolescence and adulthood, and only 5% of tumors occur in children younger than age 10 [2, 35]. There is 2:1 male/female ratio, and near 80% of these patients are present with asymptomatic cervical adenopathy [2]. Staging workup should include blood tests (complete blood count with differential erythrocyte sedimentation rate), renal and hepatic functional tests, alkaline phosphatase, and CT [2, 21, 33]. The hallmark of this disease is the Reed/Sternberg cell [2, 33]. The biopsy is indicated in all patients with Hodgkin disease, treatment is multimodal including chemotherapy and radiation therapy, and cure rate for lymphoma is approaching 90% [2, 33, 35]. NHL is more common in white persons, only 25% of cases occur in children younger than age 10, and there is male predominance (2–3:1) [2, 21]. Tumor grows rapidly, early diagnosis is critical, and NHLs are histologically generally recognized as low, intermediate, and high grade (most tumors in children) [2]. Diagnosis is made by incisional biopsy with a cervical lymph node excision as the preferred method for diagnosis in cases of cervical adenopathy (Fig. 12.7a, b) [2, 21]. Mainstay of treatment is chemotherapy [2, 33].

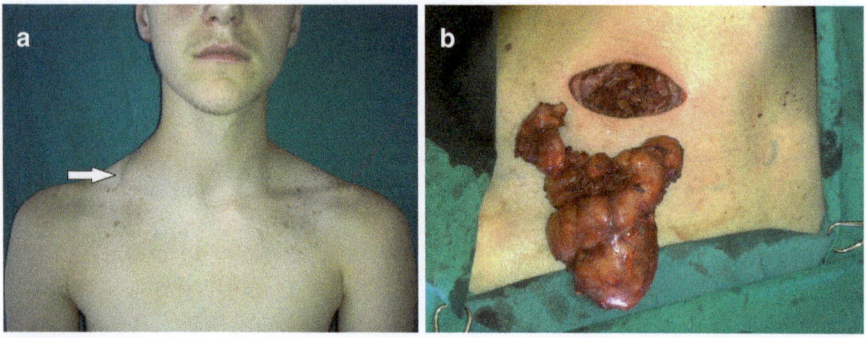

Fig. 12.7 Hodgkin lymphoma: (**a**) preoperative view; (**b**) biopsy of the supraclavicular lymph nodes

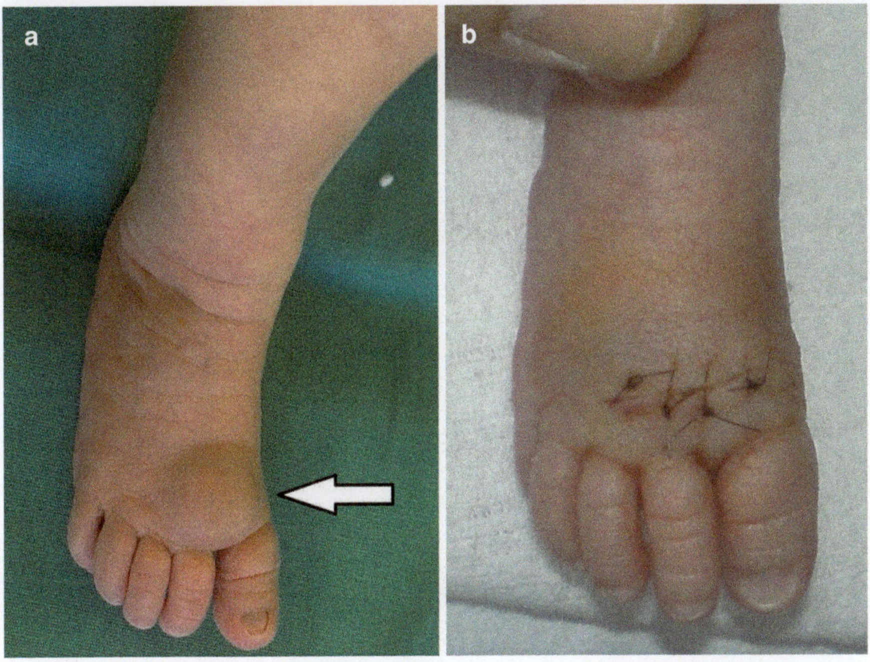

Fig. 12.8 Congenital leukemia cutis: (**a**) tumor of the right foot; (**b**) postoperative view

12.9 Congenital Leukemia Cutis

This is a extremely rare entity, and it encompasses multiple brown-red to violaceous papules and nodules [4, 36]. A skin biopsy or serum complete blood count is necessary to confirm the diagnosis (Fig. 12.8a, b) [4]. Referral should be made to a hematologist/oncologist [4, 36].

12.10 Peripheral Primitive Neuroectodermal Tumor (pPNET)

Primitive neuroectodermal tumor (PNET) is a rare tumor of pluripotent neural crest cells that includes tumors arising from the central nervous system (medulloblastoma) and from the autonomic system (neuroblastoma) [2, 37–39]. Peripheral primitive neuroectodermal tumor (pPNET) is a category of neuroectodermal tumors that involves peripheral tissues and nerves, probably originating from undifferentiated

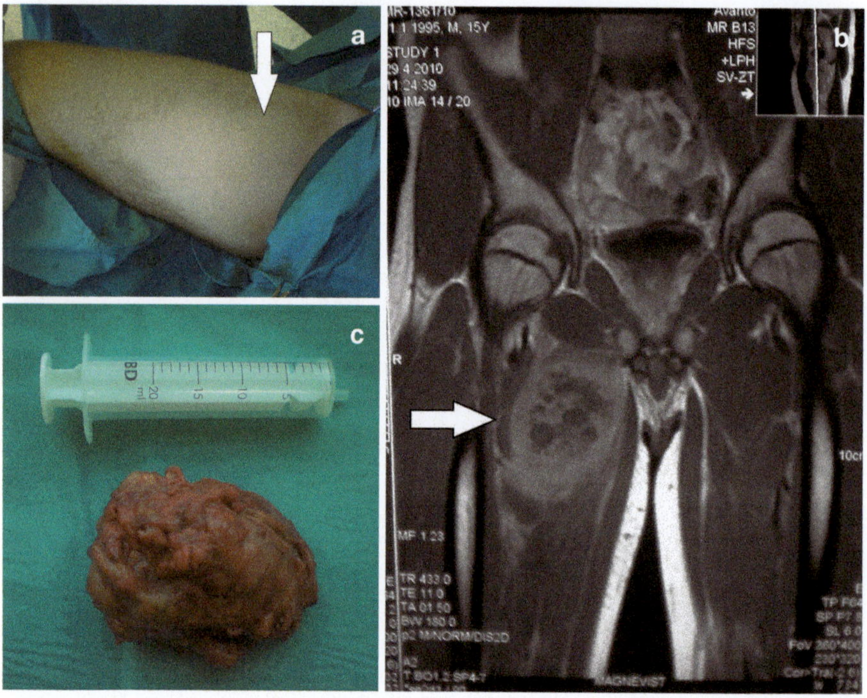

Fig. 12.9 pPNET: (**a**) tumor of the right femoral region tumor; (**b**) preoperative magnetic resonance imaging; (**c**) complete excision of the tumor

mesenchyme, and it represents 1% of all sarcomas [2, 38]. pPNET is considered to be a well-differentiated tumor, while Ewing sarcoma and Askin tumor are poorly differentiated variants [37, 38]. Treatment of pPNET includes multiagent chemotherapy, wide excision, and radiotherapy (Fig. 12.9a–c) [2, 37–39].

12.11 Langerhans Cell Histiocytosis (LCH)

This entity is characterized by abnormal proliferation of clonal CD1a-positive immature dendritic cells—Langerhans cell histiocytosis (LCH) cells, normally found in the epidermis, bone marrow, and lymph nodes [3, 5, 40]. It is one entity with different phases along a continuum, with eosinophilic granuloma representing a solitary type of LCH, Hand-Schüller-Christian disease is considered the chronic disseminated type, and Letterer-Siwe disease represents the acute disseminated type [2, 5, 40]. Nowadays LCH is classified as single-system (SS) or multisystem (MS) and unifocal or multifocal disease [40]. Cutaneous manifestations are seen in a half of patients and often are the first sign of disease (papules, erythematous rash, red nodules or papules) [5, 40]. The most common extracutaneous site of infiltration is the bone (calvarium) [2, 5, 40]. Diagnostic procedures involve biopsy-histology, radiography, CT, MRI, and immunohistochemical staining (accumulating histiocytes are positive for CD1a or langerin) [2, 40]. The prognosis is better in children

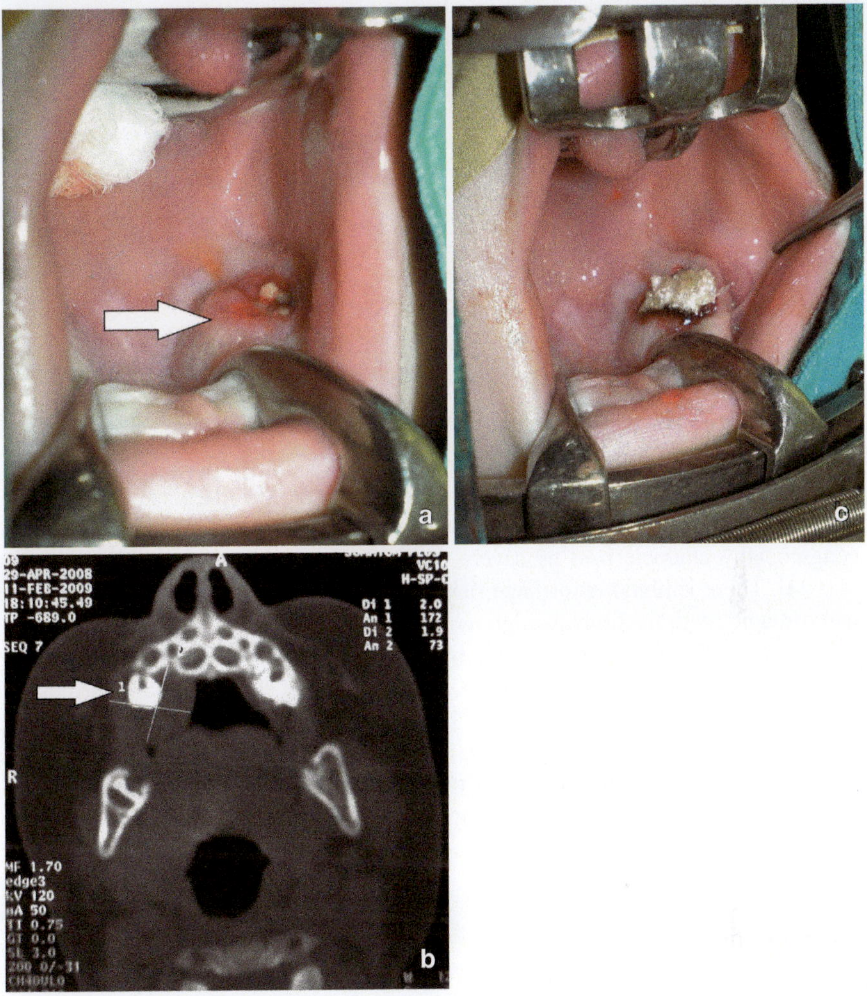

Fig. 12.10 Histiocytosis: (**a**) Intraosseous localization of the lesion; (**b**) magnetic resonance imaging; (**c**) biopsy performed

with SS disease or without risk organ involvement compare to MS disease and risk organ involvement [36]. Therapy includes enucleation, curettage, and resection for solitary self-limited lesions and chemotherapy for systemic involvement (Fig. 12.10a–c) [2, 40].

12.12 Hemangioendothelioma and Tufted Angioma

Kaposiform hemangioendothelioma (KHE) and tufted angioma (TA) are intermediate locally aggressive vascular tumors of infancy and early childhood, thought to be related entities on the same spectrum of disease [8, 20, 41–43]. They often present

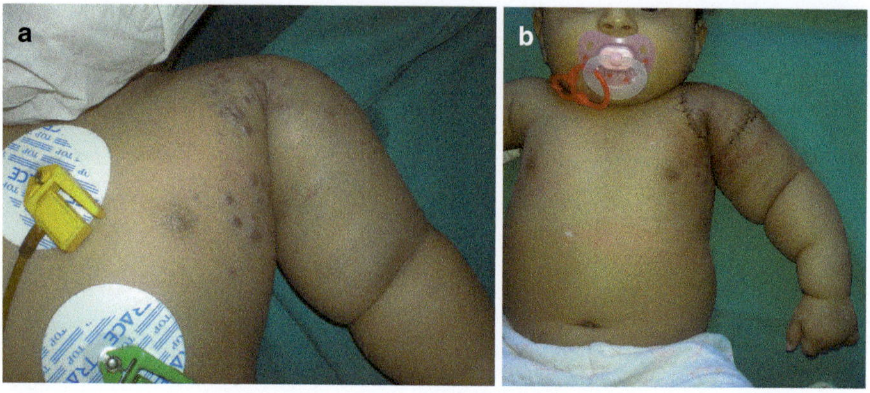

Fig. 12.11 KHE of the left deltoid and brachial region: (**a**) clinical finding; (**b**) tumor biopsy

as solitary, blue-red soft tissue tumors, with poorly defined margins [42, 43]. KHE and TA are associated with Kasabach-Merritt phenomenon (KMP), a consumptive coagulopathy characterized by severe thrombocytopenia and hypofibrinogenemia [41–43]. There is high hemorrhage risk for these children with mortality rate from hemorrhagic complications as high as 30% [5, 16]. Diagnosis is made by clinical and hematologic findings (confirmed by MRI), and biopsy is usually not indicated (Fig. 12.11a, b) [41, 42]. If they are localized, complete surgical excision KHE and TA is the treatment of choice [20, 42, 43]. Since many tumors are unresectable due to location, size, or tissue infiltration, a variety of pharmacologic treatments have been reported in the literature including corticosteroids, interferon-α, vincristine, actinomycin-D, cyclophosphamide, propranolol, and sirolimus with various successful rates [20, 41, 42].

References

1. Hamm H, Höger PH. Skin tumors in childhood. Dtsch Arztebl Int. 2011;108(20):347–53.
2. Qaisi M, Eid I. Pediatric head and neck malignancies. Oral Maxillofac Surg Clin North Am. 2016;28(1):11–9.
3. Kapur S, Bentz ML. Pediatric tumors. In: Neligan PC, Gurtner GC, editors. Plastic surgery. St Louis: Elsevier; 2013. p. 877–92.
4. Farvolden D, Sweeney SM, Wiss K. Lumps and bumps in neonates and infants. Dermatol Ther. 2005;18(2):104–16.
5. Fogelson SK, Dohil MA. Papular and nodular skin lesions in children. Sem Plast Surg. 2006;20(3):180–91.
6. Knight PJ, Reiner CB. Superficial lumps in children: what, when, and why? Pediatrics. 1983;72(2):147–53.
7. Brisse HJ, Orbach D, Klijanienko J. Soft tissue tumours: imaging strategy. Pediatr Radiol. 2010;40(6):1019–28.
8. Thacker MM. Benign soft tissue tumors in children. Orthop Clin North Am. 2013;44:657–67.
9. Sichel JY, Eliashar R, Yatsiv I, Moshe Gomori J, Nadjari M, Springer C, Ezra Y. A multidisciplinary team approach for management of a giant congenital cervical teratoma. Int J Pediatr Otorhinolaryngol. 2002;65(3):241–7.

10. Bergé SJ, von Lindern JJ, Appel T, Braumann B, Niederhagen B. Diagnosis and management of cervical teratomas. Br J Oral Maxillofac Surg. 2004;42(1):41–5.
11. Shine NP, Sader C, Gollow I, Lannigan FJ. Congenital cervical teratomas: diagnostic, management and postoperative variability. Auris Nasus Larynx. 2006;33(1):107–11.
12. Tsai YJ, Lin PY, Chew KY, Chiang YC. Dermatofibrosarcoma protuberans in children and adolescents: clinical presentation, histology, treatment, and review of the literature. J Plast Reconstr Aesthet Surg. 2014;67:1222–9.
13. Jacob LM, Dong W, Chang DW. Outcomes of reconstructive surgery in pediatric oncology patients:review of 10-year experience. Ann Surg Oncol. 2010;17:2563–9.
14. Lim SM, Yoo CJ, Han JW, Cho YJ, Kim SH, et al. Incidence and survival of pediatric soft tissue sarcomas: comparison between adults and children. Cancer Res Treat. 2015;47(1):9–17.
15. Ogawa R. Benign and malignant nonmelanocytic tumors of the skin and soft tissue. In: Neligan PC, editor. Plastic surgery. 3rd ed. St Louis: Elsevier; 2013. p. 707–42.
16. Megarbane H, Doz F, Manach Y, Fletcher C, Jaubert F, de Prost Y, et al. Neonatal rhabdomyosarcoma misdiagnosed as a congenital hemangioma. Pediatr Dermatol. 2011;28(3):299–301.
17. Chigurupati R, Alfatooni A, Myall RW, Hawkins D, Oda D. Orofacial rhabdomyosarcoma in neonates and young children: a review of literature and management of four cases. Oral Oncol. 2002;38(5):508–15.
18. Ojo R, Chen S, Pelaez L, Younis R. Pediatric rhabdomyosarcoma. Ear Nose Throat J. 2014;93(7):248–50.
19. Grundy R, Anderson J, Gaze M, Gerrard M, Glaser A, Gordon A, et al. Congenital alveolar rhabdomyosarcoma. Cancer. 2001;91(3):606–12.
20. Tranvinh E, Yeom KW, Iv M. Imaging neck masses in the neonate and young Infant. Semin Ultrasound CT MRI. 2015;36:120–37.
21. Brown RE, Harave S. Diagnostic imaging of benign and malignant neck masses in children-a pictorial review. Quant Imaging Med Surg. 2016;6(5):591–604.
22. Sulkowski JP, Raval MV, Browne M. Margin status and multimodal therapy in infantile fibrosarcoma. Pediatr Surg Int. 2013;29(8):771–6.
23. Orbach D, Brennan B, De Paoli A, Gallego S, Mudry P, et al. Conservative strategy in infantile fibrosarcoma is possible: the European paediatric soft tissue sarcoma study group experience. J Cancer. 2016;57:1–9.
24. Coffin CM. Fibroblastic-myofibroblastic tumors. In: Mitchell CW, editor. Pediatric soft tissue tumors, a clinical, pathological, and therapeutic approach. Baltimore: Williams & Wilkins; 1997. p. 133–78.
25. Alexander VR, Manjaly JG, Pepper CM, Ifeacho SN, Hewitt RJ, Hartley BE. Head and neck teratomas in children-a series of 23 cases at Great Ormond Street Hospital. Int J Pediatr Otorhinolaryngol. 2015;79(12):2008–14.
26. Moukheiber AK, Nicollas R, Roman S, Coze C, Triglia JM. Primary pediatric neuroblastic tumors of the neck. Int J Pediatr Otorhinolaryngol. 2001;60(2):155–61.
27. Haddad M, Triglia JM, Helardot P, Couanet D, Gauthier F, Neuenschwander S, et al. Localized cervical neuroblastoma: prevention of surgical complications. Int J Pediatr Otorhinolaryngol. 2003;67(12):1361–7.
28. Coffin CM. Fibrohistiocytic tumors. In: Mitchell CW, editor. Pediatric soft tissue tumors, a clinical, pathological, and therapeutic approach. Baltimore: Williams &Wilkins; 1997. p. 179–213.
29. Laor T. MR imaging of soft tissue tumors and tumor-like lesions. Pediatr Radiol. 2004;34(1):24–37.
30. Coffin CM. Synovial based tumors and synovial sarcoma. In: Mitchell CW, editor. Pediatric soft tissue tumors, a clinical, pathological, and therapeutic approach. Baltimore: Williams & Wilkins; 1997. p. 295–310.
31. Soole F, Maupain C, Defachelles AS, Taque S, Minard-Colin V, Bergeron C, De Rycke Y, Orbach D. Synovial sarcoma relapses in children and adolescents: prognostic factors, treatment, and outcome. Pediatr Blood Cancer. 2014;61(8):1387–93.
32. Stanelle EJ, Christison-Lagay ER, Healey JH, Singer S, Meyers PA, La Quaglia MP. Pediatric and adolescent synovial sarcoma: multivariate analysis of prognostic factors and survival outcomes. Ann Surg Oncol. 2013;20(1):73–9.

33. La Quaglia MP. Non-Hodgkin's lymphoma and Hodgkin's disease in childhood and adolescence. In: O'Neill JA, Rowe MI, Grosfeld JL, Fankalsrud EW, Coran AG, editors. Pediatric surgery. St Louis: Mosby; 1998. p. 461–81.
34. Locke R, Comfort R, Kubba H. When does an enlarged cervical lymph node in a child need excision? A systematic review. Int J Pediatr Otorhinolaryngol. 2014;78:393–401.
35. Freed J, Kelly KM. Current approaches to the management of pediatric Hodgkin lymphoma. Pediatr Drugs. 2010;12(2):85–98.
36. Jandali S, Kirschner RE. Congenital leukemia cutis presenting as multiple violaceous lesions in a newborn. Ann Plast Surg. 2011;66(3):310–2.
37. Jurgens H, Bier V, Harms D, Beck J, Brandies W, et al. Malignant peripheral neuroectodermal tumors a retrospective analysis of 42 patients. Cancer. 1988;61:349–57.
38. Ganugapanta L, Pendem S. Mandibular peripheral primitive neuroectodermal tumor:a rare case report with review of literature. J Maxillofac Oral Surg. 2015;14(Suppl 1):S341–7.
39. Khmou M, Malihy A, Lamalmi N, Rouas L, Alhamany Z. Peripheral primitive neuroectodermal tumors of the spine: a case report and review of the literature. BMC Res Notes. 2016;9(1):438.
40. Morimoto A, Oh Y, Shioda Y, Kudo K, Imamura T. Recent advances in Langerhans cells histiocytosis. Pediatr Int. 2014;56:451–61.
41. Margolin JF, Soni HM, Pimpalwar S. Medical therapy for pediatric vascular anomalies. Semin Plast Surg. 2014;28(2):79–86.
42. Chiu YE, Drolet BA, Blei F, Carcao M, Fangusaro J, Kelly ME, et al. Variable response to propranolol treatment of kaposiform hemangioendothelioma, tufted angioma, and Kasabach-Merritt phenomenon. Pediatr Blood Cancer. 2012;59(5):934.
43. Croteau SE, Liang MG, Kozakewich HP, Alomari AI, Fishman SJ, Mulliken JB, Trenor III. CC. Kaposiform hemangioendothelioma: atypical features and risks of Kasabach-Merritt phenomenon in 107 referrals. J Pediatr. 2013;162(1):142–7.

Hemangiomas 13

13.1 Introduction

A biological classification of vascular anomalies introduced in 1982 clearly separates two major categories of vascular anomalies, tumors and malformations [1–3]. Vascular tumors (mostly hemangiomas) are characterized by endothelial cell proliferation, and vascular malformations are inborn defects in vascular morphogenesis and rarely involute and grow in proportion to the child [1–4]. Infantile hemangiomas (IHs) have unique characteristics, consisting of a proliferating, involuting, and involuted phase [1–8]. The term hemangioma is often wrongly used to describe all types of vascular anomalies [4].

13.2 Epidemiology

Infantile hemangiomas (IHs) are the most common benign, soft tissue tumors of infancy which affect between 4 and 5% of Caucasian infants [1, 3, 5]. The incidence is 22–30% in preterm infants who weigh less than 1000 g [2–4]. The risk factors for IHs are also transcervical chorionic villus sampling, older maternal age, and multiple gestation pregnancy [1]. There is a familial history in about 12% of cases [1, 5]. IHs have female predomination 3–4:1 and mostly involve the head and neck (up to 60%), and they are solitary in 80% [1–3, 5].

13.3 Pathogenesis

The pathogenesis of IHs is still unknown [1, 5]. Angiogenic and vasculogenic factors are known as intrinsic (within the IH) and extrinsic factors (tissue hypoxia and developmental field disturbances) [1, 3, 5]. There is a theory that IHs develop from the clonal expansion of circulating endothelial progenitor cells (EPCs), resulting in de novo formation of new blood vessels (vasculogenesis) [1, 2].

A.M. Vlahovic, E.Q. Haxhija, *Pediatric and Adolescent Plastic Surgery for the Clinician*, DOI 10.1007/978-3-319-56004-5_13

Hemangioma-derived endothelial progenitor cells (HemEPCs) share similarities with placental endothelium (glucose transporter protein GLUT1, Lewis Y antigen, merosin, type III iodothyronine deiodinase); there is increased incidence of IH in association with chorionic villus sampling, placenta previa, and preeclampsia; and it has been postulated that the precursor cell for IH might have embolized from the placenta [1–3, 5, 6]. Hypoxia-induced factors (vascular endothelial growth factor, VEGF-A; matrix metalloproteinases, MMP-9) produced by endothelial cells may stimulate circulating (HemEPCs) recruitment to the growing tumor [1, 2, 5]. The mechanism for IH involution is unknown; apoptosis begins before 1 year of age and peaks at 24 months [2, 5].

There are several immunohistochemical markers for IHs (CD 31, CD 34, factor VIII-related antigen), but the most useful is GLUT1, which is strongly expressed only in IHs in all stages of evolution [1–6]. The histologic features of IHs change during rapid growth and involution [1, 3].

13.4 Clinical Features

IHs usually appear within the first 2–4 weeks of life [1–3, 5, 9]. Defined (mark-out) anatomical area of hemangioma is noted at birth as telangiectatic or macular red stain, barely visible pale area, or an ecchymotic spot [2, 3, 7]. By 5 months of age, nearly 80% of final size of IH is achieved [1, 5, 7]. IHs are classified on the basis of their soft tissue depth into *superficial* (red surface, without subcutaneous component), *deep* (under the skin surface, they appear later and grow longer compared to superficial IHs), and *mixed* (growth pattern that is intermediate between superficial and deep) (Fig. 13.1a–c) [1, 3–5, 7]. There is a specific subtype of superficial IH named abortive IHs with arrested growth phase [1].

Clinical appearance of IHs allows differentiation between focal (most common), multifocal, indeterminate, and segmental, depending on their morphology, extent, or distribution (Fig. 13.2a–c) [1, 3, 8, 9]. Focal IH arises from a single focal point, while segmental hemangioma tends to involve a larger area of the skin [1, 7–9]. Lesions between these two groups are considered indeterminate, and focal lesions occurring in more than one anatomical site are multifocal [1, 9]. Segmental IHs have more tendencies to be accompanied with other anomalies and have higher risk for complications [1, 3, 5, 8–10]. If there are more than five cutaneous hemangiomas, the child is at risk for harboring visceral, particularly intrahepatic, hemangiomas [1, 10–13].

IHs have a life cycle going through proliferation (during 5–9 months of life), plateau phase, and involution (starting from 12 months of life lasting up until 5–10 years of age) (Fig. 13.3a–c) [1–5, 7, 9]. Proliferation phase is characterized by growth of hemangioma, its elevation with surrounding pallor, and dilatation of veins [1–3, 8]. If the tumor proliferates in the lower dermis and subcutis, the lesion may not be visible until 3–4 months of age, and the overlying skin may be bluish [1, 5].

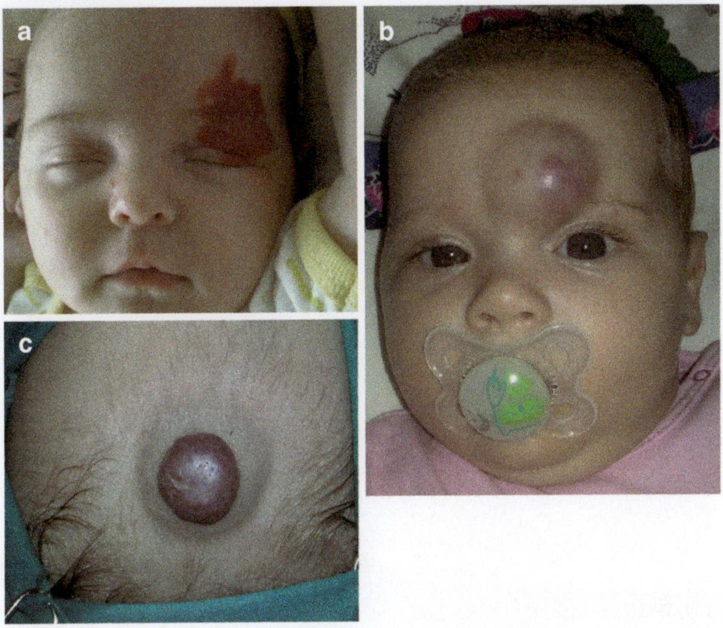

Fig. 13.1 Infantile hemangioma: (**a**) superficial; (**b**) deep; (**c**) mixed

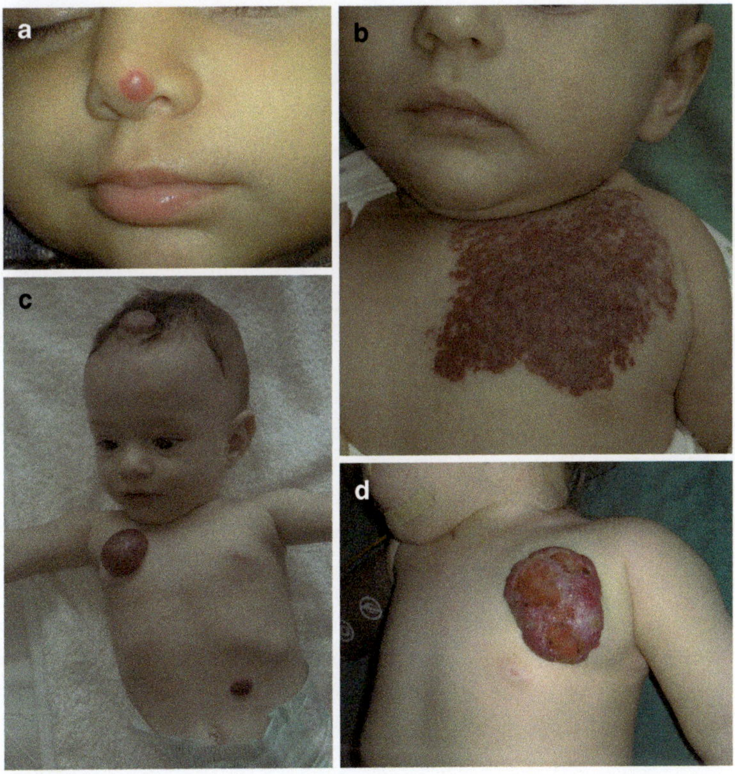

Fig. 13.2 Infantile hemangioma: (**a**) focal; (**b**) segmental; (**c**) multifocal; (**d**) intermediary

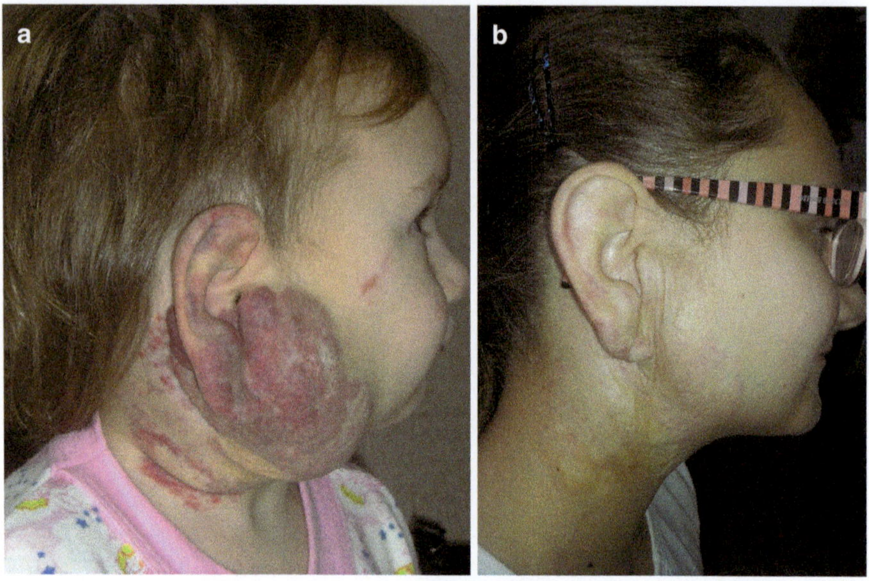

Fig. 13.3 Infantile hemangioma: (**a**) proliferative phase; (**b**) involutive phase

During involuting phase, there is fading of crimson color, central graying of the surface, and during involuted phase, there are residual skin changes including telangiectasias, crepelike laxity, scarring, or a fibrofatty residuum in a significant number of children [1, 2, 4, 5].

13.5 Complications

Approximately 24% of patients with IH experience some complication [1, 5]. Ulceration occurs in 5–21% of all cutaneous hemangiomas, leading to pain, bleeding, and infection (Fig. 13.4a–f) [1, 2, 5, 6]. Superficial and segmental hemangiomas are at higher risk, as well as hemangioma with periorbital, neck, perianal/perineal, and intertriginous localization [1, 2, 5, 9]. Treatment of ulceration includes daily application of nonadherent dressings, hydrocolloid dressing, topical antimicrobials, becaplermin gel, pulsed-dye laser (PDL), excision, and propranolol [1, 2, 5].

Bleeding from IH is rare, it stops spontaneously or with minimal pressure, and rarely it is necessary to place a mattress suture to control a local bleeding site [1, 2, 5]. Feeding impairment occurs in infants with IHs involving perioral or airway region [1].

Airway IHs can occur in a presence or absence of cutaneous hemangioma, and it can cause respiratory failure [1, 2, 5]. In case of beard distribution of hemangioma or bilateral involvement of lower facial segment, there is higher association of airway involvement [1, 5, 14]. Treatment of airway hemangioma is multidisciplinary, propranolol is first-line therapy, and tracheostomy is needed in emergent or resistant cases [1, 5, 14].

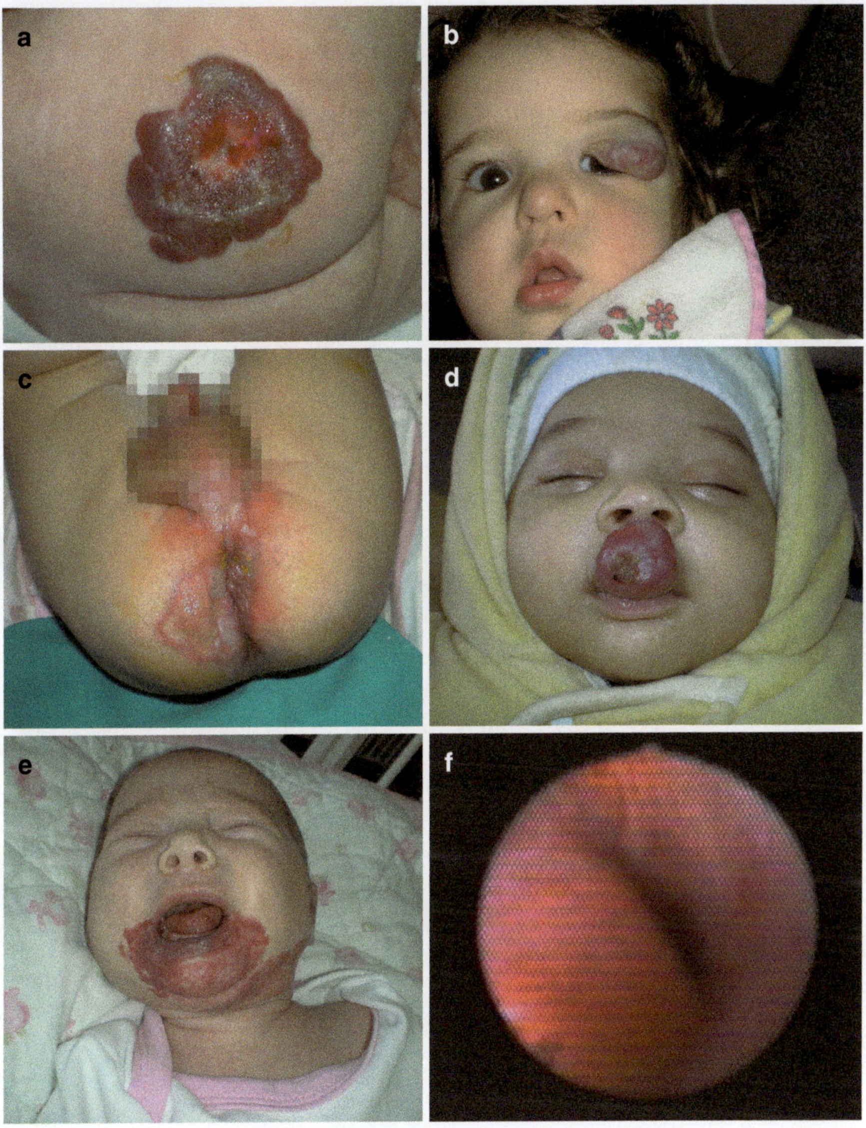

Fig. 13.4 Complication of hemangioma: (**a**) ulceration; (**b**) visual obstruction; (**c**) ulcerated hemangioma of urogenital region; (**d**) feeding problems; (**e** and **f**) airway obstruction

Child with periorbital hemangioma is in higher risk for amblyopia, and in that case evaluation of an ophthalmologist is needed [1, 2, 5]. Propranolol and surgery (in acute cases) are treatment options for periocular IHs [1, 5].

Lip hemangioma often causes distortion and ulceration of lips during proliferative phase [1, 15]. Reconstruction of the lip is indicated (usually when the growth of hemangioma ceased) [1, 5, 15, 16].

Nasal tip hemangiomas are known to cause both cosmetic and functional problem (by displacing lower lateral nasal cartilage and distorting nasal tip) [1, 2, 16, 17]. Only the hemangiomas that do not respond to propranolol, or if there is excess of the skin left, should be treated surgically [1, 16–18]. Congestive heart failure and hypothyroidism are connected as complication with large IHs and with diffuse or multifocal hepatic IHs [1, 5, 12].

13.6 Congenital Hemangiomas

Congenital hemangiomas (CHs) are less common and they are fully present at birth (Fig. 13.5a, b) [1–3]. There are three types of congenital hemangioma: noninvoluting congenital hemangioma (NICH), rapidly involuting congenital hemangioma (RICH), and partially involuting CH [2]. They have the same sex ratio, and they are negative for GLUT1 immunostaining [1–4]. NICH grows proportionately to the child and remains unchanged [1–3]. RICH goes through a rapid regression phase and may be completely gone by the time the child is 12–18 months old [1, 3].

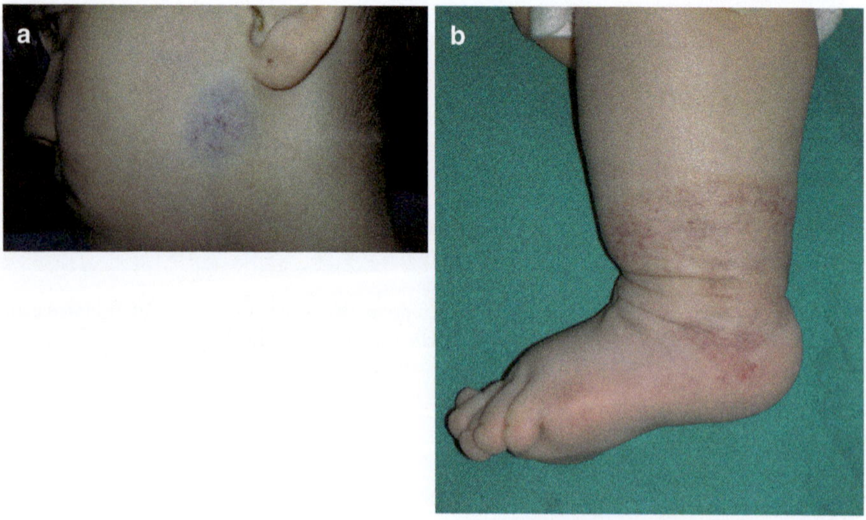

Fig. 13.5 Congenital hemangioma: (**a**) noninvoluting congenital hemangioma; (**b**) rapid involuting congenital hemangioma

13.7 Syndromes

A small subgroup of children with IHs exhibits additional associated structural anomalies like in the syndrome called PHACES (posterior fossa malformations, hemangioma, arterial anomalies, cardiovascular anomalies, eye abnormalities, and sternal clefting) [1–3, 5, 6, 8, 10, 13]. LUMBAR syndrome includes lower body IH, urogenital anomalies and ulceration, myelopathy, bony deformities, anorectal malformations, and arterial anomalies and renal anomalies (Fig. 13.6a–d) [3, 5, 6].

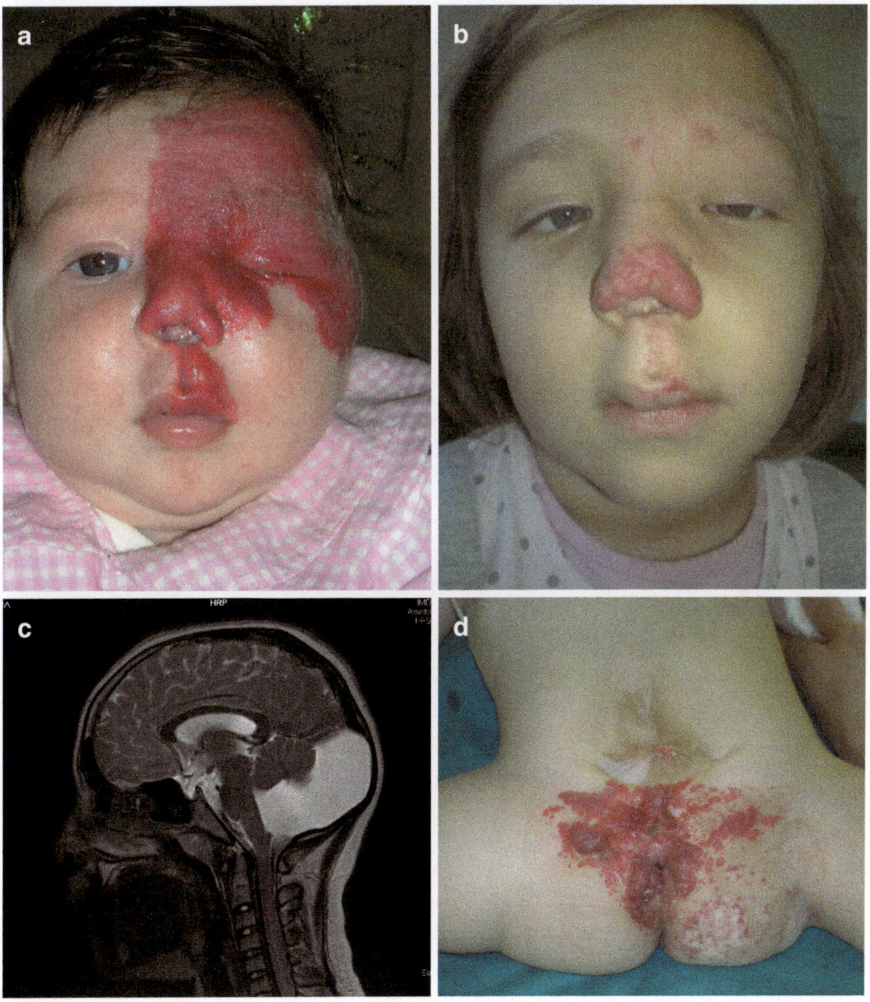

Fig. 13.6 PHACES syndrome: (**a**) beginning of the treatment with corticosteroids; (**b**) the result 4–5 years after treatment; (**c**) magnetic resonance imaging revealing intracranial anomaly; (**d**) LUMBAR syndrome

13.8 Patient Evaluation

The diagnosis of IH is possible in most cases by correlating history and physical examination [1–5]. Histologic diagnosis is gold standard, and immunohistochemically positive staining of endothelial cells in IH tumor specimens with GLUT1 presented in all stages differentiates IH from other vascular tumors and malformations [1–5, 18]. In case of deep subcutaneous, intramuscular or visceral lesions, or when there are associated anomalies, radiological evaluation is indicated including ultrasonography (US) (gray scale or color Doppler), computerized tomography (CT), and magnetic resonance imaging (MRI) with contrast, which is the gold standard diagnostic procedure for hemangioma [1, 2, 4].

13.9 Treatment Option

There are no standardized methods to measure IH growth and therapeutic response [5]. Treatment options for IHs are conservative (propranolol, corticosteroids, interferons, and chemotherapy), laser, and surgical (excision with a linear closure or circular excision and "purse-string" closure) [1, 2, 4, 18–32]. The use of propranolol for the treatment of IHs was serendipitously discovered in 2008, and it completely changed the treatment approach for IHs [1, 4, 18, 20, 23]. In 90%, IHs are small, harmless tumors that can be followed monthly through proliferative phase and on 3 months when the involution occurs [1–4]. More frequent visits are necessary whenever a hemangioma is large, ulcerated, multiple, or located in an anatomically critical area [1, 2].

13.9.1 Propranolol

Propranolol has become the first-line medical therapy for complicated IHs [1, 4–6, 17, 18, 20–23, 26, 27]. Optimal dosing, treatment timing and duration, and risk of complications have not yet been established in randomized trials [1, 18, 28]. The mode of action of propranolol in the treatment of IH is unknown (vasoconstriction, inhibition of angiogenesis, regulation of the renin-angiotensin system, and induction of apoptosis are possible mechanisms) (Fig. 13.7a, b) [1, 5, 18, 20–22, 27].

Positive responses of IHs (complete or nearly complete resolution) to propranolol are reported from 60%, 86%, and up to 98.4%, and it has most efficacies in proliferative phase [1, 20, 22–24, 26]. Lightening of the color and softening of the tumor are usually noted within hours to days of the initial dose of propranolol [1, 20]. A complete history (airway disease, lung or heart problems, and hypoglycemia), physical examination, and electrocardiography are performed, with cardiology consultation [1, 4, 20–24]. Younger infants, low heart rate, positive family history of congenital heart disease, and abnormal findings on ECG warrant echocardiogram before starting the medication [1, 4, 5, 21].

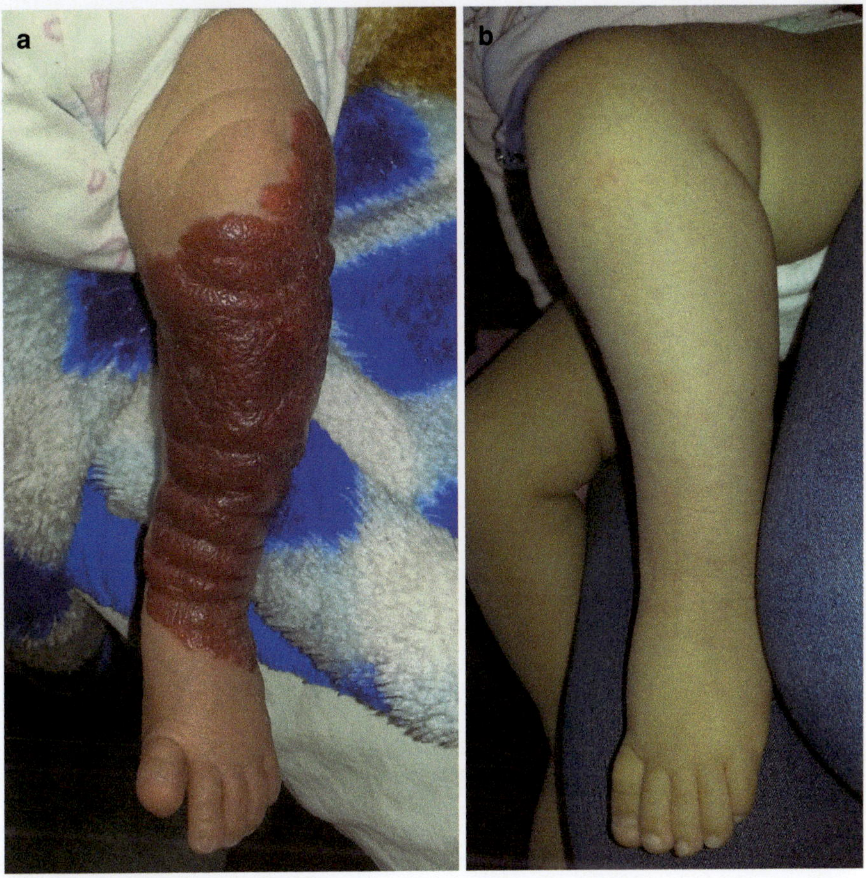

Fig. 13.7 Treatment of hemangioma with propranolol: (**a**) beginning of the treatment; (**b**) the result after 9 months

Relative contraindications to the use of propranolol for IHs include sinus bradycardia, hypotension, heart block greater than the first degree, heart failure, bronchial asthma, and known hypersensitivity to the drug [1, 4, 5, 9, 20–23]. Propranolol should be used with great precautions for patients with PHACE syndrome because theoretically there is increased risk of acute ischemic stroke [1, 2, 18, 28]. The most commonly reported adverse effects of propranolol are hypoglycemia, hypotension, bradycardia, sleep disturbance, and bronchospasm [1, 2, 5, 18, 22, 26]. Initial dose of propranolol is 0.5 mg/kg per day in three divided doses, and the target dose is 2–3 mg/kg per day [1, 5, 18, 21, 33]. Hemangeol (oral suspension of propranolol) is dosed maximally at 3.4 mg/kg per day [1]. Dosing frequency is two or three times daily (in order to reduce the risk of hypoglycemia [1, 4, 18, 20, 21, 24]. Heart rate and blood pressure measurements should be taken 1 and 2 h after the first dose and 1 and 2 h after each dosage increase [1, 18, 21]. In children with any acute illness, the dose of propranolol should be decreased, or the therapy should be ceased [1].

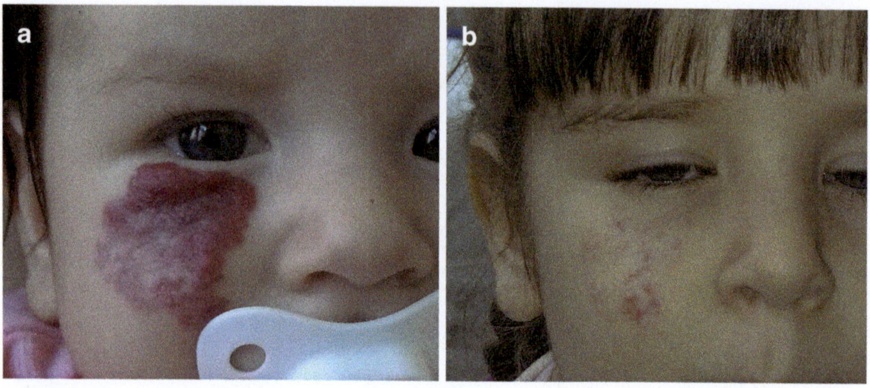

Fig. 13.8 Treatment of hemangioma with topical propranolol: (**a**) beginning of the treatment; (**b**) local finding 3 years after the treatment

Treatment duration varies from 3 to 12 months and discontinues taperly over a period of 1–3 weeks [1, 4, 21, 22]. In case of rebound growth of IH, reinitiating of therapy may be necessary [1, 24]. Topical timolol maleate (TTM) (0.5% gel-forming solution) can be recommended as an initial, and often sole, treatment modality (twice-daily topical, for more than 3 months) for many relatively superficial uncomplicated IHs (Fig. 13.8a, b) [1, 18, 25].

13.9.2 Corticosteroids

The precise mechanism of action of glucocorticoids in the treatment of IHs is unknown [1, 4, 5]. Corticosteroids can be applied as systemic, topical, or intralesional therapy [1, 2, 4–6, 18]. Oral prednisolone is still a primary treatment option for hemangioma in some centers [2]. Systemic corticosteroids are given in dose of 2–3 mg/kg/day for 4–6 weeks; thereafter the dosage is tapered slowly over several months and discontinued by 6–12 months of age [1, 2, 5, 18]. Average response rate of 84%, with an average prednisone equivalent dose of 2.9 mg/kg/day, and higher doses are associated with increased response rates but greater rates of adverse effects [1, 2, 4, 18]. Adverse effects of systemic corticosteroids are frequent, and they include cushingoid facies, temporary growth deceleration, gastric upset, behavioral changes, osteopenia, hypertension, immunosuppression, and ocular and cutaneous adverse effects [1, 2, 5, 18, 22]. Live vaccines are withheld during therapy [1, 18]. Well-localized, small cutaneous hemangioma can be treated with intralesional corticosteroid [1, 2]. Triamcinolone (25 mg/mL) (sole or as a mixture with betamethasone) is injected, and doses should not exceed 3–5 mg/kg per procedure [1, 4, 5]. Multiple (three to five) injections are needed, given at 6- to 8-week intervals [1, 5, 18]. Local complication can occur (fat and/or dermal atrophy and hypopigmentation), and special precaution has to be taken in treatment of hemangioma in periorbital region [2, 4, 5]. Topical corticosteroids are rarely used, mostly for thin, superficial hemangiomas, and their advantage is lack of systemic effects [2, 5, 18].

13.9.3 Interferons

Interferon (IFN)-2a and IFN-2b inhibit endothelial cell migration and proliferation [1, 5, 18, 33]. The empiric dose is 2–3 mU/m^2; it is injected subcutaneously, daily, for 2–12 months [5, 18]. Costs and adverse effects (spastic diplegia as the most worrisome) have made the therapy with interferons not attractive to use [1, 4–6, 18, 22, 32].

13.9.4 Chemotherapy

Chemotherapy is nowadays rarely used since propranolol has been introduced for treatment of IHs. Vincristine has been successfully used for treatment of complicated IHs, kaposiform hemangioendothelioma (KHE), and tufted angioma (TA) [1, 4–6, 18]. Cyclophosphamide can also be successful, but it is rarely given for a benign vascular tumor because of its toxicity (Fig. 13.9a–d) [32].

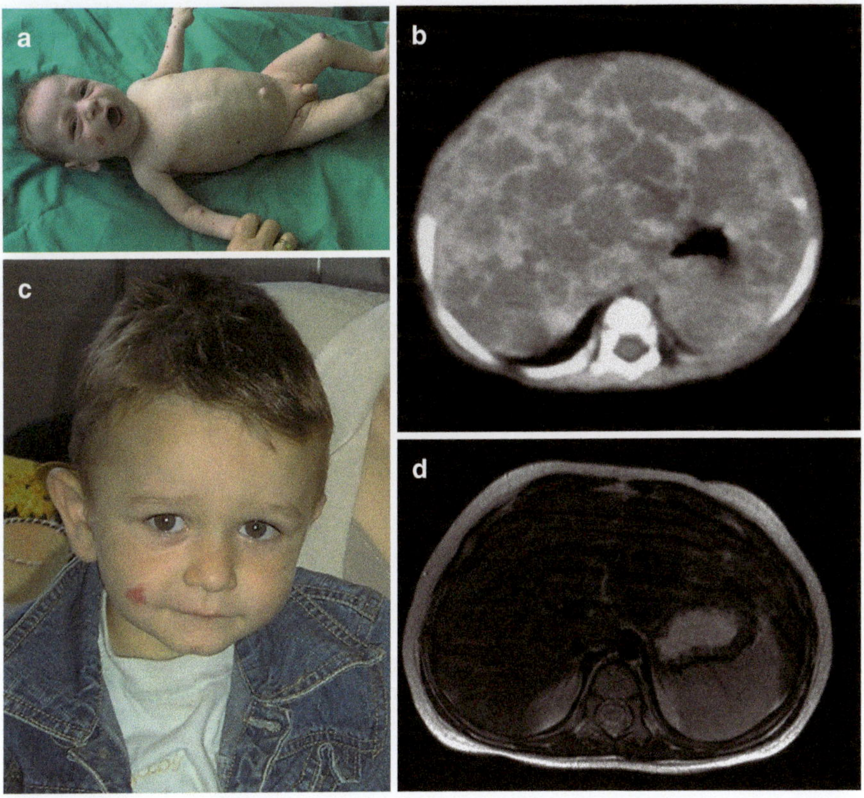

Fig. 13.9 Diffuse neonatal hemangiomatosis, treatment with cyclophosphamide: (**a**) before the treatment initiation; (**b**) computerized tomography revealed multiple hepatic hemangiomas; (**c**) after the treatment; (**d**) magnetic resonance imaging revealed no presence of hepatic hemangioma

13.9.5 Surgical Management

The role of surgery in treatment of hemangioma faded since the propranolol has been introduced, but is still important [1, 5, 17, 28, 29]. Early surgical excision during proliferative phase is rarely indicated [1, 2, 5]. Indications for surgical treatment are function-threatening lesions, failure or contraindication to pharmacotherapy, bleeding and ulceration unresponsive to therapy, well-localized tumor in anatomical area, and if the resection will be needed in the future [1, 2, 4, 5, 17, 28]. It is best to perform surgery before 4 years of age (before the child is aware of lesion) [3, 17, 28].

Since growing hemangioma acts like tissue expander, circular excision and "purse-string closure" has been proved as a good operative technique for well-selected cases (Fig. 13.10a–c) [2, 29, 30]. Transverse lenticular excision is applicable in certain locations, such as eyelids, lip, and neck, or as the final stage after circular excision (Fig. 13.11a–c) [1, 17].

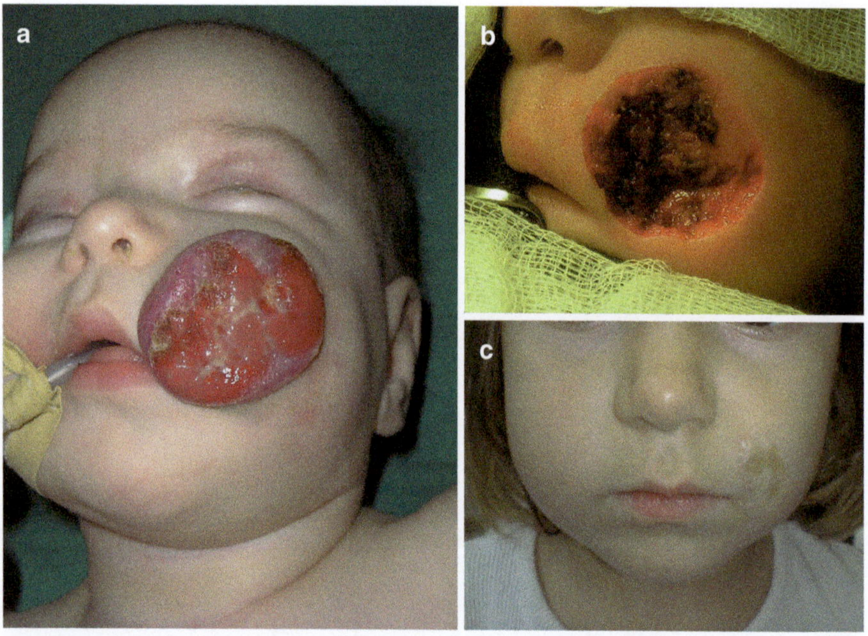

Fig. 13.10 Excision of hemangioma by circular excision and purse string suture: (**a**) large hemangioma of the left buccal region with ulceration; (**b**) circular excision of hemangioma; (**c**) the result after reconstruction of the defect with purse string suture

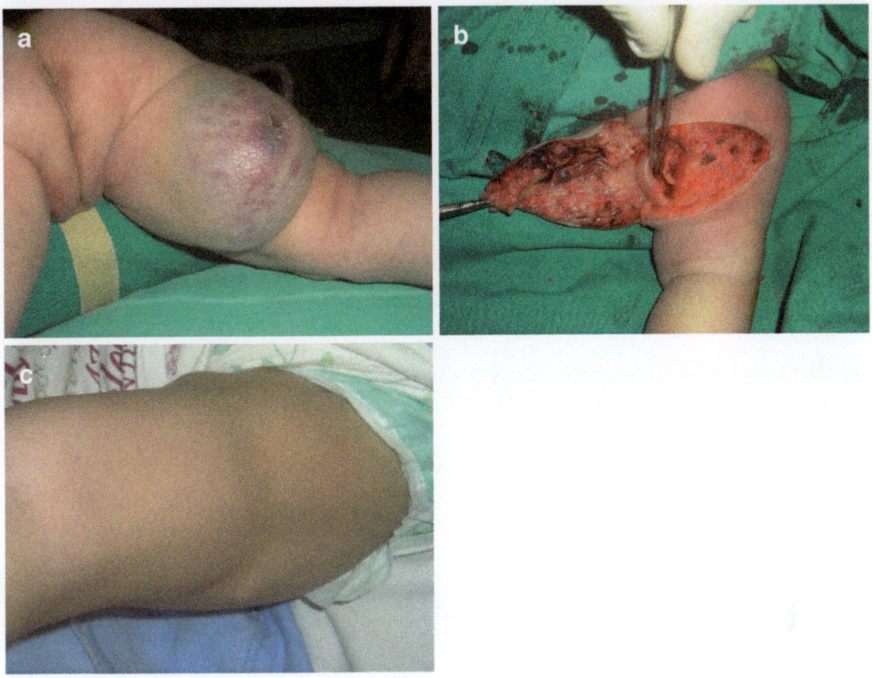

Fig. 13.11 Excision of large congenital hemangioma of the right posterior femoral region by ellipsoid excision and linear suture: (**a**) preoperative view; (**b**) intraoperative view; (**c**) postoperative result

13.9.6 Laser Therapy

The pulsed-dye laser (PDL) (wavelength 595 nm) is most commonly used for treatment of IHs, and neodymium-doped yttrium aluminum garnet (Nd:YAG) laser and CO_2 lasers are also used for treatment of IHs [1, 5, 30, 31]. Indications for laser treatment are superficial facial IHs, ulceration refractory to medical management, and residual cutaneous lesions [1, 2, 23, 29, 31]. Disadvantages of laser treatment are limited depth of penetration into the dermis (0.75–1.2 mm) and that children usually require general anesthesia [1, 2, 5, 31]. Adverse effects of laser treatment are ulceration, scarring, and hypopigmentation [1, 2, 5, 31].

13.10 Pyogenic Granuloma

Pyogenic granuloma (PG) is a benign, solitary, acquired vascular tumor of the skin and mucous membrane that grows rapidly, frequently confused with hemangioma [2, 26, 33, 34]. It is common in children, with male to female ratio of 2:1 [2, 3]. PG

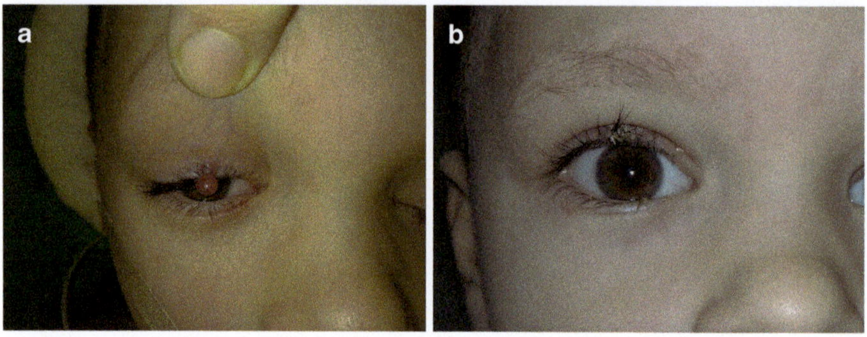

Fig. 13.12 Pyogenic granuloma: (**a**) preoperative view; (**b**) postoperative result

is mostly distributed on the head or neck and trunk, and it is commonly complicated by bleeding (64%) and ulceration (36%) [2, 26, 33, 34]. Full-thickness excision is most effective treatment [2]. Curettage, shave excision and cauterization, carbon dioxide (CO_2) laser vaporization, and topical timolol are also used for treatment of PG (Fig. 13.12a, b) [2, 26, 33, 34].

References

1. Darrow DH, Greene AK, Mancini AJ, Nopper AJ. Diagnosis and management of infantile hemangiomas. Pediatrics. 2015;136(4):e1060–104.
2. Greene AK, Mulliken JB. Vascular anomalies. In: Neligen PC, Gurtner GC, editors. Plastic surgery. Principles and practice. St Louis, MO: Elsevier; 2013. p. 677–706e7.
3. Wassef M, Blei F, Adams D, Alomari A, Baselga E, Berenstein A, et al; ISSVA Board and Scientific Committee. Vascular anomalies classification: recommendations from the International Society for the Study of Vascular Anomalies. Pediatrics. 2015;136(1):e203–14.
4. Sepulveda A, Buchanan EP. Vascular tumors. Semin Plast Surg. 2014;28(2):49–57.
5. Kwon EK, Seefeldt M, Drolet BA. Infantile hemangiomas: an update. Am J Clin Dermatol. 2013;14(2):111–23.
6. Blei F. Medical and genetic aspects of vascular anomalies. Tech Vasc Interv Radiol. 2013;16(1):2–11.
7. Chang LC, Haggstrom AN, Drolet BA, Baselga E, Chamlin SL, Garzon MC, et al. Growth characteristics of infantile hemangiomas: implications for management. Pediatrics. 2008;122(2):360–7.
8. Haggstrom AN, Lammer EJ, Schneider RA, Marcucio R, Frieden IJ. Patterns of infantile hemangiomas: new clues to hemangioma pathogenesis and embryonic facial development. Pediatrics. 2006;117(3):698–703.
9. Chiller KG, Passaro D, Frieden IJ. Hemangiomas of infancy: clinical characteristics, morphologic subtypes, and their relationship to race, ethnicity, and sex. Arch Dermatol. 2002; 138(12):1567–76.
10. Metry DW, Hawrot A, Altman C, Frieden IJ. Association of solitary, segmental hemangiomas of the skin with visceral hemangiomatosis. Arch Dermatol. 2004;140(5):591–6.
11. Waner M, North PE, Scherer KA, Frieden IJ, Waner M, Mihm MC. The nonrandom distribution of facial hemangimas. Arch Dermatol. 2003;139:869–75.

12. Christison-Lagay ER, Burrows PE, Alomari A, Dubois J, Kozakewich HP, Lane TS, et al. Hepatic hemangiomas: subtype classification and development of a clinical practice algorithm and registry. J Pediatr Surg. 2007;42(1):62–7. discussion 67–8
13. Metry DW, Garzon MC, Drolet BA, Frommelt P, Haggstrom A, et al. PHACE syndrome: current knowledge, future directions. Pediatr Dermatol. 2009;26(4):381–98.
14. Orlow SJ, Isakoff MS, Blei F. Increased risk of symptomatic hemangiomas of the airway in association with cutaneous hemangiomas in a "beard" distribution. J Pediatr. 1997;131(4): 643–6.
15. Yanes DA, Pearson GD, Witman PM. Infantile hemangiomas of the lip: patterns, outcomes, and implications. Pediatr Dermatol. 2016;33(5):511–7.
16. Waner M, Min-Jung OT. The role of surgery in the management of congenital vascular anomalies. Tech Vasc Interv Radiol. 2013;16(1):45–50.
17. Simic R, Vlahovic A, Subarevic V. Treatment of nasal hemangiomas. Int J Pediatr Otorhinolaryngol. 2009;73(10):1402–6.
18. Craiglow BG, Antaya RJ. Management of infantile hemangiomas current and potential pharmacotherapeutic approaches. Pediatr Drugs. 2013;15:133–8.
19. Guevara CJ, Alomari AI. Interdisciplinary approach to treatment of vascular anomalies. Tech Vasc Interv Radiol. 2013;16(1):55–8.
20. Leaute-Labreze C, Dumas de la Roque E, Hubiche T, Boralevi F. Propranolol for severe hemangiomas of infancy. N Engl J Med. 2008;358:2649–51.
21. Drolet BA, Frommelt PC, Chamlin SL, Haggstrom A, Bauman NM, Chiu YE, et al. Initiation and use of propranolol for infantile hemangioma: report of a consensus conference. Pediatrics. 2013;131(1):128–40.
22. Léaute-Labrèze C, Boccara O, Degrugillier-Chopinet C, Mazereeuw-Hautier J, Prey S. et al. Safety of oral propranolol for the treatment of infantile hemangioma: a systematic review. Pediatrics. 2016;138(4):pii:e20160353.
23. Elluru RG, Friess MR, Richter GT, Grimmer JF, Darrow DH, Shin JJ, Perkins JA. Multicenter evaluation of the effectiveness of systemic propranolol in the treatment of airway hemangiomas. Otolaryngol Head Neck Surg. 2015;153(3):452–60.
24. Shah SD, Baselga E, McCuaig C, Pope E, Coulie J, Boon LM, et al. Rebound growth of infantile hemangiomas after propranolol therapy. Pediatrics. 2016;137(4). Doi:10.1542/peds.2015-1754
25. Püttgen K, Lucky A, Adams D, Pope E, McCuaig C. et al. Hemangioma Investigator Group. Topical timolol maleate treatment of infantile hemangiomas. Pediatrics. 2016;138(3): pii:e20160355
26. Buckmiller LM, Munson PD, Dyamenahalli U, Dai Y, Richter GT. Propranolol for infantile hemangiomas: early experience at a tertiary vascular anomalies center. Laryngoscope. 2010;120(4):676–81.
27. Nguyen HP, Pickrell BB, Wright TS. Beta-blockers as therapy for infantile hemangiomas. Semin Plast Surg. 2014;28(2):87–90.
28. Mulliken JB, Rogers GF, Marler JJ. Circular excision of hemangioma and purse-string closure: the smallest possible scar. Plast Reconstr Surg. 2002;109(5):1544–54. discussion 1555
29. Vlahovic A, Simic R, Kravljanac DJ. Circular excision and purse string suture technique in the management of facial hemangiomas. Int. J. Ped. Otolar. 2007;71:1311–5.
30. Chinnadurai S, Sathe NA, Surawicz T. Laser treatment of infantile hemangioma: a systematic review. Lasers Surg Med. 2016;48(3):221–33.
31. Witman PM, Wagner AM, Scherer K, Waner M, Frieden IJ. Complications following pulsed dye laser treatment of superficial hemangiomas. Lasers Surg Med. 2006;38(2):116–23.
32. Vlahovic A, Simic R, Djokic D, Ceran C. Diffuse neonatal hemangiomatosis treatment with cyclophosphamide: a case report. J Pediatr Hematol Oncol. 2009;31(11):858–60.
33. Malik M, Murphy R. A pyogenic granuloma treated with topical timolol. Br J Dermatol. 2014;171(6):1537–8.
34. Pagliai KA, Cohen BA. Pyogenic granuloma in children. Pediatric Dermatol. 2004;21:10–3.

Lymphatic Malformation

14

14.1 Introduction

Vascular anomalies are divided based on endothelial characteristics in vascular tumors (mostly hemangiomas) and vascular malformation [1–3]. On the base of type of the vessel included in vascular malformation, they are divided mainly into *simple* (capillary malformation (CM), lymphatic malformation (LM), venous malformation (VM), and arterial malformation (AM)), and *combined* vascular malformation—two or more vascular malformations in one lesion, malformation of major named vessels, and malformation associated with other anomalies [1–3]. Vascular anomalies are also divided into slow-flow (CM, LM, VM) and fast-flow (AM) vascular malformation [2, 3].

14.2 Clinical Features

The lymphatic system develops during the sixth week of embryonic life [3, 4]. By the first theory, the lymphatic system is derived from the primordial endothelial buds sprouting from the developing venous system, the second theory is the theory of "centripetal" development, and the third one is the combination of these two theories [3–7].

The exact etiology of LM is unknown [4]. There are several theories for etiology of LM: failing of aberrant primordial endothelial buds to reestablish communication with venous system from which it arose, part of lymphatic channels becomes "pinched off" from the main lymphatic system, and abnormal budding of the lymphatic system with a loss of connection to the central lymph channels [3, 4]. No genetic basis has been determined for LMs [3]. LMs (traditionally called lymphangiomas) are benign vascular lesion presented as localized areas of abnormal development of the lymphatic system [3, 6, 7]. If LM is relatively large,

A.M. Vlahovic, E.Q. Haxhija, *Pediatric and Adolescent Plastic Surgery for the Clinician*, DOI 10.1007/978-3-319-56004-5_14

it can be diagnosed by ultrasound (US) prenatally by the second trimester [3, 4]. LMs are in approximately 50% of cases presented at birth and near 90% within the first 2 years of life [3, 4, 7–10]. The reported incidence of LMs varies from 0.14 to 5% of all benign soft tissue tumors, with both genders equally affected [4, 8, 10]. In up to 75% of the cases, they are localized in the head and neck region, followed by the axilla, chest, buttock, perineum, and retroperitoneum/mediastinum [3, 4, 7, 8, 10–12]. Depending on cyst diameter (there is no clear definition of the size for the lesion), LMs are divided into macrocystic, microcystic, and combined [2–5, 8, 12, 13].

Disease location, size, and depth have a major influence on prognosis [3–5, 8–13]. LM lesions are visible, nontender, soft, and compressible swellings [3, 10, 11]. Cutaneous or mucous lesions usually present as liquid-filled vesicles (blood or purulent fluid) (Fig. 14.1) [3, 8]. Deep-seated LMs can be divided into diffuse edema (microcystic) and localized multilocular cyst (macrocystic) [8].

LMs in certain anatomical regions present diagnostic and treatment challenge in the orbital region, tongue, floor of the mouth, neck, and mediastinum [4, 8]. Because of the common embryological origin, lymphatic and venous system lymphatic-venous malformation (LVM) also can occur [3, 14, 15].

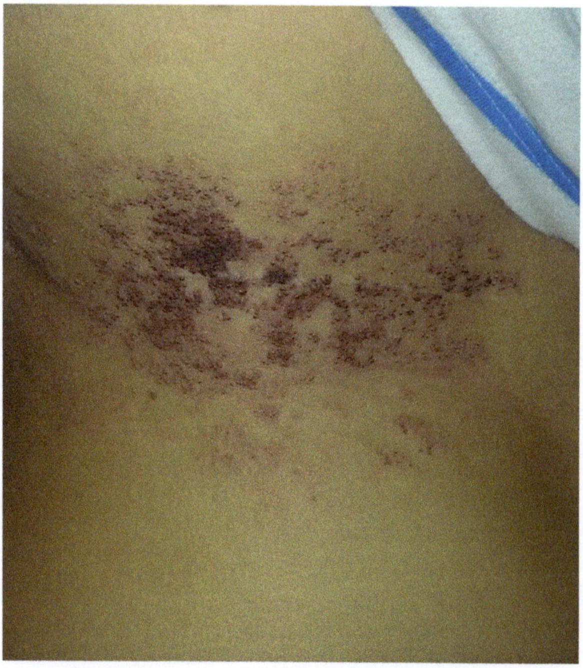

Fig. 14.1 Superficial lymphatic malformation of the abdominal wall

14.3 Complication (Symptoms) of LMs

The two most common complications associated with LM are bleeding and infection, and they result in rapid enlargement of the LM [3, 8, 10]. Intralesional bleeding occurs in up to 35% of lesions causing ecchymotic discoloration, pain, or swelling and compression of adjacent organs [3, 4]. Depending on the anatomic position of the LM, this compression can lead to acute visual disturbances, pain, headaches, respiratory distress, and dysphagia [4, 14, 15]. Infection occurs as a complication in nearly 70% of lesions [3]. Cutaneous vesicles can be associated with lymph and blood leakage [3, 4, 8].

Giant cervicofacial LM is a special group of LMs that are usually placed in multiple tissue planes and involve vital structures (Fig. 14.2) [3, 4, 15]. Oral lesions may lead to macroglossia, speech problems, poor oral hygiene, caries, and malocclusion [3, 16]. Infections and intralesional hemorrhage are the most common complication of cervicofacial LMs [14, 15]. There is a five-staging system proposed by Seeres et al. based on the location and extent of the lesions in the neck (unilateral suprahyoid, unilateral infrahyoid, unilateral supra- and infrahyoid, bilateral suprahyoid, bilateral infrahyoid, and bilateral supra- and infrahyoid) [8, 16].

There are no accepted treatment protocols for cervicofacial LMs, the management is extremely difficult, and it requires multidisciplinary approach [3, 4]. The airway is the primary concern in an infant with LM [15]. Nearly 50% of patients

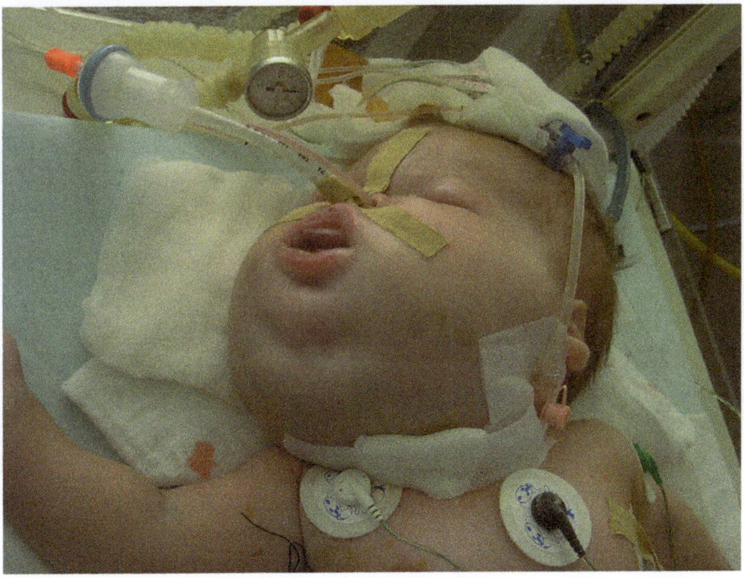

Fig. 14.2 Large lymphatic malformation of the head and neck

require tracheotomy, and it should be performed without hesitation as an ex utero intrapartum treatment (EXIT) procedure or in the first days of life [3, 4, 15]. Treatment options for LMs in cervicofacial region are resection, sclerotherapy, laser coagulation, and radiofrequency ablation [3, 8, 10, 11, 15, 16].

The surgical treatment is best performed before development of facial image (3 years old), and it is usually connected with serious complications such as nerve damage, bleeding, lymphatic drainage, and infection [8, 15, 16]. Surgical excision should be avoided for the tongue and oral floor LMs, which are better to be treated with sclerotherapy (with doxycycline, bleomycin, OK-432, and ethanol) [15]. Recently, pharmacotherapy (sirolimus) is widely used as a first line of treatment for large cervicofacial LMs [17–19].

LMs in the orbit are uncommon and they account for 3% of all orbital masses [14]. Periorbital LMs present with swelling, intraorbital hemorrhage, infection, ocular proptosis, and blepharoptosis [3, 4]. Periorbital LM causes a permanent reduction in vision (40%), and 7% of patients become blind in the affected eye [3]. Treatment options are sclerosation with doxycycline, bleomycin, OK-432, and ethanol (for extraorbital lesions only), surgical treatment, and pharmacologic therapy (sirolimus) for large LMs [14–18].

Generalized LMs present with multifocal or osteolytic bony lesions, splenic involvement, as well as pleural and/or pericardial effusions, and they are extremely difficult for treatment [18–21]. Skeletal involvement of LM is also known as Gorham-Stout syndrome, disappearing bone disease or phantom bone disease (Fig. 14.3a–c) [2, 3].

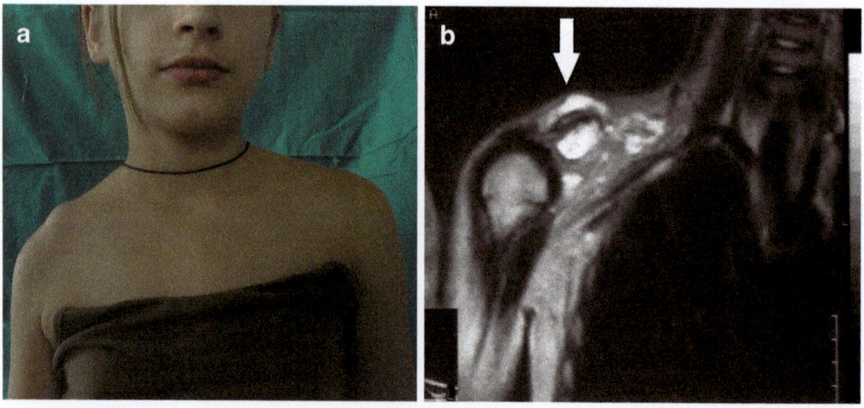

Fig. 14.3 Gorham syndrome: (**a**) deformation of the right shoulder area; (**b**) magnetic resonance imaging revealing presence of lymphatic malformation

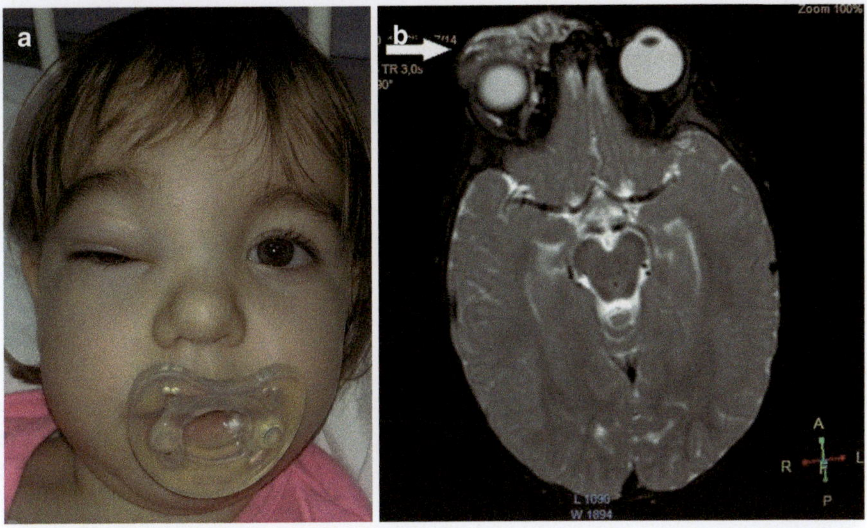

Fig. 14.4 Lymphaticovenous malformation of the right orbit: (**a**) clinical view; (**b**) magnetic resonance imaging of the head region revealing large intraorbital lymphaticovenous malformation

14.4 Patient Evaluation

Diagnosis of LM in most cases (90%) is made on the basis of history and clinical manifestations [3, 4, 7, 8]. Small, superficial lesions do not require further evaluation [3]. Radiological techniques are used to determine anatomic extent of the disease and the rheologic nature [4, 7, 9]. Ultrasonography and color Doppler study differentiate slow-flow from fast-flow anomalies and a discrete tumoral mass from the anomalous channels of a vascular malformation [7–9]. Ultrasonography is less valuable for deep-seated lesions [4]. Magnetic resonance imaging (MRI) is the best radiological technique for characterizing LM [4, 7, 8, 11, 15]. MRI with contrast can help to distinguish LM from venous malformation (VM) or lymphaticovenous malformation (LVM) (Fig. 14.4a, b) [3, 4, 9, 15].

Histologically, LMs are composed of vascular spaces filled with eosinophilic, collections of lymphocytes, and protein-rich fluid with lymphatic channels lined by a single layer of flattened endothelium [3, 4, 8, 11, 22].

14.5 Treatment Option

LM is a benign lesion and small or asymptomatic lesions may be observed [3, 21]. Spontaneous regression of LMs is rarely seen [8]. Treatment of LMs is reserved in case of symptomatic lesions that cause pain and significant deformity or if the LM is a threat to a vital structures [3, 7, 8]. An infected LM often requires intravenous antimicrobial therapy [3]. Patients and families are counseled that LM can expand following any intervention, and thus additional treatments are often required in the future [3]. Treatment option for LM is usually multimodal, and treatment algorithms are not yet created [3, 6, 8, 10–12, 16–19, 22–29, 31]. Treatment of LMs includes observation, pharmacotherapy, excision, and sclerotherapy [3–31]. Disease location has a major influence on prognosis, and outcomes are not so favorable for children with orbital, parotid, laryngopharyngeal, and oral disease [10, 14, 15].

14.5.1 Sclerotherapy

Injection sclerotherapy induces endothelial inflammation in a vascular structure with the goal of causing thrombosis, occlusion, fibrosis, and contraction within a structure [4]. Sclerotherapy has emerged during the past several decades as first-line treatment option for large or problematic macrocystic/combined LM [3, 8, 12]. Sclerotherapy is less successful and less predictive for microcystic (deep-seated) LM, the response is not instantaneous, and usually multiple procedures are needed [3, 4, 6, 13]. Different sclerosing agents have been used for sclerotherapy of LMs such as ethanol, hypertonic saline, alcoholic solution of zein (ASZ) (Ethibloc), and sodium tetradecyl sulfate (STS) [6, 8, 12, 13, 22]. Ethanol has the highest complication rate (ulceration, nerve injury, systemic toxicity) [3, 20]. The most utilized sclerosing agents for LMs are doxycycline, bleomycin, and OK-432 [3, 4, 6–8, 10–12, 16, 22, 27, 29].

14.5.1.1 OK-432

OK-432 (Picibanil) is a sclerosant developed in Japan from a low virulence strain of group A *Streptococcus pyogenes* [7, 10–12, 23, 24]. It was introduced by Ogita and coworkers for treatment of LMs in children in 1987 [11, 23, 24]. The OK-432 solution was prepared by dissolving 0.1 mg of OK-432 in 10 mL (0.01 mg/mL) of physiological saline [23, 24]. The amount of OK-432 (0.1 mg/10 mL) is the same as aspirate fluid, not more than 20 mL (Fig. 14.5a–d) [8]. The injection treatment is usually guided by US, and lymphatic fluid aspiration is followed by injection of OK-432 substance into malformation [25]. The side effects after instillation of OK-432 substance are fever and local inflammatory reaction, pain, and swelling [8, 12, 24]. OK-432 has proved itself as a safe and effective sclerosing agent; however, the use of OK-432 is limited because it is not widely available [3, 12, 25]. Surgical treatment is usually recommended after four unsatisfactory attempts of sclerotherapy with OK-432 [25].

14.5.1.2 Bleomycin (Pingyangmycin)

Bleomycin is a widely available antibiotic derivate with cytostatic properties (sclerosing effect was discovered later) [6–8, 12, 22]. Precise mechanism of bleomycin sclerosing effect is unclear (most likely produces nonspecific inflammatory process that results in fibrosis, endothelial damage, and subsequent obliteration of the

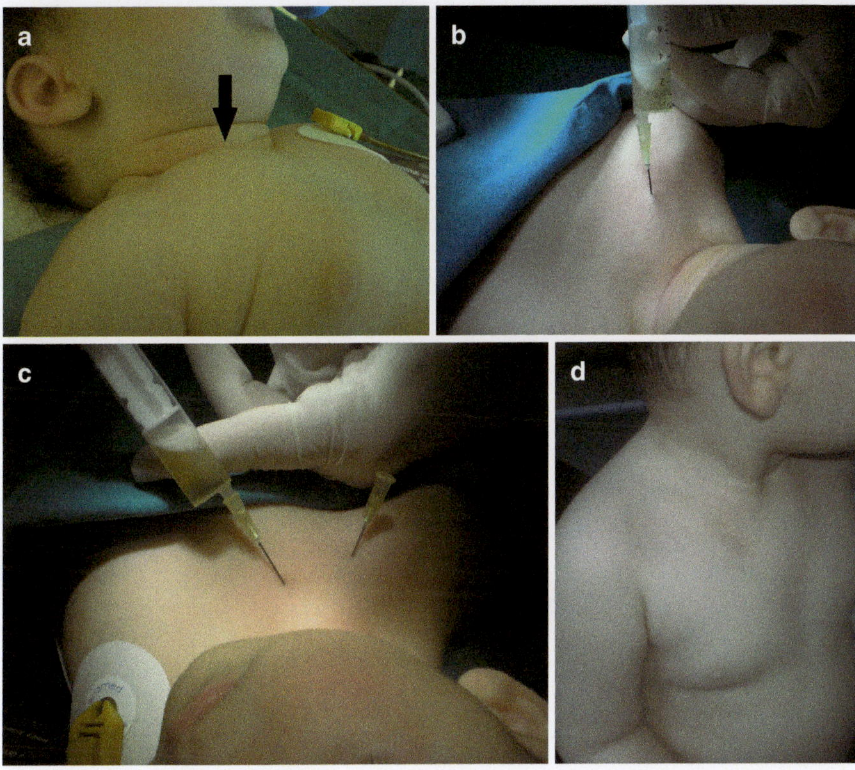

Fig. 14.5 Treatment of macrocystic lymphatic malformation with OK 432: (**a**) Lymphatic malformation of the right pectoral region; (**b**, **c**) aspiration of the cysts; (**d**) postoperative result

channels) [6, 11, 22]. It is very effective for macrocystic and superficial microcystic LM [22]. Major advantage of bleomycin is the relatively minimal inflammatory reaction and edema post injection [6]. Pediatric patients should be hospitalized; allergic status, complete blood count, and chest X-rays have to be taken, with pre-operative imaging examinations performed (US, MRI, or contrast-enhanced computerized tomography (CT)) [6, 22].

Bleomycin powder (15 U) should be diluted in concentration 1 U/mL, and maximal single session dose should be 1 mg/kg, not exceeding 15 mg [21–23, 26]. Intervention is performed under sedation or general anesthesia, with aspiration of cystic fluid under the guidance of US, followed by bleomycin injection, and pressure dressing is applied to the cyst usually for 5 min (Fig. 14.6a–c) [6, 8]. If there were no adverse reactions 24 h after treatment with bleomycin (fever, cough, dyspnea, mental confusion), the patient should be discharged [8]. If the child is older than 6 years, pulmonary function test should be performed, and for the airway LM, corticosteroids should be administrated [22]. One month after intervention, clinical and radiological reevaluation is performed, and if any residual cystic mass is found by US, a second bleomycin injection is performed [8, 22, 23]. The reported main

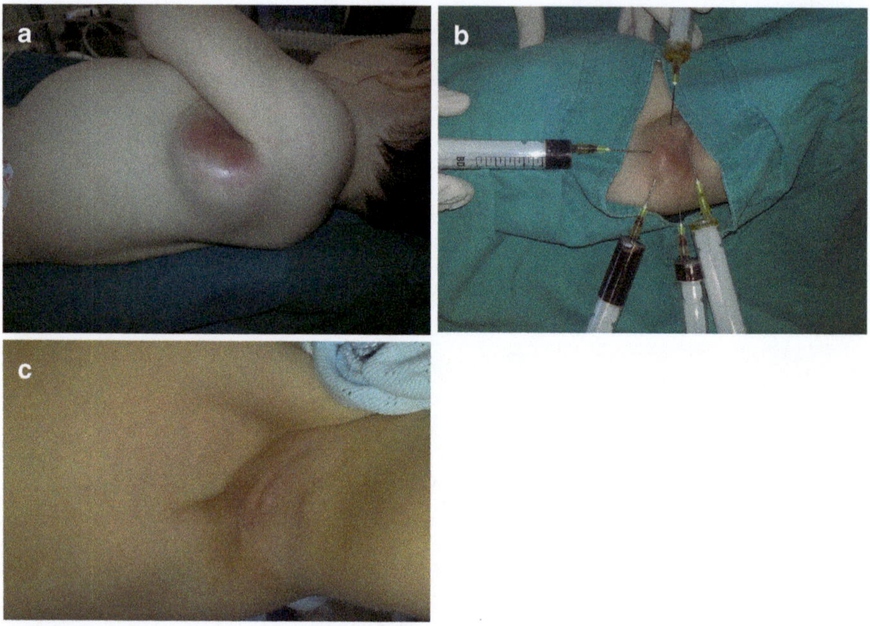

Fig. 14.6 Treatment of axillary lymphatic malformation with bleomycin: (**a**) preoperative view; (**b**) aspiration of the cysts and instillation of medicine; (**c**) the result 3 months after intervention

side effects of the intralesional bleomycin include fever, erythema, ulceration, hyperpigmentation, induration, alopecia, and scarring [6, 8, 12, 22–24, 26]. The major concern about bleomycin treatment is the association between bleomycin and pulmonary fibrosis [6–8, 12, 16, 22, 26]. The pulmonary manifestation of bleomycin toxicity is dose dependent, and there have been no documented cases of pulmonary fibrosis if the session doses do not exceed 15 mg [6, 16, 26].

14.5.1.3 Doxycycline

Doxycycline is a member of the tetracycline family of antimicrobials frequently used for sclerotherapy because it is effective, it can be used in large doses, and it has minor side effects [3, 4, 5, 7, 13, 15, 17, 27–29]. Preoperative and follow-up (6–8 weeks post intervention) imaging MRI or contrast-enhanced CT examinations should be performed [4, 13, 27]. In case of large head and neck LMs, some authors performed posttreatment MRI on day 3 to evaluate peri-airway inflammation and deviation/compression before extubation [13, 27]. Microcystic LMs do not respond well to doxycycline [5].

There is no standardized protocol for treatment of LMs with doxycycline [13]. Procedures in children are usually performed under deep sedation or general anesthesia as doxycycline injection is painful [4]. The US-guided percutaneous puncture is performed, followed by aspiration of fluid from LM and instillation of previously prepared doxycycline (100 mg of doxycycline + 5 mL of sterile water + 5 mL of water-soluble contrast making a solution of 10 mg/mL) [4, 7, 27]. If the cyst is large (greater than 30 mL of fluid), the procedure can be performed with short inpatient stay (usually 3 days) with fluid aspiration and doxycycline injection (retained for 4 h) repeated for every day until the drainage is ceased [4, 13, 27, 28]. Postoperatively, depending on the LM size, the blood level of doxycycline is measured; infants and neonates have glucose monitoring every 2 h, with baseline hearing evaluation [13, 27].

14.5.2 Surgery

Clinicians divide LMs into focal (less infiltrative) and diffuse (mostly microcystic, infiltrative) (focal lesions are easier to resect) [4]. Surgery used to be a traditional primary treatment modality for LM; however, complete surgical excision is possible in only 18–50% of patients, and there is significant morbidity with recurrence rate from 15 to 64% [3, 10, 13, 25]. Resection is usually reserved for small, well-localized LM, for symptomatic microcystic LM (with bleeding or leaking cutaneous vesicles), and for symptomatic macrocystic/combined LM that cannot be managed with sclerotherapy or pharmacotherapy (Fig. 14.7a–c) [3, 11]. Diffuse and extensive lesions are almost impossible to excise totally because they are poorly demarcated, with thin and friable walls, involving vital structures [3, 8, 10, 11, 22]. For diffuse malformations, staged resection of defined anatomical areas is recommended [3, 4, 10]. Resection of cervicofacial LM is followed by injuries of the facial nerve and hypoglossal nerve, seroma, tissue defects, heavy bleeding, and infection [8, 15].

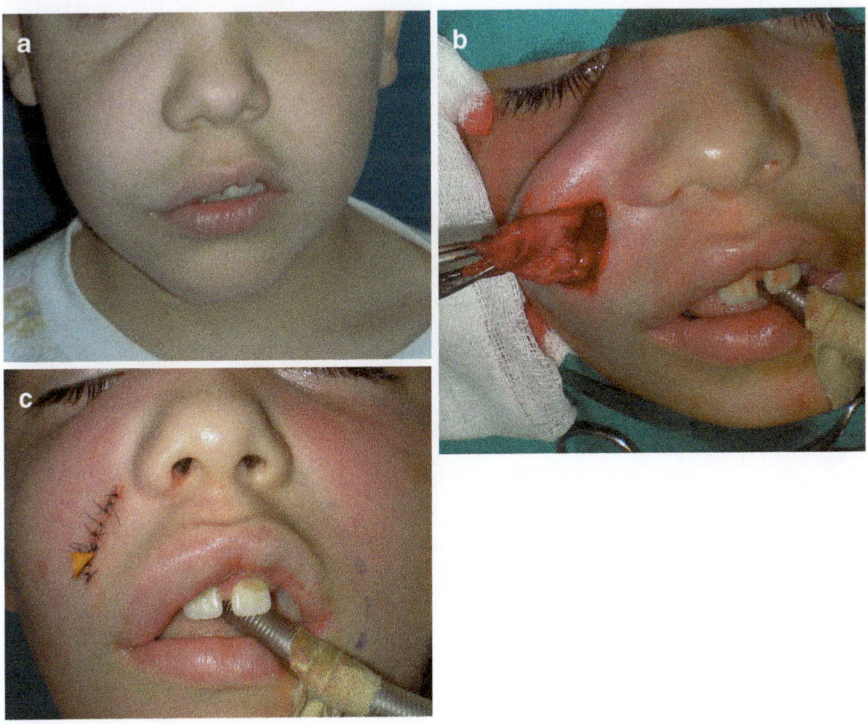

Fig. 14.7 Surgical treatment of lymphatic malformation: (**a**) preoperative view; (**b**) intraoperative view; (**c**) postoperative result

14.5.3 Laser Therapy

Lasers have been used to treat small, microcystic, and superficial lesions (carbon dioxide, neodymium-doped yttrium aluminum garnet Nd:YAG, diode lasers); however, they are not effective for deep-seated LM [8, 11].

14.5.4 Pharmacotherapy

There is evidence of successful treatment of generalized (complicated) vascular malformation with sirolimus (Fig. 14.8a–g) [17–19, 21].

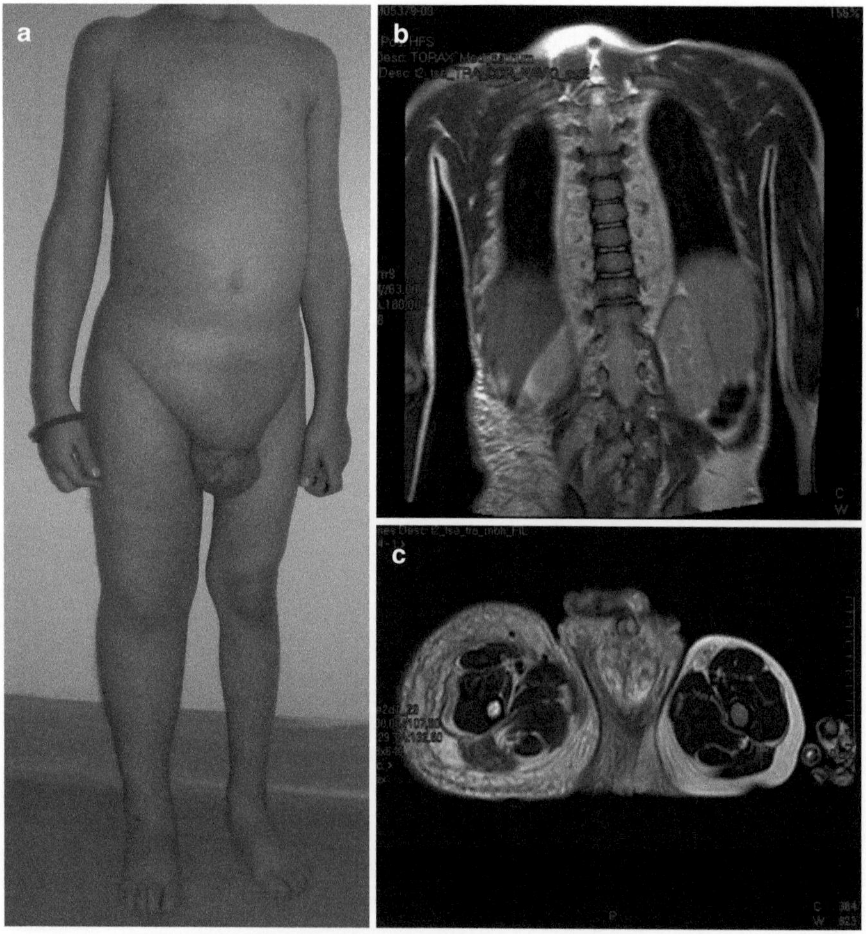

Fig. 14.8 Treatment of capillary-lymphatico-venous malformation with sirolimus: (**a**, **d**) clinical finding before the sirolimus was introducted; (**b**, **c**) magnetic resonance imaging finding in the chest and right femoral region before the treatment; (**e**) the child with significantly improved clinical finding; (**f**, **g**) magnetic resonance imaging finding in the chest and right femoral region revealing excellent result

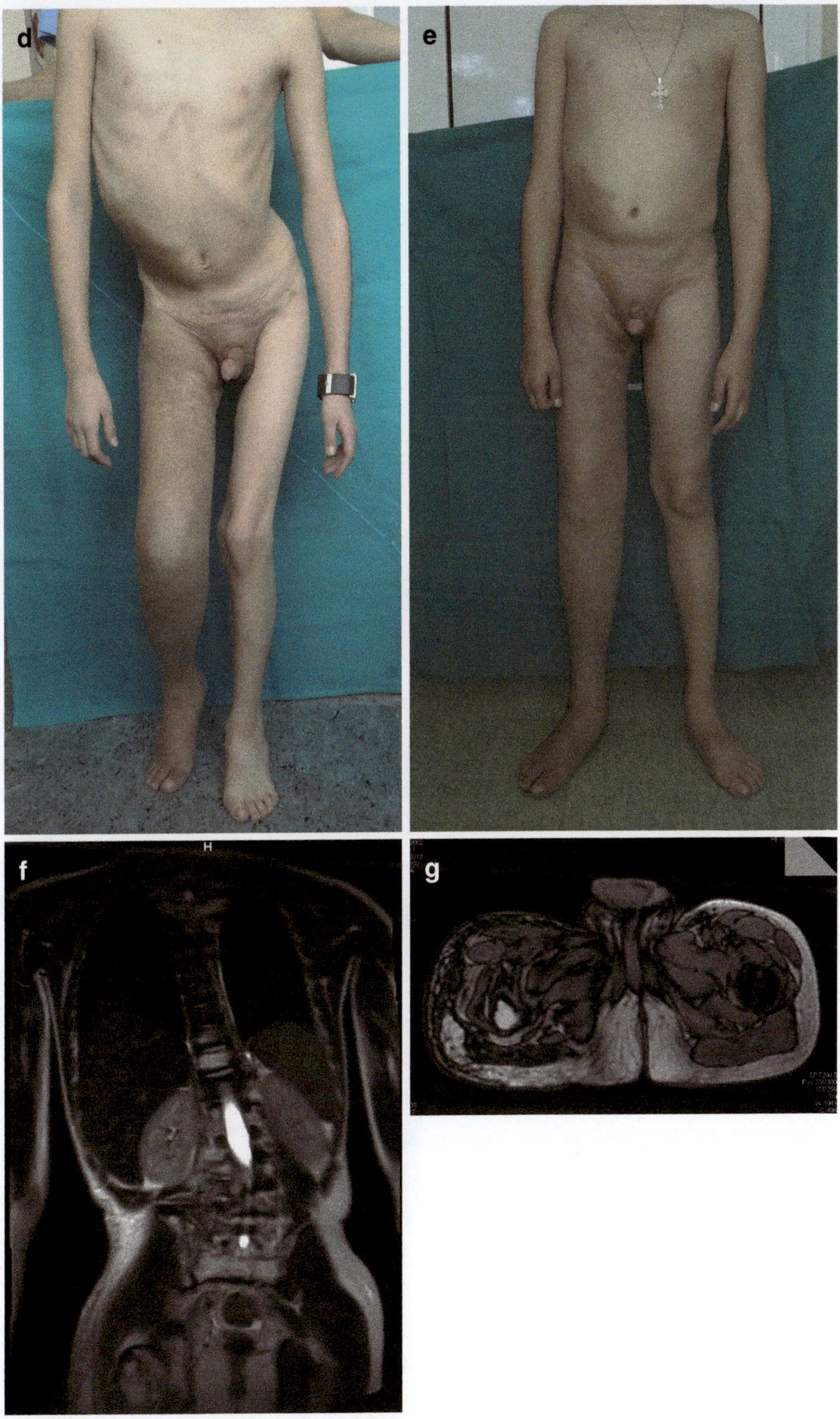

Fig. 14.8 (continued)

14.6 Lymphedema

Lymphedema is the chronic, progressive swelling of the tissue due to inadequate lymphatic function [32, 33]. It occurs primarily and secondarily (in 99% of all cases) from injury to lymph nodes and lymphatic vessels [32]. Primary lymphedemas are considered a subtype of LM due to a primary dysgenesis of the lymphatic network, and the extremities are most commonly affected, followed by genitalia (Fig. 14.9) [2, 5, 32]. Lymphoscintigraphy is the "gold standard" imaging study for evaluation of lymphatic function [32].

Most patients are treated conservatively (prevention of infection, compression, lowering of body weight, and physical activities) [32, 33]. Operative procedures

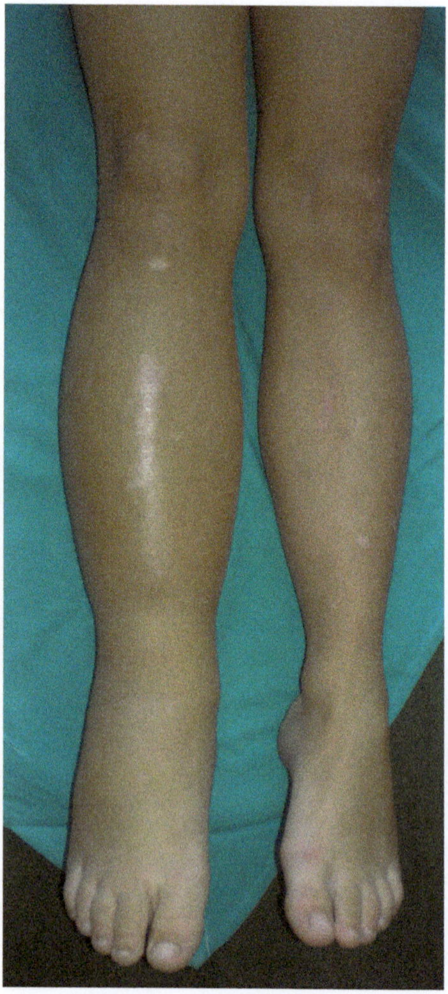

Fig. 14.9 Lymphoedema of the right crural region and foot

may include either attempt to increase drainage by creating new lymphatic connections (physiologic procedures) or to reduce the size of the area by removing excess tissues (excisional procedures) [5, 32].

References

1. Mulliken JB, Glowacki J. Hemangiomas and vascular malformations in infants and children: a classification based on endothelial characteristics. Plast Reconstr Surg. 1982;69(3):412–22.
2. Wassef M, Blei F, Adams D, Alomari A, Baselga E, et al. Vascular anomalies classification: recommendations from the International Society for the Study of Vascular Anomalies. Pediatrics. 2015;136(1):e203–14.
3. Greene AK, Mulliken JB. Vascular anomalies. In: Neligen PC, Gurtner GC, editors. Plastic surgery. Principles and practice. St Louis Missouri: Elsevier; 2013. p. 677–706e7.
4. Elluru RG, Balakrishnan K, Padua HM. Lymphatic malformation: diagnosis and management. Semin Pediatr Surg. 2014;23(4):178–85.
5. Clemens RK, Pfammatter T, Meier TO, Alomari AI, Amann-Vesti BR. Vascular malformations revisited. Vasa. 2015;44(1):5–22.
6. Chaudry G, Guevara CJ, Rialon KL, Kerr C, Mulliken JB, Greene AK, Fishman SJ, Boyer D, Alomari AI. Safety and efficacy of bleomycin sclerotherapy for microcystic lymphatic malformation. Cardiovasc Intervent Radiol. 2014;37(6):1476–81.
7. Renton JP, Smith RJ. Current treatment paradigms in the management of lymphatic malformations. Laryngoscope. 2011;121(1):56–9.
8. Zhou Q, Zheng JW, Mai HM, Luo QF, Fan XD, et al. Treatment guidelines of lymphatic malformations of the head and neck. Oral Oncol. 2011;47:1105–9.
9. Mulliken JB. Vascular anomalies. In: Thorne CH, Beasley RW, Aston SJ, Bartlett SP, Gurtner GC, Spear SL, editors. Grabb and Smith's plastic surgery. Philadelphia: Lippincott Williams & Wilkins; 2007. p. 191–200.
10. Boardman SJ, Cochrane LA, Roebuck D, Elliott MJ, Hartley BE. Multimodality treatment of pediatric lymphatic malformations of the head and neck using surgery and sclerotherapy. Arch Otolaryngol Head Neck Surg. 2010;136(3):270–6.
11. Colbert SD, Seager L, Haider F, Evans BT, Anand R, Brennan PA. Lymphatic malformations of the head and neck-current concepts in management. Br J Oral Maxillofac Surg. 2013;51(2):98–102.
12. Churchill P, Otal D, Pemberton J, Ali A, Flageole H, Walton JM. Sclerotherapy for lymphatic malformations in children: a scoping review. J Pediatr Surg. 2011;46(5):912–22.
13. Cahill AM, Nijs E, Ballah D, Rabinowitz D, Thompson L, Rintoul N, Hedrick H, Jacobs I, Low D. Percutaneous sclerotherapy in neonatal and infant head and neck lymphatic malformations: a single center experience. J Pediatr Surg. 2011;46(11):2083–95.
14. Greene AK, Burrows PE, Lois S, Mulliken JB. Periorbital lymphatic malformation: clinical course and management in 42 patients. Plast Reconstr Surg. 2005;115(1):22–30.
15. Edwards PD, Rahbar R, Ferraro FN, Burrows PE, Mulliken JB. Lymphatic malformation of the lingual base and oral floor. Plast Reconstr Surg. 2005;115(7):1906–15.
16. Lerat J, Mounayer C, Scomparin A, Orsel S, Bessede JP, Aubry K. Head and neck lymphatic malformation and treatment: clinical study of 23 cases. Eur Ann Otorhinolaryngol Head Neck Dis. 2016;133(6):393–6.
17. Nehra D, Jacobson L, Barnes P, Mallory B, Albanese CT, Sylvester KG. Doxycycline sclerotherapy as primary treatment of head and neck lymphatic malformations in children. J Pediatr Surg. 2008;43(3):451–60.
18. Adams DM, Trenor 3rd CC, Hammill AM, Vinks AA, Patel MN, Chaudry G. efficacy and safety of sirolimus in the treatment of complicated vascular anomalies. Pediatrics. 2016;137(2):1–10.

19. Lackner H, Karastaneva A, Schwinger W, Benesch M, Sovinz P, et al. Sirolimus for the treatment of children with various complicated vascular anomalies. Eur J Pediatr. 2015;174(12):1579–84.
20. Vlahovic AM, Vlahovic NS, Haxhija EQ. Sirolimus for the treatment of a massive capillary-lymphatico-venous malformation: a case report. Pediatrics. 2015;136(2):e513–6.
21. Triana P, Dore M, Cerezo VN, Cervantes M, Sánchez AV, Ferrero MM, González MD, Lopez-Gutierrez JC. Sirolimus in the treatment of vascular anomalies. Eur J Pediatr Surg. 2017;27(1):86–90.
22. Yang Y, Sun M, Ma Q, Cheng X, Ao J, et al. Bleomycin A5 sclerotherapy for cervicofacial lymphatic malformations. Vasc Surg. 2011;53(1):150–5.
23. Ogita S, Tsuto T, et al. Intracystic injection of OK-432: a new sclerosing therapy for cystic hygroma in children. Br J Surg. 1987;74:690–1.
24. Ogita S, Tsuto T, et al. OK-432 therapy for unresectable lymphangiomas in children. J Pediatr Surg. 1991;26(3):263–70.
25. Ghaffarpour N, Petrini B, Svensson LA, Boman K, Wester T, Claesson G. Patients with lymphatic malformations who receive the immunostimulant OK-432 experience excellent long-term outcomes. Acta Pediatr. 2015;104:1169–73.
26. Vlahovic A, Gazikalovic A, Adjic O. Bleomycin sclerotherapy for lymphatic malformation after unsuccessful surgical excision: case report. Acta Otorhinolaryngol Ital. 2015;35(5):365–7.
27. Burrows PE, Mitri RK, Alomari A, Padua HM, Lord DJ, et al. Percutaneous sclerotherapy of lymphatic malformations with doxycycline. Lymphat Res Biol. 2008;6(3–4):209–16.
28. Farnoosh S, Don D, Koempel J, Panossian A, Anselmo D, Stanley P. Efficacy of doxycycline and sodium tetradecyl sulfate sclerotherapy in pediatric head and neck lymphatic malformations. Int J Pediatr Otorhinolaryngol. 2015;79(6):883–7.
29. Cheng J. Doxycycline sclerotherapy in children with head and neck lymphatic malformations. J Pediatr Surg. 2015;50(12):2143–6.
30. Hamoir M, Plouin-Gaudon I, Rombaux P, Francois G, Cornu AS, Desuter G, Clapuyt P, Debauche C, Verellen G, Beguin C. Lymphatic malformations of the head and neck: a retrospective review and a support for staging. Head Neck. 2001;23(4):326–37.
31. Margolin JF, Soni HM, Pimpalwar S. Medical therapy for pediatric vascular anomalies. Semin Plast Surg. 2014;28(2):79–86.
32. Maclellan RA, Greene AK. Lymphedema. Semin Pediatr Surg. 2014;23(4):191–7.
33. Rudkin GH, Miller TA. Lymphedema. In: Thorne CH, Beasley RW, Aston ShJ, Bartlett SP, Gurtner GC, Spear SL, editors. Grabb and Smith's plastic surgery. Philadelphia: Lippincott Williams & Wilkins; 2007. p. 717–21.

Venous Malformation 15

15.1 Introduction

Vascular anomalies are classified into vascular tumors (characterized by endothelial proliferation) and vascular malformations (present the errors in morphogenesis) [1–3]. Vascular malformations are divided into *simple malformation* (capillary, lymphatic, venous malformation, arteriovenous malformation, and arteriovenous fistula), *combined malformations* (including at least two vascular malformations in one lesion), *malformation of major named vessels*, and *malformation associated with other anomalies* [1].

Venous malformations (VMs) are the most commonly treated slow-flow vascular malformation with an incidence of approximately 1–2/10,000 births [4–11]. They grow generally in proportion with the child, do not involute, and tend to enlarge disproportionately over time [3, 4, 6, 7, 10–12]. The pathogenesis of VM is unclear (TIE-2 endothelial receptor mutation is found in some of patient with sporadic VMs) [1, 2, 7, 9, 12].

VMs are classified as superficial or deep, focal, multifocal, or diffuse (Fig. 15.1a, b) [1–5]. Superficial VMs are presented as a blue skin discoloration or as a soft, nonpulsatile, compressible subcutaneous mass [2, 4, 6, 7]. Deep VMs infiltrate muscle, bone, and visceral organs and may be unrecognized for until they become symptomatic [1–4, 6, 7, 12, 13]. There is also a classification based on imaging and clinical features, dividing VMs into spongiform (most common type), phlebectatic, aneurismatic, and reticular type [6]. Dubois et al. divided VMs into four types based on the pattern of venous drainage channels, response to treatment, and rates of complication: isolated malformation without drainage, lesions draining into normal veins, lesions draining into dysplastic veins, and lesions consisting primarily of venous ectasia [6, 7]. Histologically, VMs are composed of thin-walled, dilated spongelike channels with normal endothelial lining and abnormal smooth muscle architecture [1–7, 13, 14].

A.M. Vlahovic, E.Q. Haxhija, *Pediatric and Adolescent Plastic Surgery for the Clinician*, DOI 10.1007/978-3-319-56004-5_15

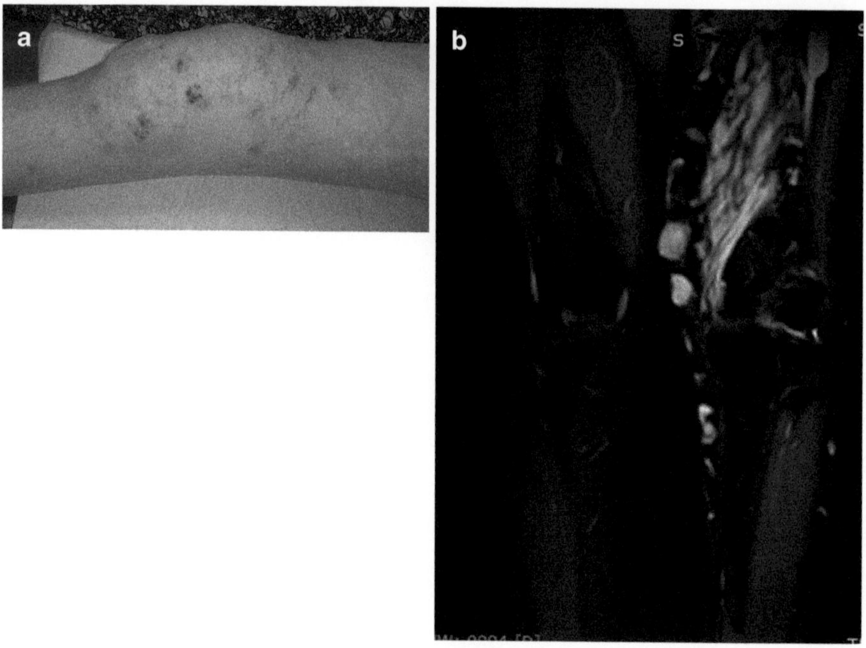

Fig. 15.1 Diffuse venous malformation of the left lower extremity: (**a**) clinical view of the knee region; (**b**) magnetic resonance imaging

Fig. 15.2 Localized venous malformation of the right foot

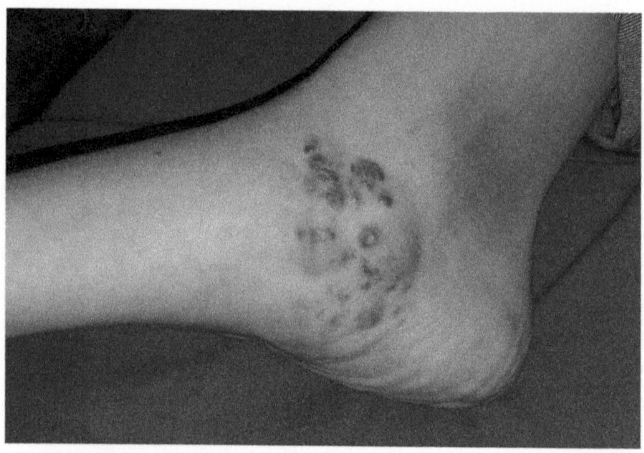

The most common types of VMs are sporadic VM, glomuvenous malformation (GVM), and blue rubber bleb nevus (BRBN) syndrome [1, 4–6]. Most VMs occur as sporadic and solitary (approximately 94% of VM) (Fig. 15.2) [1, 2, 4, 7, 14]. Sporadic VM is usually greater than 5 cm, single, and mostly located on the head and neck and extremities (Fig. 15.3a, b) [2, 8, 13].

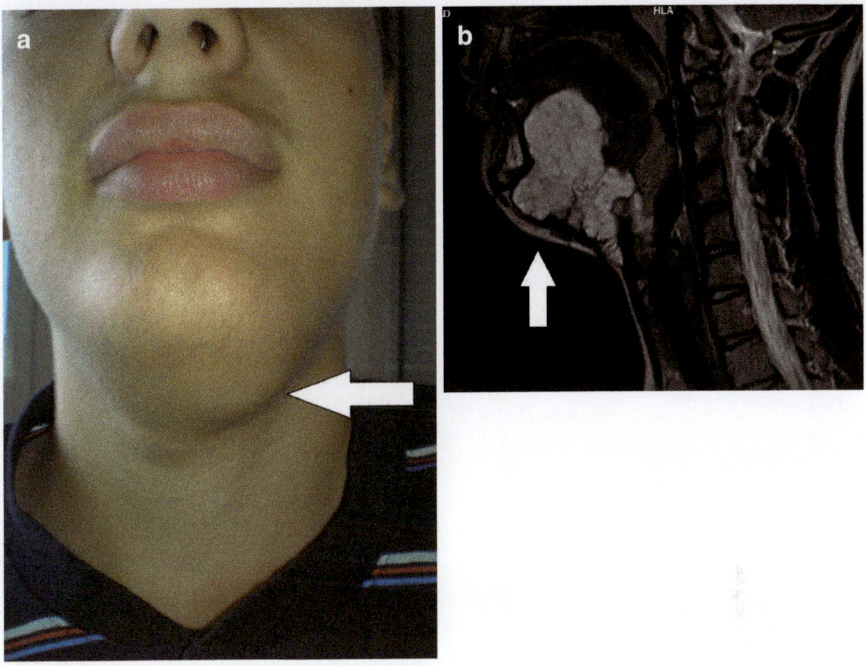

Fig. 15.3 Venous malformation of the sublingual region: (**a**) submandibular leasion; (**b**) magnetic resonance imaging of the lesion

VMs can be part of the syndromes such as capillary-lymphatic-venous malformation (CLVM) or Klippel-Trenaunay syndrome, congenital lipomatous overgrowth, vascular malformations, epidermal nevi and scoliosis or skeletal and spinal anomalies (CLOVES), mucocutaneous familial venous malformation, Maffucci's syndrome, and Proteus syndrome [6, 7, 13].

GVM is the most common familial form of venous anomaly, formerly known as glomangioma caused by mutation of the glomulin gene on chromosome 1 [1, 2, 4–6, 14]. They account for about 5% of all VM [4, 5]. GVMs form nodular or plaque-like small lesions (two thirds <5 cm), typically multiple, painful on palpation affecting the skin (rarely mucosa), and involving extremities in most cases [1, 2, 4, 5, 7, 14]. Histologically, GVMs appear as dilated venous channels with abnormal smooth muscle-like glomus cells [4, 14]. Blue rubber bleb nevus syndrome (BRBNS) or Bean syndrome is a rare condition characterized by multiple, small (1–2 cm in size) VMs, involving the skin (typically present on palmar and plantar surfaces), soft tissue, and gastrointestinal (GI) tract (Fig. 15.4) [2, 4, 6, 12, 15]. Lesions within the GI tract may be associated with significant bleeding [2, 4]. Treatment of patients with BRBNS is challenging, involving resection of skin lesions, bowel resection, and ligation of lesions, and recently, sirolimus is used for bleeding control [4, 6, 15].

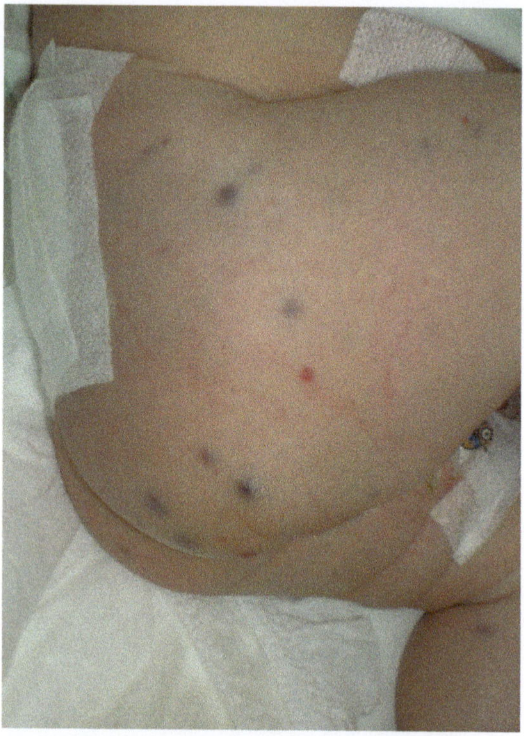

Fig. 15.4 Blue rubber bleb nevus syndrome of the right gluteal region

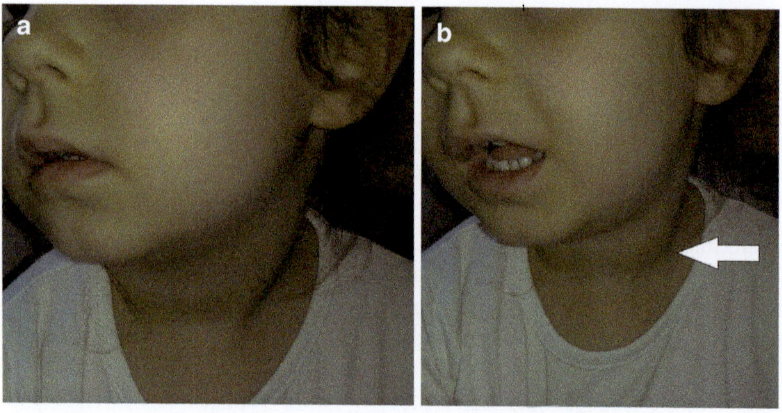

Fig. 15.5 Phlebectasia: (**a**) normal clinical finding; (**b**) neck mass enlarged with Valsalva maneuver

Differential diagnosis includes verrucous hemangioma (VH) (provisionally unclassified low-flow vascular malformation that is clinically similar to a hyperkeratotic VM); deep (subcutaneous hemangioma), lymphatic malformation; and dermal melanocytic nevi (Mongolian spot, nevi of Ota and Ito, and common blue nevus) [1, 2, 5]. Jugular vein phlebectasia is a congenital fusiform dilatation of jugular vein and is usually asymptomatic (Fig. 15.5a, b) [16].

15.2 Complications (Symptoms) of VM

The most common symptom of VM is pain due swelling, and other symptoms are usually related to localization of VMs [2, 4, 7, 12]. In head and neck region, VM can cause airway or orbital compromise due to mucosal bleeding [9, 12]. Extremity VM can cause leg-length discrepancy, hypoplasia, pathologic fracture, and hemarthrosis, and muscle VM may result in fibrosis and subsequent pain and disability [2, 12]. Gastrointestinal VM can cause bleeding and chronic anemia [2, 4, 12].

VMs are associated with spontaneous thrombosis and thrombolysis, and they are often proportional to the size of VM [4, 5, 12]. Patients with extensive VMs have been found to have elevated D-dimer levels which are sensitive marker for thrombus formation and fibrinolysis [4, 5, 7, 12, 13]. D-dimers are not elevated in GVM [6]. Stagnation within a large VM results in a localized intravascular coagulopathy (LIC), painful phlebothromboses, and pulmonary embolism [2, 4, 12]. Localized intravascular coagulopathy (LIC) is characterized by an increase in D-dimer level, normal platelet count, and decreased fibrinogen level, and patients usually well tolerate this condition LIC [4, 5]. Severe LIC can aggravate to disseminated intravascular coagulation (DIC) which is a serious life-threatening condition [5].

15.3 Patient Evaluation

VMs are in most cases diagnosed by history and physical examination [2, 4, 5, 7, 11, 14]. VMs are easily compressible and usually swell in the dependent position [2, 6]. Patients with VMs should be screened for a basic coagulation profile including complete blood count, prothrombin time (PT), partial thromboplastin time (PTT), D-dimer, and fibrinogen [4, 5, 12].

Small, superficial VMs do not require further diagnostic workup [2, 9, 12]. Large and deep VMs require imaging studying mainly performed with ultrasonography (US) (for localized lesions), Doppler US, magnetic resonance imaging (MRI), and MR venography [1, 2, 4, 9]. Conventional radiography and computerized tomography (CT) are rarely used [2, 4, 5, 9]. CT scanning is more sensitive for the detection of phleboliths and for the evaluation of osseous involvement [4, 7]. There is limitation to evaluate extensive and deep lesions with ultrasound (US) [4]. On gray scale imaging, VMs can appear as hypoechoic or heterogenous lesions, there is little to no flow on Doppler interrogation, and presence of echogenic debris or shadowing phleboliths is highly specific for the diagnosis of VM [4, 7]. Large or deeper VMs are evaluated by MRI (extent and relationship to adjacent structures) [2, 4, 7, 9]. MR venography may be performed for treatment planning to confirm the patency of a normal deep venous system and to fully assess the extent of the VM and draining venous channels [7, 12].

15.4 Treatment Options

The treatment of a patient with VMs is individualized, usually within a multidisciplinary team [4, 5, 9]. Intervention is reserved for symptomatic lesions that cause pain, deformity, obstruction, intra-articular involvement, or gastrointestinal bleeding [2, 4, 13].

Treatment options for VMs include conservative treatment (elevation, local compression, antibiotics, pain control), sclerotherapy, surgical resection, laser photocoagulation, cryotherapy, and photodynamic therapy, and they all can be used as a single procedure or as a combination [2, 4–9, 12, 14, 16–19]. The location, size, level of infiltration, symptoms (pain), and psychosocial issue are most important parameters that have to be included in the treatment plan for VMs [2, 4, 8, 9, 12]. Small, painless, and very extensive VMs can be managed conservatively, and large extensive VMs are still a therapeutic challenge [9, 12]. There is a lack of evidence for the effectiveness of different treatments of VM [8, 9, 17].

15.4.1 Conservative Treatment

Medical management of VM is an essential component to treatment, including pain control, prevention of thrombus formation, and progressive venous ectasia [4, 9]. The acute pain secondary to phlebothrombosis can be treated with anti-inflammatory medications and mild analgetics [2, 4, 5, 9, 12]. Low molecular weight heparin (LMWH) is considered for patients with significant LIC who are at risk for DIC [4, 5, 15]. Custom-fitted compression garments provide significant symptomatic relief for many patients with an extensive extremity VM, and they may prevent progressive expansion of venous lesions [4–6, 12]. Compression garments should be initiated at an early age, and they are also an important adjunct post therapy (they are contraindicated for GVM) [2, 4, 5].

15.4.2 Sclerotherapy

Sclerotherapy is first-line treatment for VMs, and most common indications are pain, disfigurement, and intra-articular involvement [2, 4, 5, 7, 12–16, 20]. Good to excellent results are obtained in 65–90% of patients, depending of the type of VM and the sclerosant [2, 4, 6, 15, 16]. Sclerosation can be used as a single therapy or in combination with surgery and laser therapy [1, 3, 4, 11, 13]. There are different sclerosants used for treatment of VM such as sodium tetradecyl sulfate (STS), polidocanol (Lauromacrogol or Aethoxysklerol), absolute ethanol, ethylcellulose-ethanol, doxycycline, OK-432, and bleomycin [2, 4–9, 12, 13, 17, 18, 19].

Most patients, especially children, are managed under general anesthesia using US, fluoroscopic imaging, or CT [2, 7, 19]. Percutaneous puncture of VM and injection of sclerosant are gold standard [6, 7]. The VM is cannulated using US guidance, the VM should be exsanguinated if possible (to achieve optimal contact between the sclerosant and endothelium), and additionally, the venous outflow into conducting veins should be prevented (by manual compression for 10 min or embolized with coil or glue prior to the sclerosant being injected) [4, 19]. Tourniquets may be required depending on the venous outflow [4, 7]. Placement of peripheral intravenous line in the affected limb is recommended for perfusion of heparinized saline to reduce the risk of secondary thrombosis [2, 7, 12]. Diffuse VMs are managed by targeting specific symptomatic areas; multiple procedures are required, combining with resection [2, 4, 12]. Patients with large VMs should be hospitalized [11, 14].

Post-procedure care for small VM includes elevation of treated area and for large VM elevation of the limb, IV rehydration, analgesics, anti-inflammatory medications, corticosteroids, and LMWH [12, 13, 19]. When it is possible, compression garments are placed post-procedure to augment the effects of sclerotherapy [4]. The patients are reassessed 6–8 weeks after the procedure, with US and MRI evaluation, and the procedure is often repeated if needed [4, 19].

Local complications observed after sclerotherapy of VMs are pain, skin necrosis, skin erythema, blistering, bleeding, and nerve injuries [2, 7–9, 12, 17–20]. Extravasation of the sclerosant into muscle can cause fibrosis and secondary contractures [2, 11]. Systemic adverse events following sclerotherapy include hemolysis, hemoglobinuria, and DIC [2, 7, 19]. Among the sclerosing agents, the highest complication rate is associated with ethanol (12%) [7, 8, 12, 19]. Conventional sclerotherapy agents combined with vascular devices such as coils, liquid embolization agents, or laser ablation may be helpful for children with rapid outflow or with lager VM [4, 7].

15.4.3 Surgical Excision

In selected patients, surgical treatment of VMs can be effective [10, 11]. Localized, accessible, small VMs that do not involve vital structures can be treated surgically (complete excision), and for more extensive lesions, subtotal resection is indicated (Fig.15.6a–e) [2, 4, 5, 9, 11, 13, 17]. If there is extensive tissue loss after resection of VM, skin grafts or flaps can be used for defect reconstruction [9]. Intra-articular VMs are also resected in most cases to prevent ongoing joint damage or pain [4]. Sclerotherapy prior to operative intervention helps to decrease the risks of intraoperative bleeding; however, scars can make it difficult to identify important nerve and vessels [2, 4, 9, 13]. Surgery is first-line therapy for GVM lesions whenever it is possible [2, 4, 5].

15.4.4 Laser Ablation

Laser can only penetrate 1–3 mm, and it can only be used for VM of this size [9]. Neodymium-doped yttrium aluminum garnet (Nd:YAG) laser (1064 nm wavelength) is mostly used for treatment of VMs, and it can also be used as an adjuvant to sclerotherapy [2, 4, 9, 13]. Laser treatment is often used in the head and neck region (multiple sessions usually required) [4]. Potassium titanyl phosphate (KTP) laser and pulsed-dye laser (PDL) are also used for treatment of VMs [9, 13]. Endovenous laser treatment (EVLT) can be used for treatment of phlebectatic and spongiform VMs in pediatric population [4, 6].

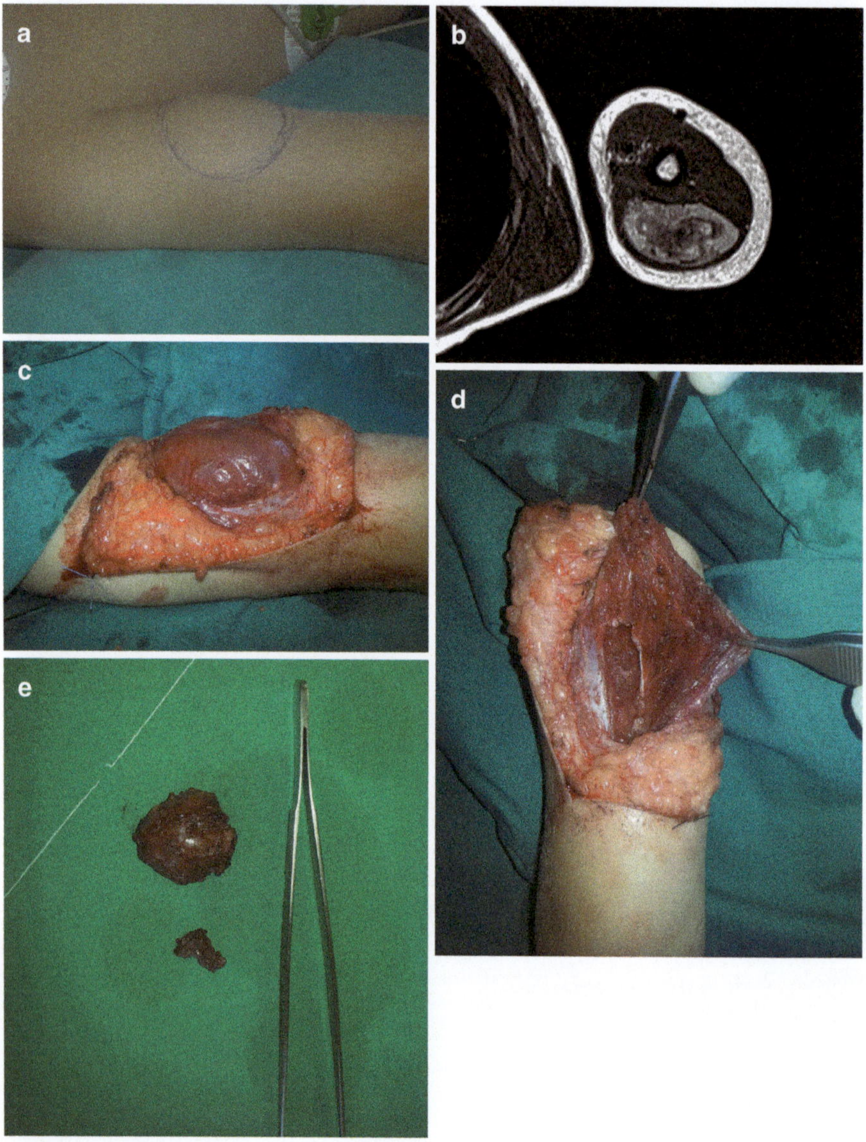

Fig. 15.6 Surgical treatment of deep localized venous malformation: (**a**) preoperative view; (**b**) magnetic resonance imaging of the left brachial region; (**c**, **d**) intraoperative view; (**e**) complete excision of venous malformation

References

1. Wassef M, Blei F, Adams D, Alomari A, Baselga E, et al. Vascular anomalies classification: recommendations from the International Society for the Study of Vascular Anomalies. Pediatrics. 2015;136(1):e203–14.
2. Greene AK, Mulliken JB. Vascular anomalies. In: Neligen PC, Gurtner GC, editors. Plastic surgery. Principles and practice. St Louis Missouri: Elsevier; 2013. p. 677–706e7.
3. Mulliken JB. Vascular anomalies. In: Thorne CH, Beasley RW, Aston SJ, Bartlett SP, Gurtner GC, Spear SL, editors. Grabb and Smith's plastic surgery. Philadelphia: Lippincott Williams & Wilkins; 2007. p. 191–200.
4. Dasgupta R, Patel M. Venous malformation. Semin Pediatr Surg. 2014;23(4):198–207.
5. Dompmartin A, Vikkula M, Boon LM. Venous malformation: update on etiopathogenesis, diagnosis & management. Phlebology. 2010;25(5):224–35.
6. Clemens RK, Pfammatter T, Meier TO, Alomari AI, Amann-Vesti BR. Vascular malformations revisited. Vasa. 2015;44(1):5–22.
7. Cahill AM, Nijs EL. Pediatric vascular malformations: pathophysiology, diagnosis, and the role of interventional radiology. Cardiovasc Intervent Radiol. 2011;34(4):691–704.
8. van der Vleuten CJ, Kater A, Wijnen MH, Schultze Kool LJ, Rovers MM. Effectiveness of sclerotherapy, surgery, and laser therapy in patients with venous malformations: a systematic review. Cardiovasc Intervent Radiol. 2014;37(4):977–89.
9. Zheng JW, Mai HM, Zhang L, Wang YA, Fan XD, et al. Guidelines for the treatment of head and neck venous malformation. Int J Clin Exp Med. 2013;6(5):377–89.
10. Steiner V, FitzJohn T, Tan ST. Surgical treatment for venous malformation. J Plast Reconstr Aesthet Surg. 2013;66:1741–9.
11. Cox JA, Bartlett E, Lee EI. Vascular malformations: a review. Semin Plast Surg. 2014;28(2):58–63.
12. Alomari A, Dubois J. Interventional management of vascular malformations. Tech Vasc Interv Radiol. 2011;14(1):22–31.
13. Berenguer B, Burrows P, et al. Sclerotherapy of cranifacial venous malformations: complications and results. Plast Reconstr Surg. 1999;104(1):1–11.
14. Nguyen HL, Boon LM, Vikkula M. Genetics of vascular malformations. Semin Pediatr Surg. 2014;23(4):221–6.
15. Margolin JF, Soni HM, Pimpalwar S. Medical therapy for pediatric vascular anomalies. Semin Plast Surg. 2014;28(2):79–86.
16. Hu X, Li J, Hu T, Jiang X. Congenital jugular vein phlebectasia. Am J Otolaryngol. 2005;26(3):172–4.
17. Qiu Y, Chen H, Lin X, Hu X, Jin Y, Ma G. Outcomes and complications of sclerotherapy for venous malformations. Vasc Endovascular Surg. 2013;47(6):454–61.
18. Zhang J, Li HB, Zhou SY, Chen KS, Niu CQ, Tan XY, Jiang YZ, Lin QQ. Comparison between absolute ethanol and bleomycin for the treatment of venous malformation in children. Exp Ther Med. 2013;6(2):305–9.
19. Burrows PE. Endovascular treatment of slow-flow vascular malformations. Tech Vasc Interv Radiol. 2013;16(1):12–21.
20. Pimpalwar S. Vascular malformations: approach by an interventional radiologist. Semin Plast Surg. 2014;28(2):91–103.

Index

A.M. Vlahovic, E.Q. Haxhija, *Pediatric and Adolescent Plastic Surgery for the Clinician*, DOI 10.1007/978-3-319-56004-5

CPI Antony Rowe
Chippenham, UK
2017-09-04 22:27